Integrative Systemic Therapy in Practice

This essential handbook provides clinicians with the tools to introduce Integrative Systemic Therapy (IST) into their practice with individuals, couples, and families.

Describing the "how to" and "how to decide what to do" aspects of IST, this book outlines a practical, problem-solving approach that considers client strengths and cultural contexts in the process of integrating interventions from various therapy models and empirically supported treatments. Chapters demonstrate how problem-solving tasks can be accomplished using the IST blueprint for therapy and include scenarios that will challenge the reader to think through the specific steps of IST, encouraging them to consider the therapeutic alliance and the use of self in therapy.

For supervisors, trainers, and clinicians familiar with IST, this book will enrich and deepen their understanding of it. The book is also relevant for practitioners of all types of therapy who seek to become more integrative and systemic in their work.

William P. Russell is a Clinical Associate Professor of psychology and the Director of Faculty of the Master of Science in Marriage and Family Therapy Program at Northwestern University.

Douglas C. Breunlin is a Clinical Professor of psychology at Northwestern University. As an author of four books and 70 articles, he is the 2020 recipient of the AFTA Lifetime Achievement Award.

Bahareh Sahebi is a Clinical Assistant Professor of psychology and the Assistant Program Director of the Master of Science in Marriage and Family Therapy Program at Northwestern University.

The Family Institute Series: Clinical Applications of the Integrative Systemic Therapy (IST) Model

Series editors: Anthony L. Chambers, Douglas C. Breunlin, William P. Russell, and Jay Lawrence Lebow

The Family Institute Series: Clinical Applications of the Integrative Systemic Therapy (IST) Model focuses on elaborating the theory and practice of Integrative Systemic Therapy (IST) and its application to various populations and contexts. Embracing empiricism, diversity, and creativity, the series distills the complex landscape of psychotherapy into clinician-friendly guidelines and strategies useful to all practitioners and students in psychology, marriage and family therapy, counseling, clinical social work and the other mental health professions.

Titles in the series:

Integrative Systemic Therapy in Practice: A Clinician's Handbook
William P. Russell, Douglas C. Breunlin, and Bahareh Sahebi

Integrative Systemic Therapy in Practice

A Clinician's Handbook

William P. Russell,
Douglas C. Breunlin, and
Bahareh Sahebi

Routledge
Taylor & Francis Group

NEW YORK AND LONDON

Cover credit: © Getty Images

First published 2023
by Routledge
605 Third Avenue, New York, NY 10158

and by Routledge
4 Park Square, Milton Park, Abingdon, Oxon, OX14 4RN

Routledge is an imprint of the Taylor & Francis Group, an informa business

© 2023 William P. Russell, Douglas C. Breunlin and Bahareh Sahebi

Library of Congress Cataloguing-in-Publication Data
A catalog record for this title has been requested

ISBN: 978-0-367-33838-1 (hbk)
ISBN: 978-0-367-33839-8 (pbk)
ISBN: 978-0-429-32227-3 (ebk)

DOI: 10.4324/9780429322273

Typeset in Times New Roman
by MPS Limited, Dehradun

"This IST Handbook is the next step in the elaboration of Integrative Systemic Therapy. With great clarity, it takes the concepts that were laid out in *Integrative Systemic Therapy* (2018) and grounds them in the specifics of practice. It details what to do, how to do it, and when to do it, from how to start the first session to how to conclude a therapeutic episode dealing with a particular problem sequence. It is a phenomenally useful guide for teachers, supervisors, and practitioners of IST, as well as an indispensable resource for clinicians wanting to expand their clinical horizons in the direction of integrative and systemic practice. Transcending the myriad models permeating psychotherapy today, this book provides a user-friendly format to guide practice, while simultaneously encouraging creativity and innovation. Read it and grow!"

William Pinsof, *PhD, LMFT, ABPP, Pinsof Family Systems*

"This is a wonderful handbook of Integrative Systemic Therapy with individuals, couples, and families. A must-read for the beginning clinician: Accessible, systematic, pragmatic step-by-step teaching of theory and technique, with lots of clinical examples and exercises. This book is also valuable for experienced clinicians looking to deepen an integrative perspective on their work. The approach is strengths-based, with a problem-solving, collaborative orientation, integrating multiple systems and approaches, and finely tuned to the therapeutic alliance. It is sensitive to socio-cultural context, addressing intrapsychic, interpersonal, and intergenerational dynamics as well as biological issues. An outstanding guide for all therapists. Highly recommended!"

Mona D. Fishbane, *PhD, author, Loving with the Brain in Mind: Neurobiology & Couple Therapy*

"Human behavior is complex. Changing it is more so. This handbook guides therapists and students of therapy through a pragmatic, step-by-step process that integrates therapy models and brings together best practices and research findings to yield a collaborative, client system-centered approach unique to each individual, couple or family and their therapist.

Thank you to Russell, Breunlin and Sahebi for a tour de force—bringing together the underlying constructs of important systemic approaches to therapy in a sophisticated yet clear and pragmatic way so that therapists and clients can identify problem and potential solution sequences, common missteps, constraints and how to lift them. The authors' attention to the therapeutic alliance, as well as the use of case illustrations, suggested exercises, and graphics at the beginning of each chapter, bring the approach to life for the reader."

Susan McDaniel, *PhD, Dr Laurie Sands Distinguished Professor of Families and Health at the University of Rochester School of Medicine*

Contents

Figures

Acknowledgments

We (Bill, Doug, and Bahareh) would like to extend our appreciation to the many clients, students, supervisors, and faculty of The Family Institute at Northwestern University who over the last 30 plus years have contributed in one way or another to the development of Integrative Systemic Therapy (IST). We acknowledge and appreciate Betty MacKune-Karrer and Dick Schwartz for their earlier contributions to Metaframeworks, many of which were subsumed into IST. We also owe a debt of gratitude to the therapy model developers, theorists and researchers whose brilliant findings, concepts and strategies are utilized within IST.

We would like to thank the supervisors and practitioners who provided input via survey or consultation to the book. They include Aaron Cohn, Carol Jabs, Adam Fisher, Shayna Goldstein, Yaliu He, Hannah Smith Lammers, Michelle McMartin, Linda Rubinowitz, Allen Sabey, David Taussig, Neil Venketramen, and Kristoffer Whittaker. Their experience contributed significantly to the knowledge base concerning the execution of the various problem-solving steps of IST. We extend our special appreciation to our colleague, Aaron Cohen, who generously advised on matters related to various therapy models and provided valuable input on the literature on sexual and gender minorities.

Two graduate students in the Master of Science in Marriage and Family Therapy Program at Northwestern University were indispensable to this project. Luca Eros and Meredith Merchant provided extensive and invaluable input on the content and voice of the book. They reviewed, formatted, and proofed the book, tracking down endless references along the way. They proved to be extraordinarily talented, dedicated, steadfast and patient, for which we are deeply appreciative.

We acknowledge the unfailing support—professional, technical, and emotional—provided by our life partners, Diane Russell, Diana Semmelhack, and Jason Shyu. That we emerge on the other side of a long journey with a book in hand is much due to the many gifts they gave us along the way.

We greatly appreciate the support and feedback of the editors of *The Family Institute Series: Clinical Applications of the Integrative Systemic Therapy Model,* Anthony Chambers and Jay Lebow, who provided invaluable feedback and support throughout the process of proposing and writing this book. Special thanks to our Routledge Editor, Heather Evans, who provided indispensable and patient guidance throughout the process of writing this book.

Finally, we extend our profound gratitude to Bill Pinsof, a leader in the field of couple and family therapy and a lead member and senior author of the team that developed IST. As a theoretician, researcher and practitioner, he developed many of the original ideas that are represented in IST and described in this book.

Foreword

Integrative Systemic Therapy in Practice: A Clinician's Handbook is the first volume in an exciting series for Routledge focused on integrative systemic therapy. The series, edited by Anthony Chambers, Doug Breunlin, Jay Lebow, and William Russell is designed to fill a unique need in the field of psychotherapy: to provide a definitive resource for the specifics of the practice of Integrative Systemic Therapy and its application to various populations and problems.

Integrative Systemic Therapy is a psychotherapeutic perspective for integrating different theories of problem maintenance/problem resolution and models of psychotherapeutic intervention. IST offers a meta-model and framework for conducting a comprehensive, efficient, integrative psychotherapy. It transcends and organizes the "tower of Babel" comprised of the myriad existent theories and treatments. As a clinical-theoretical perspective, IST aims to integrate and maximize the efficiency and effectiveness of the delivery of the plethora of different treatment methods.

IST is integrative, systemic, and empirically informed. It is integrative in that it provides an underlying set of principles for drawing upon different theories and treatments. It is systemic in having a foundation in general systems theory's understanding of the interwoven processes in biological, psychological, and social systems. Individuals cannot be understood independently of the social systems in which they are embedded. In psychotherapy, critical social systems like couples and families cannot be understood independently of the individuals that comprise them.

IST is "empirically informed" in its foundation in the best evidence from all sources having to do with individual, couple, and family processes as well as treatment processes. From this foundation, it provides a valuable framework for helping therapists decide when and how to incorporate different empirically supported treatments and intervention strategies. Its schemas are especially helpful for deciding what empirically supported strategies to use when the treatment they are currently using is not working.

Transcending traditional models, IST offers a paradigm for which empirically supported strategies and techniques can best be deployed at various points in treatment.

The IST perspective also articulates a set of principles for organizing theories and integrating psychotherapies. These principles capture the unique contributions of specific theories and models of psychotherapy, but do so in the context of language that makes these contributions accessible to therapists who have been trained or work within other models. The IST model is intended as a framework for growth and integration of new methods and ways of thinking about therapy over the professional life course. In this way, IST appeals to therapists at all stages of their professional development. Beginners like it because it helps them make sense of the field, find a simple and straightforward evidence-based way to intervene, and embrace multiple different perspectives. Intermediate-level therapists like it because it anchors them in their process of developing a coherent framework for their own personal method for employing different theories and techniques they have learned. Highly experienced therapists like it because it encourages and facilitates improvisation and creativity, and offers endless possibilities for evolving and staying vital as a therapist.

It is fitting that *Integrative Systemic Therapy in Practice* is the first volume in the series because it provides the sorts of hands-on practical information about the practice of Integrative Systemic Therapy that clinicians and clinicians in training seek. Chapter topics such as convening a client system and defining the problem, the first session, locating a problem sequence, and identifying and addressing constraints offer detailed descriptions of how to think like an IST therapist as well as a manual of specific descriptions of how to operate within its improvisational framework. *Integrative Systemic Therapy in Practice* both articulates the core principles of IST and provides very detailed descriptions of its guidelines for practice, including examples of when to say what. This book is also rich in clinical illustrations and exercises to enhance therapist skillfulness.

The authors of *Integrative Systemic Therapy in Practice* William Russell, Doug Breunlin, and Bahareh Sahebi bring endless practical experience in practicing IST and training others in IST to this book. William Russell and Doug Breunlin each bring 40 years of experience to this work and are part of the core group that developed the IST model (Pinsof et al., 2018). Together they are the principal architects of the IST training that anchors the marriage and family training program at the Family Institute at Northwestern. Bahareh Sahebi is among the foremost second-generation IST therapists and trainers, and brings the perspective of a younger generation of therapists to the model.

Integrative Systemic Therapy in Practice is a wonderful book to inaugurate this series. The reader who wants to learn more about integrative systemic therapy will find what they are looking for here. It will serve well as a text for coursework about IST in graduate programs, as a manual for the specifics of IST practice, and as a guidebook for those who wish to learn about the model and how they might use it to inform their practice. Even readers less interested in the conceptual aspects of IST will find much to learn from the authors' wisdom about the practice of psychotherapy. This impressive launch makes us certain that this series, with several volumes to follow, will become the definitive resource for the theory and practice in IST over the next decades.

Anthony Chambers, Ph.D., ABPP
The Family Institute at Northwestern University
Jay Lebow, Ph.D., ABPP
The Family Institute at Northwestern University

Reference

Pinsof, W. M., Breunlin, D. C., Russell, W. P., Lebow, J., Rampage, C., & Chambers, A. L. (2018). *Integrative systemic therapy: metaframeworks for problem solving with individuals, couples, and families*. American Psychological Association.

Preface

This book, *Integrative Systemic Therapy in Practice: A Clinician's Handbook,* expands the literature on Integrative Systemic Therapy (IST) by providing additional and highly specific explanations about the conduct of IST. It is written for supervisors, trainers and clinicians using IST, but also serves as a template for clinicians wishing to expand their practice beyond a specific model or to become more integrative and systemic in their work. It describes the "how to decide what to do" and the "how to do it" aspects of Integrative Systemic Therapy (IST). This book elaborates on the original IST book, *Integrative Systemic Therapy: Metaframeworks for Problem Solving with Individuals, Couples, and Families* (Pinsof, Breunlin, Russell, Lebow, Rampage, and Chambers, 2018). It details the operations and processes of IST in a much more granular way.

IST is a comprehensive perspective on family, couple, and individual therapy that is applicable to virtually all problems and populations. IST provides a practical, problem-solving approach that appreciates clients' strengths, provides the framework to understand a broad variety of constraints, and facilitates the planful integration of strategies and interventions from various therapeutic approaches and empirically-supported treatments.

IST helps beginning therapists organize and contain the many concepts and interventions within the field of psychotherapy. It provides practicing clinicians of varying levels of experience with a process of decision-making for integrative therapy. IST's concepts and frameworks comprise a template for the development of therapists over the course of their careers.

This book seeks to elucidate the practice of IST in four ways. First, it specifies methods of inquiry for the accomplishment of IST's essential problem-solving tasks. Second, it provides targeted case material to illustrate how these tasks can be accomplished by means of the IST blueprint for therapy. Third, it provides exercises that will aid the reader to think through and accomplish specific steps of the problem-solving process. Fourth, it challenges the reader to think carefully about the use of self and the therapeutic alliance in therapy.

The book is organized and sequenced according to IST's recursive problem-solving tasks. Decision-making about these tasks is facilitated by the use of a blueprint that integrates psychotherapeutic bodies of knowledge. The use of the blueprint to accomplish the problem-solving tasks is a process that is applicable to therapy conducted with individuals, couples, and families; hence, this book demonstrates the use of IST in all three contexts. The book does not treat each of these modalities separately in any comprehensive way as the emphasis is on the general process of IST, which applies across contexts and modalities and alters the pattern of who attends therapy depending on the issues being addressed. Future books in Routledge's *The Family Institute Series: Clinical Applications of Integrative Systemic Therapy* will focus separately on the application of IST to aspects of the work that are specific to individuals, couples, or families.

Chapter 1 presents an overview of IST including its pillars, core concepts, essential problem-solving steps, blueprint for decision-making, and the hypothesizing and planning metaframeworks used in ongoing case formulation. Chapters 2 through 10 each describe a step in IST's problem-solving process which is represented in a flow chart at the beginning of each of these chapters. Chapters 2 and 3 present the process of conducting the initial phone call and first session. Included are considerations about who to invite to the initial session, how to begin forming alliances and how to define a presenting problem. Chapter 4 details the process of understanding the systemic context in which presenting problems are embedded through the use of a concept called the problem sequence. Chapters 5 and 6 move to the next steps in the process of change, which are defining and then implementing a solution sequence. When successfully implemented, the solution sequence utilizes new actions, meanings and/or emotions that resolve the presenting problem. Chapter 7 elaborates on what happens when clients are unable to implement the solution sequence. IST posits that this failure derives not from some deficit in the client system, but from the presence of constraints that prevent the solution sequence from working. Working with constraints enables the integrative therapist to transcend the conceptual underpinning of the various models of individual, couple, and family therapy. Chapter 8 presents the integrative means by which IST proceeds to lift constraints utilizing its six planning metaframeworks. This chapter makes it clear how IST transcends and integrates the various models of individual, couple, and family therapy. Chapters 9 and 10 illustrate how to evaluate progress in IST and how to end an episode of therapy. Chapter 11 describes the various pathways IST can take given special client circumstances, particular contexts of therapy, therapist preferences, and person-of-the-therapist issues. Throughout the book, case material with details modified to protect clients' confidentiality is used to illustrate specific steps or phases of the therapy.

Each chapter includes a set of exercises designed to promote understanding and facilitate the application of the content covered in that chapter. Some of the exercises are thought experiments. Others invite the reader to apply specific concepts and procedures to their own cases. Although designed for an individual reader, most of the exercises can easily be converted to discussion questions for small groups or dyads.

Contributors

William P. Russell, MSW, LCSW, LMFT, BCD, is a Clinical Associate Professor of Psychology and Director of Faculty of the Master of Science in Marriage and Family Therapy program at Northwestern University. He has practiced, taught and supervised systemic, integrative therapy for over 35 years and has held leadership positions in both academic and clinical programs. Mr. Russell is an approved supervisor of the American Association for Marriage and Family Therapy and a board-certified diplomate in clinical social work. He has authored articles and book chapters on systemic therapy as well as a variety of other topics related to the practice of couple and family therapy, and he is co-author of the book, *Integrative Systemic Therapy: Metaframeworks for Problems Solving with Individuals, Couples, and Families*. He is co-editor of *Routledge's Family Institute Series: Clinical Applications of Integrative Systemic Therapy.*

Douglas C. Breunlin, MSSA, LCSW, LMFT is a Clinical Professor of Psychology at Northwestern University. His previous books include: *Metaframeworks: Transcending the Models of Family Therapy* (with Schwartz and Mac Kune Karrer), *The Handbook of Family Therapy Training and Supervision* (coedited with Liddle and Schwartz), *Integrative Systemic Therapy: Metaframeworks for Problems Solving with Individuals, Couples and Families* (with Pinsof, Russell, Lebow, Rampage, and Chambers), and *The Encyclopedia of Couple and Family Therapy* (coedited with Lebow and Chambers). He is the co-editor of *Routledge's Family Institute Series: Clinical Applications of Integrative Systemic Therapy.* He has authored over 70 articles and served on the Editorial Boards of four journals. He has served as secretary, treasurer, and board member for the American Family Therapy Academy (AFTA). He is the 2020 recipient of the AFTA Lifetime Achievement Award.

Bahareh Sahebi, PsyD, LMFT, is a Clinical Assistant Professor of Psychology and an Assistant Program Director of the Master of Science in Marriage and Family Therapy program at Northwestern University. As an Approved Supervisor of the American Association of Marriage and Family Therapy, she has trained graduate-level students in marriage and family therapy, counseling, and clinical psychology. Her integrative, systemic clinical practice addresses a broad range of client concerns and includes a specialty in the treatment of trauma. Dr. Sahebi has extensive experience in program development and is the recipient of the 2018 Dr. Christine Bard Compassion and Skill in Rehabilitation Practice Award. Her scholarship has focused on clinical supervision, couples' health, teletherapy, multicultural issues and intersectionality, and immigrant parenting practices. She is an associate editor of the *Encyclopedia of Couple and Family Therapy*.

Chapter 1

Integrative Systemic Therapy

Introduction

The field of psychotherapy contains an overwhelming amount of information about human functioning, theories of change, common factors, clinical models, evidence-based treatments, and clinical competencies. Therapists face the significant challenge of determining how to effectively utilize the extant ideas, models and interventions available to them. They do so in the context of their work with unique client systems that present a broad variety of problems that are maintained by factors ranging from mere lack of information to complex and challenging networks of constraints. Therapists struggle with how to organize and utilize the available knowledge and interventions, as well as how to plan and sequence therapy. Therapists who practice within a specific model struggle with what to do when the strategies and interventions of that model do not address the concerns of their clients. Eclectic therapists struggle to find a coherent means of organizing their work—a set of principles to help them decide what to do and when to do it.

This confusing and sometimes overwhelming experience that individual clinicians face presents, in the collective, a developmental challenge for the field. Integrative Systemic Therapy (IST) is a meta-level systemic perspective that addresses this challenge by providing a means of integrating the vast and diverse field of knowledge about human systems, their problems, and the therapeutic models and interventions that have emerged to address them (Russell & Breunlin, 2019; Pinsof et al., 2018; Breunlin et al., 2018). IST is an integrative and systemic perspective for individual, couple, and family psychotherapy that provides a framework for transcending the specific models of therapy and accessing their concepts and interventions to meet the particular needs of specific cases. It is a comprehensive perspective in that it can be applied to a wide range of client concerns (problems, aspirations, symptoms, and disorders).

IST has its roots in the work of Douglas Breunlin and his colleagues on Metaframeworks (Breunlin et al., 1992) and the work of William Pinsof on Integrative Problem Centered Therapy (Pinsof, 1995). It was also

DOI: 10.4324/9780429322273-1

influenced by the work of Jay Lebow on psychotherapy integration and common factors (Lebow, 1997, 2014). IST was developed at The Family Institute at Northwestern University where, for over 20 years, Pinsof, Breunlin and William Russell taught the evolving perspective in graduate and post-graduate training programs in marriage and family therapy. Prior to the perspective's designation as IST, it was called Integrative Problem Centered Metaframeworks (Breunlin et al., 2011; Pinsof et al., 2011; Russell et al., 2016).

Anthony Chambers and Cheryl Rampage joined Pinsof, Breunlin, Russell, and Lebow to formulate a complete description of IST's theoretical framework and its clinical application, which can be found in Pinsof et al. (2018). To grasp the theory of IST and understand the depth and breadth of its application, we recommend that this book be read carefully before reading and working with this handbook. This chapter serves as a review of that material.

Recent publications have focused on IST with African American couples (Chambers, 2019), managing clinical complexity with an integrative, systemic perspective (Russell & Breunlin, 2019), supervision in IST (He et al., 2021), and IST with couples (Breunlin et al., in press).

Empirically Informing IST

The blueprint is the basis for empirically informing IST, as it provides a clinical-experimental process for incorporating information and interventions into the therapy. It views each case as a single case study, informed both by feedback from the clients and by bodies of knowledge relevant to the case. The blueprint empirically informs the process of therapy in two ways. First, the therapist draws on empirical findings about human problems and therapy methods that can be organized into blueprint components (hypothesizing, planning, conversing, and feedback). Second, IST encourages the use of standardized progress instruments (completed by clients) which provide empirical data on the progress of therapy that informs the therapist on how to modify and improve the quality of intervention (Pinsof et al., 2015).

As a broad-spectrum, meta-perspective for integrative, systemic therapy, IST has not sought to demonstrate efficacy through randomized clinical trials of a manualized treatment. Two studies have lent support to the effectiveness of IST. In a naturalistic investigation of the first eight sessions of IST (then called IPCM) therapy with 125 couples, Knobloch-Fedders et al. (2015) found that IST was effective in treating problems of both individual functioning and relationship adjustment. A second, larger study (Pinsof et al., n. d.) in a randomized clinical trial examined the use of a progress research instrument, the Systemic Therapy Inventory of Change (STIC) (Pinsof et al., 2015), with over 700 clients in individual and couple therapy.

Although this was not a manualized study of IST, the therapists in the study were trained in IST and the cases were assigned to IST and IST-plus-STIC conditions. The results showed that IST-trained therapists were effective in treating individuals and couples with and without the use of the STIC and were significantly more effective with cases in which the therapist used the STIC system.

Theoretical Framework: Integrative and Systemic

As IST's name states, it is an integrative and systemic therapy. The commitment to integration rests on the observation that specific therapy models are based on assumptions and viewpoints that limit, with good effect for some clients, the terrain of their psychotherapy. Consequently, the various models describe different and often complementary aspects of the therapeutic terrain, each in their model-specific languages, ignoring and sometimes depreciating other explanations of human problems and strategies for change (Fraenkel, 2009, 2018; Lebow, 1997, 2014). IST moves beyond the confines of a model-driven approach and toward a comprehensive and guideline-informed perspective for integrating existing and yet-to-be-developed concepts, strategies, and interventions.

To provide a perspective that integrates therapy models, IST's theoretical framework transcends the theories of the various models and substantively incorporates what the models have to offer. IST accomplishes this in three ways. First, it provides a set of theoretical pillars on which its conceptual framework and practice guidelines are built (Pinsof et al., 2018); second, it prioritizes common factors such as the therapeutic alliance, client readiness, goal consensus, and collaboration (Sprenkle et al., 2009); and third, it utilizes a set of metaframeworks that capture the breadth of human experience relevant to the practice of family, couple and individual psychotherapy (Breunlin et al., 2011). Each metaframework addresses an important aspect of human experience that can be integrated into the conceptualization of cases and utilized in the selection of strategies and interventions. Importantly, the application of concepts and frameworks with particular clients is not driven by the concepts or frameworks themselves, rather it is based on the actual patterns revealed in the collaborative conversation with the clients. In this sense, IST is tailored to fit each case. It is client system-centered.

The Pillars of IST

IST rests on five theoretical pillars that describe the presuppositions of the approach and provide the basis for the *systemic* in the name, IST. At first glance, the pillars may seem impractical or overly philosophical, but they are the presuppositions of IST and find expression in any number of

IST's concepts and procedures. All models of therapy rest on pillars, but they are often not explicitly articulated.

The *epistemological* pillar addresses the human capacity to know reality by asserting that there is an objective reality, but that human knowledge of that reality is unavoidably partial and limited by the perspective of the observer. As we engage with our clients over time, our knowledge about them can become more accurate but is never definitive or complete. The *ontological* pillar addresses the nature of social reality by adopting a multilevel view of human systems that includes the subsystems of person, relationship, family, community, and society (von Bertalanffy, 1968). Systems concepts and principles, such as wholeness, self-regulation, and feedback are seen as applicable to each level of the system and to the interaction between the levels. IST's *causality* pillar addresses cause and effect in human systems by viewing the interaction among systems and subsystems as a web of mutual influence with various systems contributing differentially to the variance in any process or outcome. The *sequences* pillar holds that pattern exists in human systems, and that it is useful to describe patterns in terms of recurrent sequences of events that play out over various intervals of time and include actions, meanings, and emotions. The *constraint* pillar provides a general theory of change as the identification and removal of constraints that prevent problem-solving (Breunlin, 1999; Pinsof et al., 2018). IST focuses on identifying adaptive solutions and removing or mitigating the factors that constrain the implementation of those solutions.

Based on the systemic presuppositions of its pillars, IST conceptualizes all psychotherapeutic practice within a multi-systemic context. Given the properties of systems, all forms of therapy intentionally or unintentionally intervene in a *client system*, which consists of all the people who may be involved in the maintenance or resolution of the presenting problems (Pinsof, 1995). IST divides the client system into direct and indirect systems. The clients attending therapy on a given occasion comprise the direct client system and those members who are not directly involved in the therapy are designated as the indirect client system. Therapists typically view their work as intervening solely with those in the room (the direct system). IST views interventions with individuals or subsystems of a family as interventions into the whole client system, including direct and indirect client systems. The therapy affects and is affected by all members of the system, whether or not they attend sessions. IST proposes that the field of psychotherapy should move beyond its predominant focus on individuals toward a perspective that views human behavior and therapeutic intervention in the context of multiple systems—biological, psychological, couple, family, community and society—regardless of who is physically present for therapy. The concept of the multisystemic context suggests that we more carefully consider who should attend the therapy with a preference, unless contraindicated, for involving multiple members of the client system in the therapy. Further, the boundary between the direct and indirect client systems is permeable so that clients in the indirect system may, under many circumstances, be invited to attend therapy. The direct system at any given point in therapy ideally consists of those members who are needed to address the therapy tasks at hand.

Widening the systemic lens, IST constructs therapy as the inter-relationship of two systems: the client system and the therapist system (Pinsof et al., 2018). The client system is discussed above. The therapist system consists of a direct therapist system that conducts the sessions (the therapist) and an indirect therapist system that consists of the therapists and professionals who influence the therapy but are not directly involved in the session (supervisor, consultant, other therapists who consult, agency policymakers). The boundary between the direct therapist system and the indirect therapist system is somewhat permeable. For example, a supervisor may decide to attend a session, thus entering the direct therapist system. The client and therapist systems form the therapy system, which is depicted in Figure 1.1. The arrows between the systems depict the mutual influence between the two systems and the arrows within each system depict the mutual influence between the direct and indirect subsystems.

The Essence of IST

The essence of IST is a collaboration of therapist and clients in the effort to resolve or improve the clients' presenting problems and concerns. This collaboration, led by the therapist, focuses on the biopsychosocial context in which the problem is embedded. An initial, partial understanding of

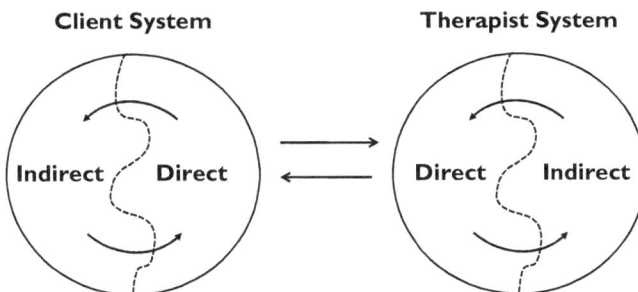

Figure 1.1 The therapy system. Adapted from Integrative systemic therapy: Metaframeworks for problem-solving with individuals, couples, and families (p. 46), by W. M. Pinsof, D. C. Breunlin, W. P. Russell, J. L. Lebow, C. Rampage, and A. L. Chambers, 2018, American Psychological Association. Copyright 2017. Adapted with permission.

the context is established by convening the clients, defining the presenting problem, and agreeing on a description of a problem sequence. A problem sequence is the set of recurring behaviors, thoughts, and feelings in which the problem is embedded. Approaching clients with a curiosity about sequences locates the problem in time and space and clarifies what is happening before, during, and after the problem occurs. A problem may be described as marital conflict, but the problem sequence provides a description of what is happening in that conflict and suggests how it fits in the lives of the couple. A problem sequence is a practical and partial understanding of the client system.

Change is initiated when clients and the therapist identify a solution sequence that would modify or replace the problem sequence and may, if enacted, resolve or begin to resolve the problem. Once a solution sequence is agreed upon, the therapist encourages the clients to enact it. If the clients try the solution and it improves the problem, then they may be on the way to accomplishing their goal for therapy. If the clients report that they did not implement and maintain the agreed-upon solution (which is often the case), the therapist works with the clients to identify the constraints that have prevented the solution sequence from being implemented. As the constraints are identified, the therapist collaborates with the clients to remove the constraints so they can enact the solution sequence or a modified version of it based on the continuing therapeutic collaboration.

The factors that constrain clients range from lack of information (at the simplest level), to fears about proposed solutions, to differences in cultural expectations, to illness, to the sequelae of traumatic experiences that occurred in early childhood (at the most complex and remote level). IST's problem-solving process—defining a problem, locating the problem in a problem sequence, identifying and implementing a solution sequence, identifying and lifting constraints that block a solution sequence, and maintaining a solution sequence—is depicted in the flow chart (see Figure 1.2) known as the *essence diagram* (Russell et al., 2016). As a problem is solved, the therapy moves on to additional presenting concerns or toward termination. In IST the collaboration on the essence tasks strengthens the therapeutic alliance as the therapist addresses what is of concern to the clients (the problem) and works carefully to establish an agreement with clients at each essence step. The general description of problem-solving provided in the essence diagram draws its real-life specificity from the clients' experience and from the therapist's use of the IST blueprint.

The Blueprint

The essence diagram serves as a roadmap that sequences the general problem-solving steps of therapy, whereas the IST blueprint for therapy (Breunlin et al., 1992; Pinsof et al., 2018) provides both the bodies of

Intake ↓

Convene a Direct Client
System and Define the
Problem(s)

Terminate

Locate a
Problem in a
Problem
Sequence

Identify the
Constraints

Implement and
Maintain the
Solution
Sequence

unsuccessful

successful

Attempt to Lift the
Constraints

Identify a
Solution
Sequence

Evaluate
Outcome
(Feedback)

Implement the
Solution
Sequence

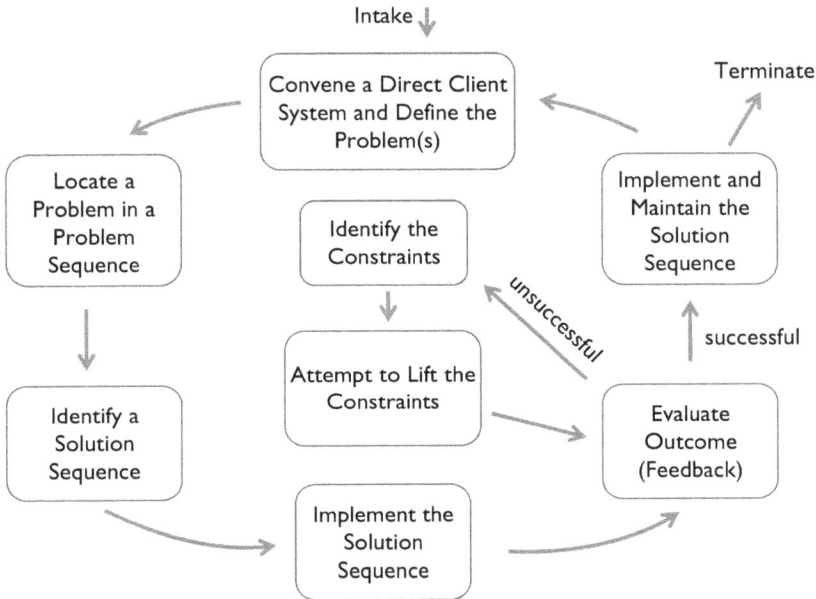

Figure 1.2 Essence of integrative systemic therapy. Reprinted from "Integrative Problem Centered Metaframeworks (IPCM) Therapy," by W. P. Russell, W. Pinsof, D. C. Breunlin, and J. Lebow, in T. L. Sexton and J. Lebow (Eds.), Handbook of Family Therapy (p. 531), 2016, Routledge. Copyright 2016 by Taylor & Francis. Reprinted with permission.

knowledge and the decision-making process required to determine how the *essence* tasks are accomplished and how therapeutic strategies are selected. The blueprint replaces the clinical logic of the various models of therapy that are integrated into IST. It has four components: *Hypothesizing, planning, conversing,* and *reading feedback.* The IST Blueprint for therapy (see Figure 1.3) depicts an iterative decision-making and decision-evaluating process that repeats throughout each session and in larger planning arcs throughout the therapy. It guides the therapist in dealing with any and all issues related to the essence steps and the therapeutic alliance. Unlike the traditional notion of assessment, hypothesizing—a way of progressively understanding the client system—can reveal new and critical information at any time in the course of therapy. Similarly, plans are never final, as new pathways for change derive from new hypotheses that develop in relation to conversation and feedback.

Comprehensive integration requires both the incorporation of what therapy models have to offer and the freedom to operate beyond their

Hypothesizing   Conversing

Planning   Feedback

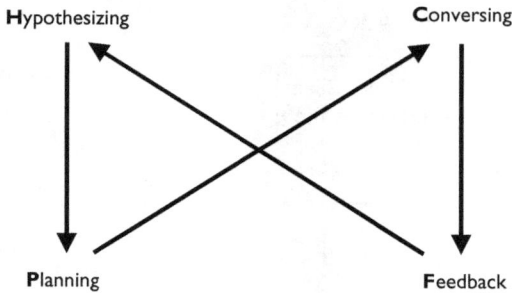

Figure 1.3 Blueprint for therapy. Reprinted from "Integrative Problem-Centered Metaframeworks (IPCM) Therapy I: Core Concepts and Hypothesizing," by D. C. Breunlin, W. Pinsof, W. P. Russell, and J. Lebow, 2011, Family Process, 50(3), p. 300. Copyright 2011 by John Wiley & Sons. Reprinted with permission.

logic. In IST, hypothesizing utilizes hypothesizing metaframeworks to transcend the logic of the specific models. The seven hypothesizing metaframeworks, described below, provide frameworks and information about the domains of human experience most often addressed in psychotherapy. Hypothesizing metaframeworks provide the ideas used to formulate hypotheses about solution sequences, client strengths, factors that constrain solutions, and nuances of the therapeutic alliance. The blueprint also provides a set of planning metaframeworks that contain interventive strategies, originally developed within therapy models and empirically supported treatments.

For the conversing component of the blueprint, IST therapists use a set of tools that facilitate attending closely to therapeutic conversation, as they purposefully construct what they say in sessions to meet the tasks of each step of the essence and maintain a good working alliance with the clients. The blueprint component of reading feedback is facilitated by careful attention to the nuances of verbal and nonverbal communication as well as the content and process dimensions of communication. This attention yields information that serves as feedback that informs hypothesizing and, in turn, the selection of interventions.

The Hypothesizing Metaframeworks

IST's seven hypothesizing metaframeworks (organization, development, mind, culture, gender, biology, and spirituality) organize and contain a wealth of information drawn from models of therapy and from other relevant fields of knowledge. In sessions and between sessions, the therapist can "open" specific metaframeworks in order to interpret and utilize feedback (client report, therapist observations, progress instrument data). A brief description of the hypothesizing metaframeworks follows (Breunlin et al., 2011; Russell et al., 2016).

- *Organization*: Concepts that describe how the components of a system fit together and function as a whole (e.g., boundaries, leadership, harmony)
- *Development*: Information concerning developmental issues and competencies within families, relationships, and individuals
- *Mind*: Analysis of cognitions, emotions, and intentionality, at three increasingly complex levels: sequence, organization, and development
- *Culture*: Framework for understanding contexts of membership such as race, ethnicity, class, economic status, education, sexual identity, and sexual orientation, including their relationship to issues of inclusion and social justice
- *Gender*: Information related to gender identity, gender-based power, and views on gender roles
- *Biology*: Medical, physiological and neurobiological factors (e.g., illness, disability, brain chemistry, physiology of emotions)
- *Spirituality*: Perspectives on religious beliefs and spiritual resources, including faith, prayer, transcendence, and acceptance

The hypothesizing metaframeworks are used to understand all the levels of the multi-level biopsychosocial system. A human system is a nested hierarchy of subsystems that include the person, dyadic and triadic relationships, family, community, society, and global context. The *IST web of human experience* combines the system levels and the hypothesizing metaframeworks to form a diagram (see Figure 1.4). In the diagram, the metaframeworks (the straight lines) cut across the various levels of systemic organization (concentric circles). The web is a heuristic device the therapist uses to generate hypotheses about the client system, including hypotheses about client strengths, solution sequences, constraints, and the alliance. The web helps the therapist consider both the nature (described by a metaframework) and location (in the biopsychosocial system) of factors that constrain the client system from solving its concerns. For example, if parents seem to be split on how to deal with an adolescent with acting-out behavior, an IST therapist would hypothesize that there could be a constraint of organization at the level of the family.

The Planning Metaframeworks

In planning, IST distinguishes strategies and interventions. Strategies state a general direction for solving a problem or removing a constraint.

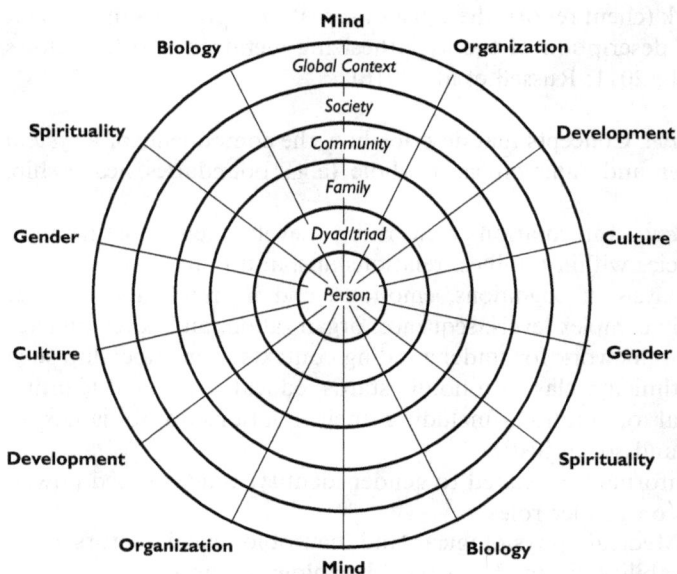

Figure 1.4 Web of human experience. Reprinted from "Integrative Problem-Centered Metaframeworks Therapy I: Core Concepts and Hypothesizing," by D. C. Breunlin, W. Pinsof, W. P. Russell, and J. Lebow, 2011, Family Process, 50(3), p. 301. Copyright 2011 by John Wiley & Sons. Reprinted with permission.

Interventions are specific ways of accomplishing the strategies. As an integrative perspective, IST draws its strategies and interventions from a variety of sources. Common sense ideas that are part of everyday life and the clinical experience of the therapist are often sources of initial solution sequences. More formalized strategies for identifying solution sequences and addressing constraints are drawn from the models of psychotherapy, mechanisms of change that are common to all effective therapy (common factors; Sprenkle et al., 2009), and research on the process and outcome of therapy. Integration in IST is facilitated by organizing interventive strategies into a set of planning metaframeworks, positioning the metaframeworks on a planning matrix, and providing guidelines for their utilization. The planning metaframeworks are containers of various types of therapeutic strategies and their associated interventions. The planning matrix depicts a set of guidelines for the selection of strategies and interventions.

The planning metaframeworks contain strategies that describe general plans for establishing solution sequences or removing constraints. The strategies are meta to the models in that they each typically have a place in multiple psychotherapy models. The strategies, described in model-neutral language, extract the strategies from the various models and group them according to their foci and mechanisms of change. Based on a hypothesis, the therapist selects a strategy from a planning meta-framework to facilitate the implementation of a solution sequence or address a constraint that prevents its implementation. Each strategy may be accomplished by means of a variety of interventions. The interventions associated with the strategies were typically developed within various models of therapy. Each IST therapist fills their own planning meta-frameworks with interventions they learn in support of the strategies. A brief description of each of the six planning metaframeworks follows (Pinsof et al., 2011; Pinsof et al., 2018; Russell et al., 2016).

- *Action*: These strategies and associated interventions are primarily aimed at helping clients modify their patterns of action and interaction. Establishing an action plan requires a collaborative understanding between therapists and clients. This understanding is accomplished in the realm of cognition and emotion, but the central focus of an action strategy is to initiate change through action. Action strategies are accomplished by interventions drawn from social learning (Bandura, 1991), behavioral and cognitive-behavioral approaches (Barlow et al., 1989; Baucom et al., 1990; Craske, 1999; Jacobson & Margolin, 1979; Patterson et al., 1992), dialectical behavior therapy (Linehan, 2015; Linehan & Wilks, 2015), structural family therapy (Minuchin & Fishman, 1981), strategic therapy (Haley, 1987; Watzlawick et al., 1974) and solution-focused therapy (Berg, 1994).
- *Meaning/Emotion*: These strategies and interventions are primarily focused on modifying thoughts and feelings. They seek to regulate constraining emotions, heighten adaptive emotions, or develop adaptive cognitions, meanings, or narratives. The meaning/emotion strategies include interventions drawn from cognitive behavioral (Beck, 1996; Beck, 2011), integrative behavioral (Baucom et al., 2002; Christensen et al., 1995), emotion-focused (Greenberg, 2011), emotionally focused (Greenberg & Johnson, 1988), narrative (White & Epston, 1990; McAdams & Janis 2004), dialectical behavioral (Linehan, 2015; Linehan & Wilks, 2015), acceptance and commitment (Hayes et al., 1999), psychoeducational, and experiential (Safran et al., 1988; Greenberg, 2004) approaches.
- *Biobehavioral*: These strategies are targeted to modify underlying biological processes that seem to be constraining a solution sequence. Biobehavioral interventions include medication, biofeedback (Rogers, 1981), eye movement desensitization and reprocessing (Shapiro, 1995; Shapiro, 2001), mindfulness meditation (Tang, 2017); acupuncture (Chon & Lee, 2013); and physical exercise.

- *Family of Origin*: These strategies address adult clients' relationships with their families of origin and, in doing so, facilitate differentiation of self and mature interdependence. The focus can be on developing insight into how the family of origin patterns impact current relationships, or on direct work with the family of origin to modify relational patterns that constrain the client. The family of origin metaframework draws strategies and specific interventions from the work of family therapy pioneers Murray Bowen (Bowen, 1974), Ivan Boszormenyi-Nagy (Boszormenyi-Nagy & Spark, 1973), and James Framo (Framo, 1992), as well as the work of Mona Fishbane (Fishbane, 2016, 2015) and Monica McGoldrick (McGoldrick et al., 2008).
- *Internal Representation*: These strategies address internalized mental representations of early relational experiences and family figures that appear to be constraining problem resolution. They seek to modify internal objects or parts of mind, the relationships among them, and/ or the relationship between the objects/parts and other people. The internal representation strategies utilize interventions derived from internal family systems (IFS) therapy (Schwartz, 2013), object relations theory (Guntrip & Rudnytsky, 2013; Scharff, 1995), and other psychodynamic approaches.
- *Self*: This metaframework targets change in the therapeutic relationship as the means of helping a client develop a stronger, more flexible self. When the therapist has worked extensively with the other planning metaframeworks, but constraints of mind persist, individual therapy to strengthen the self may be recommended. Approaches to this work include functional analytic psychotherapy (Kohlenberg & Tsai, 2007), which applies clinical behavioral analysis to the therapeutic relationship, and self psychology (Kohut, 1977; 1984), which focuses on the analysis of transference and on as ruptures and repairs of the therapeutic alliance. If the client is self-harming, highly impulsive, profoundly reactive to criticism or rejection, or satisfies the diagnostic description of borderline personality, the preferred treatment is dialectical behavior therapy (Linehan, 2015).

The action, meaning/emotion, and biobehavioral metaframeworks focus primarily on the here-and-now, dealing with constraints that can be directly addressed without intensive focus on historical events. The family-of-origin, internal representation, and self planning metaframeworks are the historical or there-and-then planning metaframeworks, which focus on constraints that originate in the past, but currently impede problem resolution. Typically, IST works first with strategies from the here-and-now planning metaframeworks and moves, if necessary, to strategies located in the historical planning metaframeworks. A more extensive discussion of each of the planning metaframeworks can be found in

Pinsof et al. (2018). Examples of strategies associated with each of the planning metaframeworks, along with intervention resources for fulfilling the various strategies, are found in Appendix A.

The Contexts of Therapy

IST specifies three intervention contexts within which strategies from the planning metaframeworks can be applied. The *family/community context* includes two or more family members (excluding couples) and may include members of the community. It often involves members of more than one generation, but may comprise adult siblings or important friends within the same generation. The *couple context* involves two people who are in a committed partnership—a relationship with a past and possibly a future. This context includes married couples, dating couples, and unmarried cohabitating couples. A couple may include members of any gender identity or sexual orientation. In the *individual context* one person from the client system attends therapy.

Figure 1.5 depicts the IST matrix, which consists of the contexts of therapy and the planning metaframeworks. With the exception of the self

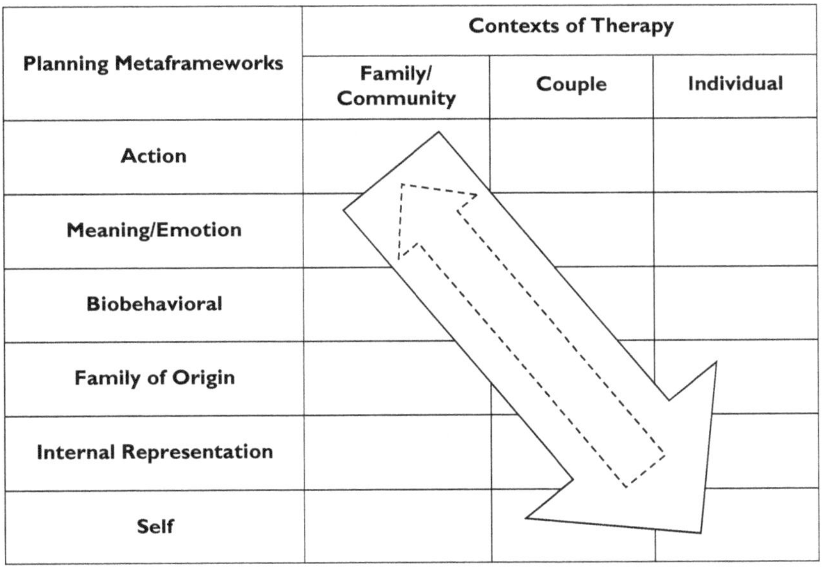

Planning Metaframeworks	Contexts of Therapy		
	Family/ Community	Couple	Individual
Action			
Meaning/Emotion			
Biobehavioral			
Family of Origin			
Internal Representation			
Self			

Figure 1.5 Planning matrix. Adapted from "Integrative Problem-Centered Metaframeworks Therapy II: Planning, Conversing, and Reading Feedback," by D. C. Breunlin, W. Pinsof, W. P. Russell, and J. Lebow, 2011, Family Process, 50(3), p. 318. Copyright 2011 by John Wiley & Sons. Adapted with permission.

planning metaframework, which is generally associated with individual therapy, IST's intervention strategies are not tied to particular contexts and can be applied within each of the intervention contexts. For example, action or family-of-origin strategies can be used in individual, couple, and family contexts. Thinking in terms of individual, couple, or family *contexts* contrasts with the conventional terms of individual, couple or family *therapy*, which tend to link who is in the room (modality) with certain models and strategies that have traditionally been practiced with that modality. The planning metaframeworks along with the therapy contexts establish IST as a post-model and post-modality perspective.

Guidelines for Intervention: What to do When?

As we have seen, decision-making in IST is governed by the blueprint as hypotheses and plans are tested in conversation (intervention) and feedback suggests how the hypotheses or plans may need to be revised. A set of planning guidelines (Breunlin et al., 2011; Pinsof et al., 2011) also guides decision making as they suggest therapists privilege certain hypotheses at certain points in therapy and approach intervention in a generally preferred, but ultimately flexible way. A complete list of IST guidelines is provided in Appendix B. Those that apply to the matrix comprise IST's principle of application and are described briefly here and illustrated by the arrows on the *IST planning matrix*, depicted in Figure 1.5.

The *interpersonal guideline* asserts that whenever possible and appropriate, therapy should begin in an interpersonal context and progress, as necessary, to the individual context. To illustrate this guideline, the large arrow originates in the family and couple contexts. This indicates a general preference, though therapy may also begin in the individual context. The *temporal guideline* asserts that therapy begins with a here-and-now focus and progresses, if necessary, to interventions that address the there-and-then (distant-past events and related patterns). This is depicted by the arrow originating in the upper half of the matrix which contains the here-and-now planning metaframeworks. The *cost-effectiveness guideline*, also illustrated by the origin of the arrow, asserts that the therapist should use the most direct, simplest, and least expensive interventions before moving to more indirect, complex, and expensive interventions which are in the lower half of the matrix. The *strength guideline* assumes that, unless proven otherwise, the client system has the strengths and ability to solve their problems with limited therapeutic intervention. Only when clients are too constrained to use strategies from the here-and-now metaframeworks do therapists hypothesize a more complex web of constraints requiring interventions drawn from lower on the matrix. The *failure-driven guideline* asserts that the movement from left to right and from top to bottom depicted by the matrix arrow occurs as strategies involving a further left context or those from a metaframework located higher in the matrix have been ineffective. "Failure" in IST is seen as an opportunity to learn more about the system and search for effective solutions. Still, failure is a loaded word, so it is not used in conversation with clients. Rather, IST approaches intervention as a set of "experiments" from which clients and their therapists learn more about what it will take to solve the problems presented for therapy.

The smaller arrow within the matrix's larger arrow points back up which signifies that the purpose of intervention at the lower level of the matrix is to facilitate changes in the way clients behave with each other and how they establish solution sequences that address what they have sought to accomplish in therapy (solving the presenting problem). Along the road of therapy, clients and their therapist may agree to work on new problems or issues, but until they do, the primary goal of therapy is to successfully address the initial presenting concerns and related problem sequences. The smaller arrow continually reminds the therapist not to get lost in the exploration of remote constraints for their own sake at the expense of the therapy's problem-centered focus. The plans drawn from the matrix and tested in the blueprint are always in service of the essence tasks.

The arrows are not meant to depict a rigid or ideal order of application. IST therapists are strongly committed to the guidelines, but flexible in their actual application. Flexibility with the guidelines is necessary for three reasons. First, the therapist will override the interpersonal guideline when physical or emotional safety may be at stake. For example, a therapist receiving a request from a woman for a conjoint session with her step-father to discuss his past sexual abuse of her will convene individual sessions with both the woman and her step-father prior to scheduling a conjoint session in order to assess risks, maximize the likelihood of a safe and manageable process, and minimize re-traumatization. Second, a compelling hypothesis developed from feedback may lead a therapist to bypass a therapy context or a planning metaframework level of the matrix. For example, in a case of a person presenting with symptoms of psychosis that seem an obvious constraint to working with action or meaning/emotion strategies, the therapist may require an evaluation for medication (biobehavioral planning metaframework) prior to working more intensively with strategies drawn from higher on the matrix. Third, maintaining the therapy alliance will require the therapist to be flexible in the application of the guidelines as the client may not be on board with the plan that results from a particular level of the matrix. For example, some clients resist beginning therapy with a focus on their patterns of action. For them, patterns of mind and the meaning/emotion planning metaframework may be more central to the therapy from the very beginning.

Although IST's principle of application, as represented by the matrix arrows, suggests that action strategies be considered before strategies that focus on meaning and emotion, IST therapists track and converse in the language of action, meaning, and emotion in every session. Straightforward action interventions require a mutual understanding of the purpose of the intervention (meaning) and attunement to clients' emotions. Conversely, changes in meaning or emotion often lead to immediate opportunities for work in the realm of action. As constraints are identified, their nature along with client feedback suggests the preferred and proportionate focus on action, meaning and/or emotion.

All of what is done in IST rests on the creation of a therapeutic alliance. The therapeutic alliance has three dimensions within IST: Goals, tasks, and bonds. The goal dimension has to do with whether the therapist and clients are in alignment on the goals for therapy. The task dimension of the alliance describes the degree to which the therapist and clients are in alliance with respect to specific tasks (strategies and their interventions) of therapy. The bond dimension describes a connection that develops over time, which transcends specific goals and tasks. The bonds that develop may, in time, give the therapist more room to challenge a client, but attention to goal and task alignment is essential in maintaining, as well as building, the therapeutic alliance. IST posits an *alliance priority guideline*, which asserts that creating and maintaining a good therapeutic alliance takes priority over both the therapist's hypotheses and the general guidelines for how therapy progresses that are depicted in the matrix. If maintaining the alliance with the client system requires suspending a hypothesis or guideline, the IST therapist will do so unless doing so fundamentally compromises the effectiveness or integrity of the therapy.

An additional guideline supports the alliance and acknowledges the societal and community forces that are oppressive to clients. The social justice guideline posits that the therapist attends to cultural contexts of membership (intersectionality), inclusion, and social justice issues at each step of the problem-solving process. Particular attention is paid to how questions and suggestions impact clients and whether the direction of therapy feels fitting and respectful to them.

Conversing and Reading Feedback

The execution of all essence tasks, including specific plans for intervention, occurs in the context of a series of collaborative conversations. IST therapists are the leaders of these conversations which are the vehicle for establishing an alliance, developing an understanding of the client system, engaging clients in the process of change, and structuring the therapy. The clients bring their expertise concerning their experience, circumstances, and context. The therapist brings expertise in therapeutic conversation, problem-solving and therapeutic methods. IST therapists attend carefully to what they say during sessions and make a study of conversing and the use of self. This requires attention to the conscious use of language to accomplish the tasks of therapy and awareness of one's own internal experience (countertransference) that could otherwise be a constraint to the conversation.

The IST therapist also pays careful attention to the feedback that results from conversations and interventions. Feedback is any information that informs the therapist about the client system or suggests a direction for therapy. Sources of feedback include what clients report, the therapist's observations of behavior and interaction, the therapist's emotional responses, conversations with other providers, documents such as intake forms or the results of psychological testing, and data from empirical progress instruments. Feedback is a primary source of material for hypothesizing, planning, and conversing. Attending closely to the feedback affords the therapist the opportunity to chart a course that fits the client system and monitors progress.

The essence orients the therapist to the problem-solving process. The blueprint facilitates decision-making about the essence steps and the alliance. Feedback grounds the conversation in the client's concerns, goals, circumstances, and actual patterns of behavior. Although IST includes guidelines, frameworks and heuristic devices that inform practice, it is not a manualized approach. "IST views therapy as an idiosyncratic, idiographic and improvisational process. Every episode of therapy is unique and requires improvisation and clinical judgement. The metaphor of jazz seems appropriate, as IST involves a structured, planful and disciplined process that plays out differently and uniquely with each client system and episode of therapy. And, just as every master jazz musician has his or her unique sound, IST therapists adapt the model to their personality and values to create a unique 'sound' that makes their therapy real and genuine" (Breunlin et al., 2018, p. 10).

Therapist Development

Experienced IST practitioners have acquired knowledge and skills from a variety of models as well as the important meta-model skills in hypothesizing, planning, conversing, reading feedback, and maintaining alliances. Beginning IST practitioners who are also beginning therapists will not yet have acquired extensive knowledge of the various models of therapy. They will be tasked with learning the strategies and interventions of the various models of therapy over a period of time. Experienced therapists who decide to expand or organize their work with IST will already have learned a variety of concepts and interventions that they use in their work. They are tasked with learning IST's meta-model concepts and skills that are discussed in this book.

Importantly, a therapist can never fully master IST as there is always more to learn and integrate into one's practice. IST is not just a perspective for conducting therapy; it is also a framework for growth and learning for therapists over the course of their careers. Each of the blueprint components (hypothesizing, planning, conversing, and reading feedback) can symbolically house the information, interventions, and techniques that a therapist learns over many years of practice. The therapist calls upon these stores of information and skills when utilizing a component of the blueprint. For example, when *hypothesizing* the therapist calls on the knowledge stored in the web of human experience, including knowledge about various hypothesizing metaframeworks. Or, when *conversing* the therapist calls upon principles of communication and the art of asking questions and making statements that advance the therapeutic conversation.

Growth and learning for therapists include the acquisition of specific knowledge and skills. Since IST proposes drawing that knowledge and those skills from a broad variety of approaches, it follows that IST therapists will be hard-pressed to become experts in all of the models of therapy from which they draw. IST takes the position that expert knowledge of specific models is not necessarily required and that it is reasonable to be "good enough" at the interventions selected, and that developing a solid alliance and being careful to read the feedback can substitute for the higher level of model-specific expertise (Russell & Breunlin, 2019). Many interventions can be adopted with limited study and practice. Other interventions require a level of knowledge and skill that results from more formalized training in a model or method. Given such training, complex interventive strategies can be brought into IST as modules of intervention. For example, a therapist may incorporate a module of an exposure therapy protocol to address a fear or phobia. Alternatively, an IST therapist who has not attained sufficient knowledge of a formal intervention protocol can refer a case for a specific intervention. Distinguishing which skills require formal training and which require only informal study is a responsibility that is handled by supervisors during training and assumed by the therapist in consultation with other professionals after the completion of formal training.

IST provides a variety of tools to understand and assist client systems, but all of what therapists do happens in the context of who they are, how they are affected by the work, and how they use themselves as an instrument for building relationships, understanding client systems, and initiating change. Growth of the person-of-the-therapist (Aponte & Kissil, 2016) results both from pursuing psychological understanding of self and seeking critical awareness of one's own cultural contexts and privilege. Training programs provide a variety of classroom-based or group-based experiences that help trainees become more aware of who they are and what their personal growth edges are. In IST, the most direct impetus for growth in the person-of-the-therapist results from two primary sources, both located in the context of clinical work and supervision. First, trainees are encouraged to access and express their unique selves in the process of conducting therapy sessions. Second, supervisors work with trainees to help them reflect on their work and identify the emotional responses and cultural assumptions that constrain how they function in therapy (He et al., 2021).

Conclusion

Integrative Systemic Therapy (IST) is not a model of therapy. It is a meta-level systemic perspective that provides a structure for integrating the vast field of knowledge about human systems, their problems, and the therapeutic models and interventions that have emerged to address them. It provides a framework for individual, couple, and family psychotherapy that transcends the models of therapy and accesses their concepts and interventions, as well as common factors and best practices, to meet the particular needs of specific client systems. Within its guidelines and frameworks, IST is an improvisational process that addresses a set of essential problem-solving tasks by means of hypothesizing, planning, conversing, and reading feedback. As a comprehensive approach to a wide variety of problems and situations, IST is necessarily complex. As such, its concepts and frameworks comprise a substrate not just for practice but for the lifelong learning and growth of integrative, systemic psychotherapists.

This chapter provided an overview of IST. Chapter 2 will explore the first step in the process of therapy, the initial phone call. Subsequent chapters will explore each of the problem-solving tasks delineated in the essence diagram (Figure 1.2). Along with addressing the practical issues associated with these tasks, careful attention will be paid to the use of the blueprint to accomplish these tasks and maintain the therapeutic alliance.

Exercises

1   Think about a recurrent challenge or problem in your life. Consider (or discuss) one or more solutions for it. Select one and imagine enacting it. Do you feel hesitant? Is there something that would get in the way of your doing it? If so, review the solution again to make sure it is a reasonable course of action. If so, think about the thing that would get in the way of the solution again (the feeling or the anticipation). Consider what can be done about it in order to allow yourself to enact the solution.
2   Consider (or discuss) the pillars of IST. Are there some that you readily agree with? Are there any that you do not understand or feel

resistant to? If so, review pages 41–52 in Pinsof et al. (2018) to see if you can get a new understanding of any that you struggle with.

3   Review the IST guidelines (Appendix B). Re-read the interpersonal guideline. Consider (or discuss) your reactions to the following scenario.

A man calls a therapist to initiate therapy for the anxiety he experiences at work. During the phone call, the therapist discovers that the man is partnered. The therapist suggests that the partner attend the first session with the man.

Why would the therapist make this suggestion? If you were to suggest this, how would you present it and explain it? What would you do, if the man said he preferred not to attend with his partner?

References

Aponte, H. J., & Kissil, K. (Eds.). (2016). *The person of the therapist training model: Mastering the use of self*. Routledge.

Bandura, A. (1991). Social cognitive theory of self-regulation. *Organizational Behavior and Human Decision Processes*, *50*(2), 248–287.

Barlow, D. H., Craske, M. G., Cerny, J. A., & Klosko, J. S. (1989). Behavioral treatment of panic disorder. *Behavior Therapy*, *20*(2), 261–282.

Baucom, D. H., Epstein, N. B., & Norman, B. (1990). *Cognitive-behavioral marital therapy*. Brunner/Mazel.

Baucom, D. H., Epstein, N. B., LaTaillade, J. J., & Kirby, J. S. (2002). Cognitive-behavioral couple therapy. In A. S. Gurman & N. S. Jacobson (Eds.), *Clinical handbook of couple therapy* (3rd ed., pp. 31–72). Guilford Press.

Beck, A. T. (1996). Beyond belief: A theory of modes, personality, and psychopathology. In P. M. Salkovskis (Ed.), *Frontiers of cognitive therapy* (pp. 1–25). Guilford Press.

Beck, J. S. (2011). *Cognitive behavior therapy: Basics and beyond* (2nd ed.). Guilford Press.

Berg, I. K. (1994). *Family-based services: A solution-focused approach*. W. W. Norton.

Boszormenyi-Nagy, I., & Spark, G. M. (1973). *Invisible loyalties: Reciprocity in intergenerational family therapy*. Harper & Row.

Bowen, M. (1974). Toward the differentiation of self in one's family of origin. *Georgetown family symposium*, *1*, 222–242.

Breunlin, D. C. (1999) Toward a theory of constraints. *Journal of Marriage and Family Therapy*, *25*(3), 365–382. 10.1111/j.1752-0606.1999.tb00254.x

Breunlin, D. C., Pinsof, W., & Russell, W. P. (2018). Integrative systemic therapy. In J. Lebow, A. Chambers & D. Breunlin (Eds.), *Encyclopedia of couple and family therapy*. Springer.

Breunlin, D. C., Pinsof, W. M., Russell, W. P., & Lebow, J. L. (2011) Integrative problem centered metaframeworks (IPCM) therapy I: Core concepts and hypothesizing. *Family Process*, *50*(3), 293–313. 10.1111/j.1545-5300.2011.01362.x

Breunlin, D. C., Russell, W. P. Chambers, A., & Solomon, A. (In Press). Integrative systemic couple therapy. In Snyder, D. & Lebow (Eds.), *Handbook of couple therapy*.

Breunlin, D. C., Schwartz, R. C., & Mac Kune-Karrer, B. M. (1992). *Metaframeworks: Transcending the models of family therapy*. Jossey-Bass.

Chambers (2019). African American couples in the 21st century: Using integrative systemic therapy (IST) to translate science into practice. *Family Process, 58*(3), 595–609.

Chon, T., & Lee, M. (2013). Acupuncture. *Mayo Clinic Proceedings, 88*(10), 1141–1146. 10.1016/j.mayocp.2013.06.009

Christensen, A., Jacobson, N. S., & Babcock, J. C. (1995). *Integrative behavioral couple therapy*. Guilford.

Craske, M. G. (1999). *Anxiety disorders: Psychological approaches to theory and treatment*. Basic Books.

Fishbane, M. D. (2015). Couple therapy and interpersonal neurobiology. In A. S. Gurman, J. Lebow, & D. Snyder (Eds.), *Clinical handbook of couple therapy* (5th ed.). Guilford.

Fishbane, M. D. (2016). The neurobiology of relationships. In J. Lebow & T. Sexton (Eds.), *Handbook of family therapy* (4th ed.). Routledge.

Fraenkel, P. (2009). The therapeutic palette: A guide to choice points in integrative couple therapy. *Clinical Social Work Journal, 37*(3), 234–247.

Fraenkel, P. (2018). Integration in couple and family therapy. In J. Lebow, A. Chambers, & D. C. Breunlin (Eds.), *Encyclopedia of couple and family therapy*. Springer. 10.1007/s10615-009-0207-3

Framo, J. L. (1992). *Family-of-origin therapy: An intergenerational approach*. Psychology Press.

Greenberg, L. (2004). Being and doing in psychotherapy. *Person-Centered & Experiential Psychotherapies, 3*, 52–64. 10.1080/14779757.2004.9688329

Greenberg, L. S. (2011). *Emotion-focused therapy: Theory and practice*. American Psychological Association.

Greenberg, L. S., & Johnson, S. M. (1988). *Emotionally focused therapy for couples*. Guilford Press.

Guntrip, A. S., & Rudnytsky, P. L. (2013). *The psychoanalytic vocation: Rank, Winnicott, and the legacy of Freud*. Routledge.

Haley, J. (1987). *Problem-solving therapy* (2nd ed.). Jossey-Bass.

Hayes, S. C., Strosahl, K., & Wilson, K. G. (1999). *Acceptance and commitment therapy: An experiential approach to behavior change*. Guilford Press.

He, Y., Hardy, N., & Russell, W. P. (2021). Integrative systemic supervision: Promoting supervisees' theoretical integration in systemic therapy. *Family Process, 61*, 58–75. 10.1111/famp.12667

Jacobson, N. S., & Margolin, G. (1979). *Marital therapy: Strategies based on social learning and behavior exchange principles*. Brunner/Mazel.

Kohlenberg, R. J., & Tsai, M. (2007). *Functional analytic psychotherapy: Creating intense and curative therapeutic relationships*. Springer.

Kohut, H. (1977). *The restoration of the self*. International Universities Press.

Kohut, H. (1984). *How does analysis cure?* The University of Chicago Press. 10.72 08/chicago/9780226006147.001.0001

Knobloch-Fedders, L. M., Pinsof, W. M., & Haase, C. (2015). Treatment response in couple therapy: Relationship adjustment and individual functioning change processes. *Journal of Family Psychology*, *29*, 657–666. 10.1037/fam0000131

Lebow, J. L. (1997). The integrative revolution in couple and family therapy. *Family Process*, *36*, 1–17. 10.1111/j.1545-5300.1997.00001.x

Lebow, J. L. (2014). *Couple and family therapy: An integrative map of the territory*. American Psychological Association. 10.1037/14255-00

Linehan, M. M. (2015). *DBT skills training manual* (2nd ed.). Guilford Press.

Linehan, M. M., & Wilks, C. R. (2015). The course and evolution of dialectical behavior therapy. *American Journal of Psychotherapy*, *69*(2), 97–110. 10.1176/appi.psychotherapy.2015.69.2.97

McAdams, D. P., & Janis, L. (2004). Narrative identity and narrative therapy. In L. E. Angus & J. McLeod (Eds.), *The handbook of narrative and psychotherapy: Practice, theory, and research* (pp. 331–349). Sage. doi:10.4135/9781412973496.d13

McGoldrick, M., Gerson, R., & Petry, S. S. (2008). *Genograms: Assessment and intervention*. W. W. Norton.

Minuchin, S., & Fishman, H. C. (1981). *Family therapy techniques*. Harvard University Press.

Patterson, G. R., Reid, J. B., & Dishion, T. J. (1992). *Antisocial boys: A social interactional approach*. Castalia.

Pinsof, W. M. (1995). *Integrative problem centered therapy: A synthesis of biological, individual and family therapies*. Basic Books.

Pinsof, W. M., Breunlin, D. C., Russell, W. P., & Lebow, J. L. (2011). Integrative problem centered metaframeworks (IPCM) therapy II: Planning, conversing, and reading feedback. *Family Process. 50*(3), 314–336. 10.1111/j.1545-5300.2011.01361.x

Pinsof, W. M., Breunlin, D. C., Chambers, A. L., Solomon, A. H., & Russell, W. P. (2015). Integrative, multi-systemic and empirically informed couple therapy: The IPCM perspective. In A. Gurman, J. Lebow, & D. K. Snyder (Eds.), *Clinical handbook of couple therapy* (5th ed., pp. 161–191). The Guilford Press.

Pinsof, W., Breunlin, D., Russell, W., Lebow, J., Chambers, A. L., & Rampage, C. (2018) *Integrative systemic therapy: Metaframeworks for problem solving with individuals, couples, and families* (1st ed.). American Psychological Association. 10.1037/0000055-000

Pinsof, W., Zinbarg, R. E., He, Y., Goldsmith, J., Latta, T., & Hardy, N. (Unpublished manuscript). The Family Institute at Northwestern University.

Rogers, K. (1981). Biofeedback. Reference Section, Science and Technology Division, Library of Congress.

Russell, W. P., Pinsof, W., Breunlin, D. C., & Lebow, J. (2016). Integrative problem centered metaframeworks (IPCM) therapy. In T. L. Sexton and J. Lebow (Eds.), *Handbook of family therapy* (4th ed.). Routledge. 10.4324/9780203123584

Russell, B., & Breunlin, D. (2019). Transcending therapy models and managing complexity: Suggestions from integrative systemic therapy. *Family Process*, *58*(3), 641–655. 10.1111/famp.12482

Safran, J. D., Greenberg, L. S., & Rice, L. N. (1988). Integrating psychotherapy research and practice: Modeling the change process. *Psychotherapy Theory Research & Practice*, *25*(1), 1–17. 10.1037/h0085305

Scharff, M. E. D. (Ed.). (1995). *Object relations theory and practice: An introduction*. Jason Aronson Inc.

Schwartz, R. (2013). *Evolution of the internal family systems model*. Center for Self Leadership.

Shapiro, F. (1995). *Eye movement desensitization and reprocessing: Basic principles, protocols and procedures*. Guilford Press.

Shapiro, F. (2001). *Eye movement desensitization and reprocessing: Basic principles, protocols and procedures* (2nd ed.). Guilford Press.

Sprenkle, D. H., Davis, S. D., & Lebow, J. L. (2009). *Common factors in couple and family therapy: The overlooked foundation for effective practice*. Guilford Press.

Tang, Y. (2017). *The neuroscience of mindfulness meditation: How the body and mind work together to change our behaviour* (1st ed.). Springer International Publishing. 10.1007/978-3-319-46322-3

von Bertalanffy, L. (1968). *General systems theory: Foundations, development, applications*. Braziller.

Watzlawick, P., Weakland, J. H., & Fisch, R. (1974). *Change: Principles of problem formation and problem resolution*. Norton.

White, M., & Epston, D. (1990). *Narrative means to therapeutic ends*. Norton.

Chapter 2

Convening a Client System and Defining a Problem: The First Phone Call

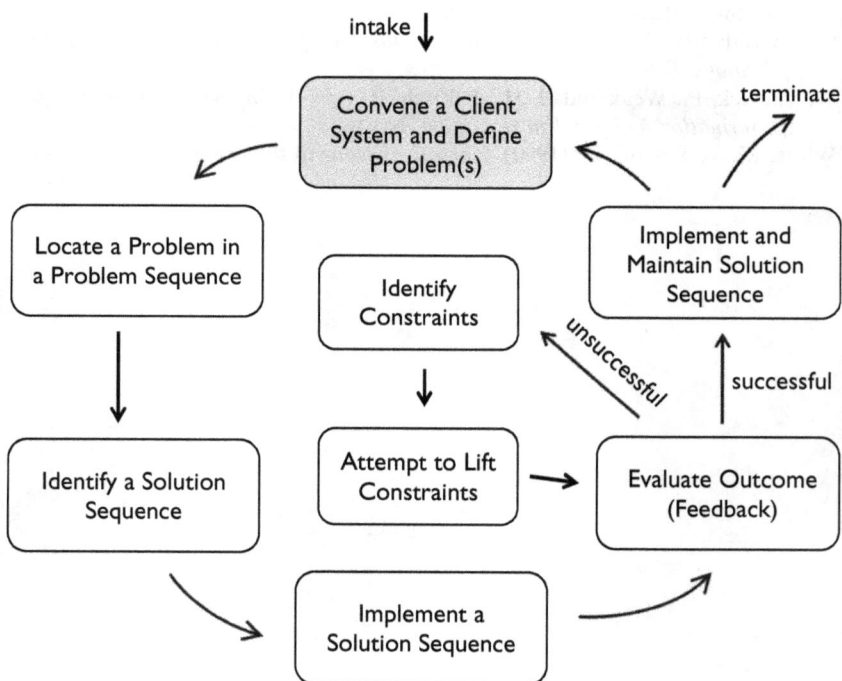

intake ↓

Convene a Client System and Define Problem(s)

terminate

Locate a Problem in a Problem Sequence

Implement and Maintain Solution Sequence

Identify Constraints

Identify a Solution Sequence

Attempt to Lift Constraints

Evaluate Outcome (Feedback)

unsuccessful

successful

Implement a Solution Sequence

IST Essence Diagram.

Objective

This chapter discusses the objectives of the first phone call with a prospective client. These objectives include: making a connection with the caller, understanding the reason for their call (presenting problems), identifying the members of the household and other people involved with

DOI: 10.4324/9780429322273-2

the problem, identifying any imminent danger or risks, briefly describing the IST approach, deciding who will be invited to the first therapy session, and scheduling the first session. It is worth noting that what is called a first phone call in this chapter may also be accomplished by means of HIPAA-compliant video conferencing.

Introduction

Depending on the therapeutic context (agency, private practice, hospital, etc.), a caller's initial contact can occur in a variety of ways. Some agencies have intake departments that handle initial calls from potential clients. These agencies handle the initial contact, screen the caller to ascertain fit with agency mission and level of care, and then assign the client to a therapist. When therapists working in such contexts contact the caller, much of the information that is needed may have already been collected; hence, the therapist is typically ready to schedule an initial session and begin the work. In other contexts, the caller's initial contact is with the person who will ultimately be the therapist. In this case, the therapist assumes the intake role. In this chapter, the assumption is that the caller's first substantive contact is with the person who will likely conduct the therapy. IST therapists believe this initial contact is far more impactful than an information-gathering exercise. The initial phone call is the beginning of therapy. What transpires during the call sets the stage for how the therapy will progress.

In IST, the first phone call between the therapist and a member of the client system is an important initial step with objectives that far exceed the goal of scheduling the first therapy session. The person who contacts the therapist is often the one most motivated to enter therapy. Usually, that motivation derives from the caller's distress about the presenting problem. For example, "My wife's parents always interfere in our marriage, and I don't think I can take it much longer." Or, "My daughter isn't eating much, and I am concerned that she might be developing an eating disorder."

Importantly, the caller's impressions of the initial phone call will likely be taken back to other members of the client system. Thus, the call is not just the first contact with the caller, it is the first contact the therapist has with the client system. The call provides the opportunity for the therapist to decide which members of the client system to invite for the first session. It also provides the therapist with feedback (information and observations) that is useful for initial hypothesizing about the case. For example, when a caller who presents with depression seems very anxious about or resistant to their partner being invited to attend the first session with them, the therapist may wonder if the caller feels ashamed about the depression, or has limited trust in the partner, or harbors a secret. The feedback will prompt the therapist to ask the caller to share their concerns about the partner attending.

For experienced therapists, there may be minimal conscious preparation for the call, as many repetitions of calls with clients have established a level of expertise in the process. For newer therapists, it is best to carefully prepare. Preparation for the first phone call involves a thoughtful review of any intake information, a review of some of the key questions to ask, and the cultivation of a therapeutic presence characterized by empathy, curiosity, and respect.

The therapist will need to attend to a number of tasks including but not limited to: (1) introducing oneself and joining with the caller, (2) hearing and understanding the caller's concerns, (3) asking who is in the family and whether there are others involved in the concerns being presented, (4) ruling out immediate danger or risks that require a higher level of care, (5) informing the caller about the limits of confidentiality in therapy, (6) acclimating the client to paperwork and screening tools they will need to complete before the first session, (7) confirming the fee and answering their questions about insurance coverage, if applicable, (8) reading the client feedback to form initial hypotheses about the client system, (9) determining who will attend the first session, and (10) ensuring they are aware of how to get to the office and/or understand the technology required for teletherapy sessions. Many of these tasks are common to any form of therapy, and some vary according to the procedures established in various practices. This chapter focuses primarily on the aspects of the first call that are associated with IST.

Method

Initiating a call to a therapist or agency and committing to attend the first session can be exciting and hopeful for some, but oftentimes it is a confusing process that has generated some fear or anxiety. The therapist remains mindful of the client system's ambivalence and makes the space to normalize their feelings, acknowledge the courage it has taken to seek help and solicit the caller's questions. It is important to attend carefully to questions about the process of therapy, as well as questions about the therapist's background. Answering these questions openly will be a significant step in building the therapeutic alliance.

IST encourages therapists to attend carefully to the clients' struggles and dilemmas as well as the process by which they are communicated in the first call. The content of what they say and the way in which they say it comprise the feedback that can be read (observed and considered) during and after the first call. This feedback supports hypothesizing about how to respond within the call and how to begin to think about the problems being presented. How are they telling their story or describing their dilemma? What seems particularly important to the caller? What emotions accompany the story? The therapist attends to the emotions directly expressed and the latent emotional content of the caller's story, acknowledging the caller's feelings and expressing genuine concern.

The caller may offer responses that serve as a good barometer of the sensitivity of certain topics and the level of initial trust or mistrust placed in the therapist. The therapist must be aware that the caller may fear being judged or have concerns about confidentiality. This may especially be the case for some clients who seek therapy to work on traumatic experiences, for clients who are concerned that therapy is a sign of weakness, or for clients faced with decisions that they feel will carry some community or societal judgment, such as whether to seek a divorce. IST therapists value the feedback callers provide with respect to their readiness to disclose information about trauma, dilemmas, perceived failures, or other aspects of their lives that carry sensitivity or concerns about privacy.

Callers may be anxious about the call, and they are understandably unsure about how much to share during the call. Arranging a time to talk can help the client feel more prepared for the conversation. To clarify what needs to happen in the call, the therapist begins with a brief orientation on what will be covered. In the orientation, the therapist establishes expectations for the conversation and shares that they may focus it so that it is not more detailed than necessary. Therapists often develop a personal style for opening the phone conversation. There may be incidental things to comment on, such as the process of making contact, but assuming the time and circumstances are convenient for the client, the therapist begins the conversation. An example of an initial orienting statement for a phone call follows:

Therapist: I appreciate the opportunity to talk with you today. I want to hear about the reason for your call, and I will have some questions that will help me determine how to proceed. During the call, we can each consider whether I am a good fit for your needs. I will just need a brief description of the issues that concern you, and we can dive more into the details of the situation if we decide to meet and work together. I should mention that sometimes the things that bring folks to therapy are stressful or painful to discuss. If I ask something that is uncomfortable for you, please let me know and we can pass on that question for now.

Setting the expectations upfront will hopefully help reduce the caller's apprehension, demonstrate respect for their autonomy, and begin to build the therapeutic alliance. Then, with the caller's assent, the therapist asks for a description of the concerns that led to the call.

As the caller describes the reason for seeking therapy, the therapist carefully attends to what is being said and follows up by respectfully asking questions that address such issues as when the problem started, why the caller is seeking therapy at this time, and whether there was a precipitating event that led to the call. The therapist guides the conversation to what needs to be known to convene a direct system for the first session where the work will begin. As such, this is not the time for giving suggestions or advice about the caller's presenting concerns. The therapist will advise on who should attend the first session and how to encourage family members to attend a session, or where to seek help if the therapist believes a different level of care or expertise is required.

One distinction is whether the caller is the one seeking therapy or the representative of a larger group of people seeking therapy (i.e., spouse seeking couple therapy, parent seeking family therapy, etc.). In the case of a caller who represents others, the therapist will be interested in whether the other family members know about the call, and whether they agree with the idea of therapy and would attend a session. Regardless of who the therapy is for, the therapist seeks to learn who is in the immediate family, and whether there are other people significantly involved in the presenting problem. This information will help determine who will be invited to the first session.

There are times when the caller is simply trying to get an initial appointment scheduled and may not be prepared to speak to the presenting concern or provide information about the client system. Typically, the therapist will propose a designated time to talk by phone before the meeting but may decide to have the first substantive contact in person, especially if the client is concerned about the privacy of the call. How this is handled will vary according to agency policies and procedures.

Some callers have difficulty providing the information the therapist seeks. When this is the case, the caller may answer questions with cryptic responses, respond without addressing a question, or tell stories that are difficult to track. The therapist can respectfully try to draw the caller out, summarize what has been said, or interrupt to ask questions, but as the call continues the therapist may still be at a loss to know why the caller is seeking therapy. In such scenarios, the therapist can make a calculated guess at an understanding of the caller's narrative. For example, if the caller's narrative suggests considerable anxiety about many life matters, the therapist might say: "From what you have told me, it sounds like you have several life challenges, and these challenges can make you feel anxious. Is that something you were hoping to work on in therapy?"

Assessing Risk and Level of Care

It is essential that therapists ascertain from the outset that they possess the competence (autonomously or with supervision) required to provide therapy to the client system. In other words, the case as presented by the caller must fit within the scope of the therapist's practice. The therapist must also ascertain that the setting in which they work can provide the level of care required to meet the severity of the client system's needs. If the client system needs a higher level of care or a provider with certain expertise, the therapist provides the caller with the appropriate resources and referrals. For example, a parent calls seeking outpatient individual therapy for a daughter recently discharged from a hospital following her second serious suicide attempt. As the conversation progresses, the therapist concludes that outpatient psychotherapy would not provide the level of care necessary for the teenager at this time; therefore, an evaluation for a day hospital program is suggested, and the therapist provides the contact information.

When the caller is the client, the therapist can directly assess the level of risk and, therefore, determine the appropriate level of care. Risk assessment and management are governed by state law, professional ethics, best practices and specific agency policies and procedures. The therapist will need to be knowledgeable about these requirements. Rather than attempting to specify a risk assessment protocol in this chapter, the authors acknowledge that IST can integrate and accommodate various protocols for risk assessment. If the caller is calling on behalf of the family or couple system or a member of the client system such as a child or adolescent, the therapist assumes a broader view and asks the caller about any risks they see for members of the system. With the information collected, the therapist can make an initial determination about whether to convene the client system, convene part of the client system, or refer a member for a more intensive level of care such as intensive outpatient care, partial hospitalization, or hospitalization.

Deciding Who to Invite to the Initial Session

In the initial phone call, goals include discovering why the caller is seeking therapy and deciding how best to meet that need. As the caller answers the therapist's questions, the therapist uses the hypothesizing component of the IST blueprint to conceptualize the presenting issue and consider who in the client system is involved in the problem. This process enables the therapist to determine who should attend the initial session. While the therapy hasn't yet formally begun, this phone activity involves both assessment and intervention. As noted in Chapter 1, assessment and intervention in IST are inseparable. In a first phone call, the assessment includes a focus on both content (what information the caller is providing) and process (how the caller provides that information). For example, Amanda placed a call for couple therapy. During the discussion, she disclosed that she and her partner had a history of pushing each other during arguments. The content of the call—that partner violence was an issue—required consideration. In addition, Amanda's tone of voice and hesitation in providing this information made the therapist wonder if she had fears that would keep her from openly discussing domestic violence in a session with her partner. The therapist mentioned to her that she seemed hesitant to disclose this information and asked her if that meant anything. Amanda paused, and it was clear that she was crying. The therapist read this nonverbal feedback and spent some time exploring whether she or her partner had ever been injured, and whether she felt physically safe in the relationship. Amanda shared that there had never been any injuries, and that she did feel safe. She then disclosed that she wanted to give couple therapy a try, but she wasn't sure she wanted to stay in the relationship. The therapist explored whether she felt safe in attending a session with her partner and discussing the pushing incident, as well as whether her partner was aware that she may not want to stay in the relationship. As the answer to both of these questions was yes, the therapist felt comfortable inviting the couple to the first session. Feedback that Amanda did not feel safe, evidence of more severe violence, or information that her partner was not aware of her ambivalence about staying in the relationship would have led the therapist to begin therapy with an individual session for Amanda.

As discussed in Chapter 1, IST divides the client system into direct and indirect systems (see Figure 1.1). For review, the clients attending therapy comprise the direct client system and those members who are not directly involved in the therapy are designated as the indirect client system. Some combination of members of the client system come to the initial session, but subsequent sessions can alter that composition. In the example above, the therapist convenes the couple as the direct client system. The children would be in the indirect client system in that they would not be attending sessions. As the couple works in therapy, they report that their 10-year-old daughter is highly anxious about the parents divorcing and their 14-year-old son has become withdrawn. The therapist and couple might decide to bring the children into the direct client system for one or more sessions in order to talk about their fears and concerns. The concepts of direct and indirect client systems support a systemic view of the members and their problems that keeps the therapist thinking about the members who are in the room and those who are not.

The IST therapist will invite the largest appropriate group of family members to the session. The process of invitation will require proposing, negotiating as necessary, attending to the alliance, and being transparent about what therapy will look like. Despite their strong preference for convening relational systems, IST therapists need to be judicious about situations in which conjoint sessions are contraindicated. Such situations include concerns about physical and emotional safety, conjoint sessions that require scaffolding with prior individual sessions, and a firm preference by the caller for an individual session. An example of the need for scaffolding as a precondition of conjoint sessions is the adult woman who requested to schedule a session with her stepfather to confront him on his sexual abuse of her when she was a child. In this case, the therapist cannot afford to schedule that session without scaffolding the work with individual sessions with both parties. First, the risk of damage, including re-traumatization for the woman, is too high. Second, the likelihood of success without the careful staging of sessions is too low.

Given IST's alliance priority guideline (see Appendix B) that establishes the primacy of the alliance, any decision about the composition of the direct client system for the initial session must not damage the incipient alliances that are yet to be solidly formed. Sometimes the caller and therapist are immediately aligned on who should be in the direct client system. For example, the caller is a man seeking couple therapy for himself and his partner. In this instance, it would be straightforward to invite both partners to the initial session. At other times, the caller is seeking individual therapy for couple distress. Unless safety is an issue, the IST therapist begins with the preference for both partners to attend the initial session. The therapist would highlight the benefits of treating couple issues with both partners present, but the caller may still want to come to the first session alone. In this case, given IST's alliance priority guideline, the therapist would defer to the caller and agree to begin with an individual session while still hoping to engage the partner at a later time.

Describing the IST Approach

The caller will likely be interested in how the therapist works or what to expect in the therapy, so the therapist should be prepared to describe IST. This description will be repeated in the first session, but callers often will ask about it during the first call. Here is an example of a description:

Therapist: I base my work on a collaboration between myself and my clients. I focus on what they are concerned about and look for patterns in how they cope and interact. I believe in beginning with straightforward solutions that we agree on. They either lead toward what you want to accomplish or help us learn more about what we need to know to achieve your goals. When we run into obstacles, I will consider a variety of approaches and look for those that fit best for you.

Explanations such as this set expectations for how therapy will work and guide the therapist in the first steps of establishing a common purpose and vocabulary for therapy. The therapist develops a style of describing the work and may adapt the language of it to the caller. IST practitioners vary in their degree of formality, their expressiveness, and their use of language. Each therapist develops their own unique ways of being genuine, curious, respectful, and collaborative.

Specific Requests for Therapy

Although each client situation is unique, it is important to consider common presenting circumstances and corresponding recommendations concerning who will attend the first session (direct system). Below are several classic scenarios IST therapists encounter in initial phone calls. Of course, there are many variations to these scenarios, so what is offered below is intended to provide a starting place for how to think about the types of requests made during the first call.

Requests for Individual Adult Therapy

Adults typically present for individual therapy when they are encountering a problem or concern. Sometimes their concern is about a relationship, in which case they may not be surprised that the IST therapist explores the possibility of the other person or people in the relationship attending the therapy. The therapist explores this and shares the rationale that it is generally more effective to work on a relational issue when the other party or parties are present and can contribute to the work. The therapist understands, however, that some people have strongly held reasons for not attending with a partner.

Some callers present with problems that, on the surface, do not seem to be relational. For example, a man feels anxious and has difficulty sleeping at night. The problem is initially presented without a context or a reference to a relationship. When an adult is partnered, an IST therapist will suggest that the caller and partner attend the first session together. The therapist might say something like, "I find that these kinds of issues impact partners. Partners are often more involved in the problem than it would appear. And, they can often help. Would you be open to attending the first session with your partner?" When the adult is not partnered, the therapist explores whether there is a family member or someone else in the caller's life that might be impacted by the problem or be able to help facilitate improvement in it. In some cases, the caller's parents or siblings may be very involved in the issues and can attend the first session or join the direct client system at a later point in time. Although the caller may live a great distance from their family of origin members, the advent of teletherapy suggests that geographical distance may no longer be an insurmountable constraint to family of origin participation.

An individual adult may also seek therapy to work on a problem for which they require privacy. The therapist will need to understand and support this and begin the therapy with individual sessions. For example, a young adult with issues related to gender identity may fear their family will judge them or reject them. Individual sessions can be utilized to work with the client on their thoughts and feelings about their identity and prepare for discussing it with the family if the client agrees to do so. Another example of the need for privacy would be a client who has been arrested for a crime that hasn't been divulged to the family. The client may feel the need to work through feelings of guilt and shame in individual sessions before informing the family. When the client feels ready to divulge the crime to family members, they can be invited to sessions.

Requests for Couple Therapy

When a caller requests couple therapy, typically both partners will attend most sessions. The exception to this rule would be the presence of intimate partner violence or concerns by one party that there is a risk of violence. For this reason, the therapist asks if there is a history of violence and whether the caller has any safety concerns. If there is doubt about the safety issue, the therapist can convene each partner separately for the first sessions and assess whether to recommend couples therapy or refer each partner to an appropriate therapeutic setting for their respective position within the cycle of intimate partner violence.

The caller may reveal a secret. It may be an affair, a plan to divorce or an undisclosed financial transaction. It is essential that the therapist establishes on the call and in the first session whether the therapist will keep secrets communicated by one of the parties. Thus, the caller can make a judgment on what to disclose based on that knowledge. The authors of this book and those of other IST writings have generally adopted a *no secrets policy* in which the couple is treated as a unit with the expectation that what is shared by one party should be known by the other, with the caveat that the burden to share the secret lies with the client. Once this policy is adopted, there could come a time when a secret being held by one client compromises the integrity of the therapeutic alliance and leads to the termination of the therapy. IST does not rule out that there are special circumstances for which a different policy on secrets would be established, but clients must be informed of how the information will be handled and whether what they say privately to the therapist can be expected to remain private.

Requests for Family Therapy

An IST therapist who prefers to convene families talks with a caller who asks that their family be seen in therapy. On the surface, this would seem like a perfect match. That may be the case, but concerns about safety, a client's request for privacy, or the therapist's decision to scaffold the work with individual or subsystem sessions will result in the family as a whole not being convened for the first session. For instance, a 30-year-old woman calls to request family therapy with her parents. The therapist asks if she has siblings, to which the caller responds that she has an older brother. She states that she does not want him to be part of the therapy because he had recently sided with her ex-husband during the process of a divorce and painful custody dispute. In this situation, convening all parties for a first session would be contraindicated, since the caller is firmly against it and since doing so without preparing all parties would seem to carry more risk than reward (hypothesis). At this point, the therapist can convene the woman and her parents, define the presenting problem, and ask about the relationship with the brother and whether it is related to what they want to work on in therapy.

Requests for Child Therapy in Single-Parent and Two-Parent Families

IST operates with the belief that a child exhibiting a problem should be seen in the family context. This may be with the whole family present, which is generally preferred, but may also consist of sessions with the parent(s) and child. It is not always easy to guide the caller to a plan for family therapy, as many parents believe the child needs a private place to talk with a professional. If the identified patient is a child and the parent is calling, at some point in the conversation the therapist can say something like the following:

Therapist: I believe in the strengths of families to solve problems. My approach to children in therapy is to identify their patterns of thinking, feeling and acting in the family context and to work together with family members to solve their problems. Parents and often siblings are such an important part of the process. You know your children better than I ever will and you will be helping them far longer than I will, so I would like to partner with you (and your family) to address the issues that led you to make this call.

Not all parents will entirely buy into this approach at that time, but most parents will agree to be part of the process. The approach with adolescents is similar in terms of scheduling the first session, though depending on the presenting problems and circumstances, the course of therapy may include individual sessions with the adolescent as well as family sessions.

Requests for Child or Family Therapy with Binuclear Families (Divorced, Remarried)

A binuclear family (Ahrons, 1994; Pinsof, 1995) is an extended family typically consisting of the two households created by divorce or the dissolution of an unmarried partnership. These are complex cases that require careful attention to decisions about who attends the initial sessions. When the focus is on the behavior or adaptation of a child, the IST ideal would be to convene as many of the members of both households as possible, but this may be contraindicated by an elevated level of stress between households or between parents. And, conducting such a session may take an advanced level of skill, especially in the case of remarriages. Given these factors, it is usually best to conduct separate sessions with each household. That being said, in some cases, the divorced parents may have a good co-parenting relationship and it may be reasonable to convene them together for a parents-only first session. All this involves the judgment of the therapist based on information gathered about the co-parenting relationship in the first phone call. As the therapist proceeds with the case, the identification of a problem sequence and later the constraints will be the ultimate determinants of who attends the sessions, as the therapist hypothesizes about who needs to be present to solve the problem or alleviate the concern.

When the caller is requesting family therapy for one of the households without identifying a child as having a problem, the first session would likely be with that household, though the children's parent in the other household would be asked to agree to the therapy. These requests typically are focused on communication within the family, improvement of relationships, or the development of greater cohesion. As with any case involving children, the therapist must follow agency policy and state law with respect to verifying the custodial arrangement and soliciting custodial approval of children to be involved in the therapy.

Requests for Mandated Therapy for a Child

In the case of mandated therapy for a child, the first phone call is the first step in determining how therapy will proceed in a complex multi-system context. It is essential for the therapist to fully understand the reasons for the mandated therapy (e.g., abuse and/or neglect by a caregiver), who is entitled to know about therapeutic assessment and progress (i.e., the caregivers and/or the court system), and whether reports to the court are required. This means that there is work to do before convening the clients and the therapist will need to attend carefully to agency policies, state law and court orders in proceeding with the case. Typically, the therapist will need to see both the child custody documents as well as the report mandating therapy. Next, the therapist will get parental permission to talk with the guardian ad litem, social worker, or other representatives of the court in order to understand more about the situation. Then the therapist can convene the first session consistent with the court order and what has been learned about the case thus far. These cases are complex and fraught with potholes for a therapist not sufficiently prepared to manage them. For this reason, it is recommended that these cases be seen by therapists who specialize in them or by therapists who are supervised by therapists who have expertise with them.

Conclusion

IST therapists consider the initial phone call to be the beginning of therapy, so it is handled thoughtfully through a systemic lens. The phone call constitutes an encounter with a caller who may be representing a couple or family system and facilitating their entry into therapy. In the case of the caller initiating individual therapy, the therapist is mindful that the caller is a member of a client system consisting of members who may at some point participate in the therapy. During the phone call, the therapist must achieve the following goals: Establish a connection with the caller, understand the problem the caller wants to address in therapy, identify the members of the household and other people involved with the problem, identify the presence of any imminent danger or risks that may require a more intensive level of care, briefly describe the IST approach, and, if the therapist and caller agree to schedule a session, decide which members will attend the initial session.

Regardless of the type of therapy requested, from the very first phone call, the therapist pays particular attention to what the caller is seeking and is mindful that the opportunity for a therapeutic alliance begins with the first sound of the therapist's voice. From the first moment of the call, the therapist is gathering information and reading the feedback that supports hypothesizing about clients' strengths as well as patterns of behavior, thought and emotion in the client system. Hypothesizing is facilitated by careful attention to the content and process of the phone conversation, commitment to the IST interpersonal and alliance predominance guidelines (see Appendix B), and knowledge about IST's hypothesizing metaframeworks.

Exercises

1   Callers will ask you about your approach to therapy. Construct and practice a very brief description of IST.

2   Review the case scenarios provided below. Answer the following questions, write or record your responses, and save them, as you will be asked to refer to them in the next chapter.

   a   *Caller is the father:* Parents (ages 47 and 45) request family therapy to discuss a recent increase in the acting-out behavior of their middle son, who is nine years old.

   i   Determine what you will say to open the phone conversation. Consider practicing it out loud or role-playing it.

   ii How will you explore the presenting problem? What questions will you ask?

   In conversation, you learn the following: These mixed-sex, cis gender parents also have a 13-year-old son and a 4-year-old daughter. The parents moved to the United States 10 years ago from Uruguay. They do not have extended family members in town and report feeling isolated. The female partner is contemplating moving back to Uruguay with the children.

   iii Determine who you will invite to the first session and why.

   iv   Which hypothesizing metaframework(s) do you think will be relevant to the case? Why?

   b   *Caller is the mother:* Mixed-sex co-parents are looking to work on co-parenting skills after their recent divorce.

   i   Determine what you will say to open the phone conversation. Consider practicing it out loud or role-playing it.

   ii How will you explore the presenting problem? What questions will you ask?

   In conversation you learn the following: Marriage ended because of an affair; however, the caller is interested in rekindling their relationship. She has shared this interest with her ex-husband. He is not thinking about getting back together as a couple but states that he has an interest in co-parenting counseling. The couple would like to include their two children, ages five and eight, in therapy. No risk factors were reported at intake.

   iii Determine who you will invite to the first session and why.

   iv   Which hypothesizing metaframework(s) do you think will be relevant to the case? Why?

   c   *Caller is a 35-year-old woman:* She would like couple therapy with her 40-year-old same-sex partner and would like to discuss her partner's recent infidelity.

i   Determine what you will say to open the phone conversation. Consider practicing it out loud or role-playing it.

ii   How will you explore the presenting problem? What questions will you ask?

In conversation you learn the following: Couple has been together almost seven years and wants to address the trust issues in their relationship. Attempts to discuss infidelity have not been successful. Both partners have a history of being sexually assaulted outside of their current relationship. No current risk factors were reported.

iii   Determine who you will invite to the first session and why.

iv   Which hypothesizing metaframework(s) do you think will be relevant to the case? Why?

d   *Caller is a 44-year-old man*: His presenting concerns are anxiety and grief.

i   Determine what you will say to open the phone conversation. Consider practicing it out loud or role-playing it.

ii   How will you explore the presenting problem? What questions will you ask?

In the conversation, you learn the following: The client is a cis gender, straight, married father of four who has been highly anxious in recent years. He wants to work through grief about the death of his father three years ago. He also wants to work on being more attentive to his wife and kids. He denies risk factors.

iii   Determine who you will invite to the first session and why.

iv   Which hypothesizing metaframework(s) do you think will be relevant to the case? Why?

e   *Caller is a 19-year-old nonbinary person*: The caller requests individual therapy for anxiety.

i   Determine what you will say to open the phone conversation. Consider practicing it out loud or role-playing it.

ii   How will you explore the presenting problem? What questions will you ask?

In conversation you learn the following. At the suggestion of a parent, the caller is seeking therapy for the anxiety they are experiencing. The client has difficulty defining a presenting problem other than some general anxiety that is not particularly associated with any specific thing in their life. No risk factors have been reported.

iii   Determine who you will invite to the first session and why.

iv   Which hypothesizing metaframework(s) do you think will be relevant to the case? Why?

References

Ahrons, C. (1994). *The good divorce*. Harper Collins.

Pinsof, W. M. (1995). *Integrative problem centered therapy: A synthesis of biological, individual and family therapies*. Basic Books.

Chapter 3

Convening a Client System and Defining a Problem: The First Session

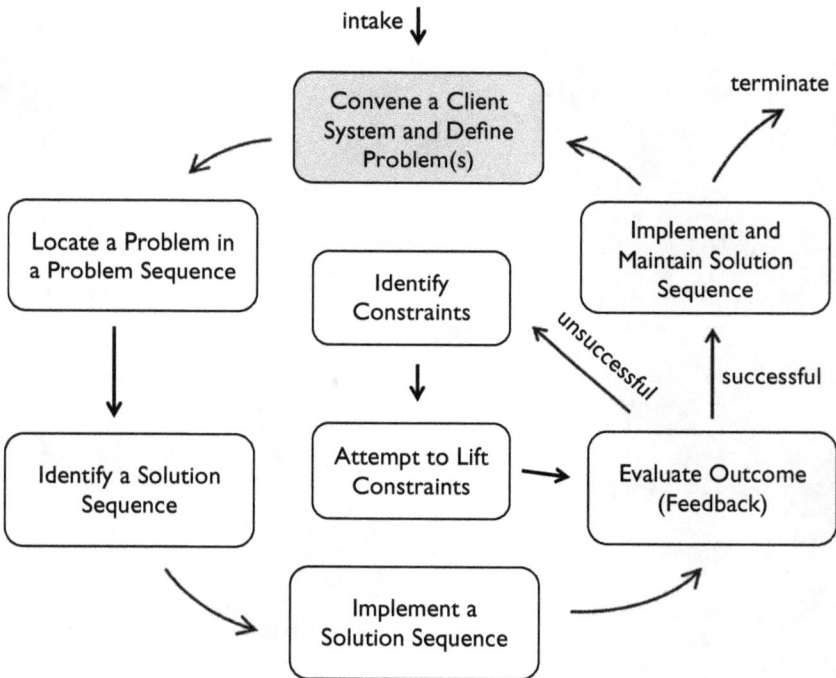

intake ↓

Convene a Client System and Define Problem(s)

terminate

Locate a Problem in a Problem Sequence

Identify Constraints

Implement and Maintain Solution Sequence

Identify a Solution Sequence

Attempt to Lift Constraints

Evaluate Outcome (Feedback)

unsuccessful

successful

Implement a Solution Sequence

IST Essence Diagram.

Objective

This chapter discusses the objectives of a first therapy session. Although there are universal aspects of a first session that an IST therapist will accommodate (e.g., getting acquainted, dealing with administrative issues, and assessing for risk and appropriate level of care), this chapter

DOI: 10.4324/9780429322273-3

focuses primarily on IST-specific aspects of the first session which include describing therapy as a problem-solving process, defining the presenting problem, locating the problem in a problem sequence, obtaining information about the context of the client system, and beginning to form an alliance with all members of the direct client system.

Introduction

In his classic book, *Problem Solving Therapy* (1976), Jay Haley included a chapter on conducting the first session. Haley argued that the structure of the first session had specific goals that, when accomplished, set the tone for all the sessions that followed. Breunlin et al. (1992) asserted that the goal of the first session is to get a second session. Through the ways the therapist interacts with the clients, a positive tone is set that inclines the clients present for the first session to want to continue therapy. Therapists cultivate their own style of guiding the session and demonstrating genuine interest, acceptance, and respect. In IST the therapist leads the collaborative process of addressing the universal and IST-specific objectives of the first session. These objectives, discussed in this chapter, comprise a protocol for the session. From the very first moments of the session, the therapist makes a significant impression on the clients and begins to build a therapeutic alliance.

Method

As is the case with virtually any approach to therapy, the IST therapist will obtain information about the members of the client system, describe the approach to therapy, and assess risk and the level of care needed. Readers who are experienced therapists have established ways of fulfilling these objectives. Particularly useful for beginning therapists, Patterson et al. (2018) specify four stages of an initial interview: Introductions, administrative issues (including a description of the therapy process, confidentiality, and fee policy), defining client goals, and beginning assessment. Staging the first session in this order fits well within IST, with the provision that the assessment that begins in the first session continues throughout the therapy as assessment and intervention are co-occurring and continuous in IST. In addition to Patterson's four stages, there are IST-specific aspects of a first session that clarify the approach to goal setting and alliance-building.

Five objectives for the initial session are IST-specific or have IST-specific implications. These objectives are to describe therapy as a problem-solving process, to define the presenting problem, to locate the problem in a problem sequence, to obtain information about the context of the client system, and to begin forming an alliance with all members of the direct client system. Facility with these objectives comes with experience, so therapists-in-training often need more than one session to accomplish them. An additional objective—to initiate a solution sequence—is sometimes possible for experienced practitioners in a first session, but is contingent on having made sufficient progress with the first five objectives.

Universal Aspects of the Initial Session

Experienced therapists have highly developed skills and their own personal style of engaging clients in the first session, orienting them to the process, asking what the client wants from therapy, and screening for risk. When adopting IST, their task is to integrate the IST-specific objectives for the first session into their existing pattern of engagement. On the other hand, therapists-in-training will need to learn and incorporate both the universal first-session objectives and the IST-specific objectives as they begin their journey of developing the skills and personal touch they will ultimately bring to their practice.

The first step of the initial session is to get acquainted in a developmentally appropriate way with all clients attending (the direct client system). The therapist greets all members in attendance in a friendly way. Incidental comments about such things as the circumstances of the clients finding the office, the access to the teletherapy platform, or the weather are appropriate. Getting acquainted will typically include asking each participant about themselves (their school or work involvement and, in the case of children and adolescents, their interests). This is not idle talk, however, as the therapist is attempting to put the clients at ease and beginning the process of getting to know them. And reading feedback this early in the process of therapy may lead to initial hypotheses. For example, in a first family session, when invited by the therapist to introduce themselves, one parent says to the other, "You're the one who thinks we need to be here. You go first!" This at once makes a demand on the other parent and also says something about the commitment to participate in therapy. The therapist is beginning to learn about the family system.

In getting acquainted with the clients, the therapist will need to be mindful of the developmental level of the participants. This is particularly salient for therapists seeing families with children. A forthcoming book in the IST book series will focus on the complexities of working with children in family therapy, but a few initial comments on getting acquainted with children are offered here. If children are present in the first session, attending to their level of comfort with the space, providing age-appropriate toys or supplies for drawing, and sharing something of interest can be the first steps in establishing an alliance and orienting them to therapy. For example, here are a few things a therapist might say as a way of getting acquainted with a 7-year-old child attending a first therapy session:

Therapist: So nice to meet you, Tara. I am happy to see you here today. I think your mom told you about me. (The ensuing conversation can establish what the child understands about the therapy.)

Therapist: I like to meet with kids and parents and find new ways to talk together. Sometimes we draw or play a game together. I hope you will like doing that. Do you have any questions about me?

Therapist: I see that you have a dog keychain. I have a dog named Lucky! Would you like to see his picture?

The examples above suggest how a therapist may begin a conversation with a child, determine whether she knows the reason for the meeting, and provide an initial description of the therapy process. Searching for mutual interests also contributes to alliance-building (e.g., the shared love of dogs). The therapist can extend some autonomy to the child by providing the option of drawing with crayons and paper as a means of buffering the experience of being in a new environment and helping with the management of any anxiety. The therapist attends to the process as well as the content of the child's engagement in the conversation. For example, does the child make eye contact? At what points does the child look toward a parent for guidance, reassurance, or permission to respond? How does the parent respond? Even in the getting-acquainted stage of the session the therapist is reading the feedback and learning about the family. As can be seen from this brief discussion of welcoming a child to therapy, the developmental level of participants in the direct client system can have a significant impact on the process of therapy and thus, the therapist's knowledge about developmental stages is essential.

Once the therapist and clients have become acquainted, it is wise to address administrative issues such as explaining and completing required forms, discussing fee policy, and explaining confidentiality and its limits. This is also a good time to briefly explain the therapeutic process and answer clients' questions and concerns about it. Then, the therapist can move on to a discussion of the clients' presenting concerns. It is recommended that the therapist briefly acknowledge the conversation that occurred with the caller and then invite all members present to talk about why they have come to therapy. The therapist listens carefully to the themes and stories of the clients' concerns and begins to understand the reasons the clients are seeking therapy. The therapist is empathic with all members and demonstrates unconditional positive regard for them

(Rogers, 1965). The problem definition stage of the first interview will be more thoroughly discussed below in the IST-specific section of this chapter.

Assessing Risk and Level of Care Required

Continuing with a theme established in the initial phone call, it is essential that therapists ascertain that they possess the competence (autonomously or with supervision) required to provide therapy to the client system. In other words, the case as presented in the first session must fit within the scope of the therapist's practice. The therapist must also confirm or disconfirm that the setting in which they work can provide the level of care required to meet the severity of the client system's needs. If the client system needs a higher level of care or a provider with certain expertise that the therapist does not have, the therapist provides them with the appropriate resources and referrals.

Risk assessment and management, as well as abuse reporting requirements, are governed by state law, ethical standards, best practices and specific agency policies and procedures. The therapist will need to be knowledgeable about these requirements. Rather than attempting to specify protocols for risk assessment and requirements for abuse reporting in this chapter, the authors acknowledge that the therapist must place the highest priority on safety (including the risks of self-harm, suicidality, danger to others, domestic violence, human trafficking, sexual assault, and elder abuse or neglect) and the protection of children from abuse and neglect. Various protocols for risk assessment and abuse reporting can readily be incorporated within IST.

IST-Specific Aspects of the Initial Session

Building an Alliance

Establishing a therapeutic alliance is a requirement for any successful therapy. It is discussed in this section due to the implication of IST-specific concepts such as the alliance guideline (see Chapter 1) and the dimensional approach to the therapeutic alliance adopted within IST. Research on psychotherapy outcome has repeatedly demonstrated that the therapeutic alliance accounts for a significant portion of the variance toward a positive clinical outcome (Fife et al., 2013; Sprenkle et al., 2009; Sprenkle & Blow, 2004). Further, there is compelling evidence that the "early treatment alliance is highly predictive of how therapy will unfold" (Sprenkle et al., 2009, page 95). It is incumbent on the therapist, therefore, to have the alliance in mind in the first phone call, during the initial session, and throughout the course of therapy. IST utilizes the integrative psychotherapy alliance model

(Knobloch-Fedders et al., 2007; Pinsof, 1995; Pinsof & Catherall, 1986) that asserts that the alliance includes the dimensions of goals, tasks, and bonds. Hence, to build an alliance it is vital to achieve goal consensus with the client system, collaboratively arrive at mutually agreed upon tasks (solution sequences) and begin to build bonds with all members of the client system. A starting point within the first session includes welcoming clients, making introductions, and providing a statement on what to expect in the session. Following is an example of a therapist's initial statement about what will happen in the session. It can follow the introduction (i.e., getting acquainted) stage and precede the administrative (i.e., forms and procedures) stage. Importantly, it acknowledges that the therapist and the client(s) will both have agency in a decision to work together.

Therapist: We have a few forms and procedures to review today, but beyond that the goals of this first session are for me to begin to get to know you, learn about what is bringing you into therapy at this time, and see if I am a good fit for you. I will ask you some questions about yourselves and your concerns, but this is also a time when you can begin to get to know me, so I will tell you about how I work and save some time for your questions about me or the therapy process. I hope you will feel comfortable working with me, but I will be open to hearing whether or not that feels right for you.

Therapists can do things in a session that inadvertently damage a nascent alliance. Statements or questions that have an undertone of judgment may cause a client to feel shame or experience resentment toward the therapist. Therapists must also guard against agreeing with the negative views a client in the direct system has about a client in the indirect system because the latter may at some point become part of the direct client system. For example, a woman insisted on seeing the therapist alone for the first session. In that session, she indicated that her partner is a narcissist. She asserted that she had read books about narcissism, and they all clearly depicted her partner. What the woman asserted put the therapist in a dilemma. Challenging the woman's statement might damage the newly forming alliance with her. Agreeing with her would risk damaging the unformed alliance with the partner who may ultimately come into the therapy. The therapist must use the conversational skills of IST to strike a middle ground so as to preserve the potential for forming an alliance with both partners. There is no one right way to respond to this dilemma, but the therapist might say: "I hear your concerns. You certainly are reporting some things that would lead you to wonder why a person would act in that way. I also hear that you are hoping to avoid a divorce, so I suggest that I learn more about your situation and perhaps we can see if there are some things you appreciate about your partner." The prospects of productively convening the couple together are reduced if the woman goes home and tells her partner that the therapist agrees with the label of "narcissist."

Cultural Humility, Cultural Competence and the Therapeutic Alliance

Fostering an alliance with clients requires that the therapist acknowledge important cultural factors such as race, ethnicity, sexual orientation, sexual identity, and ability/disability, and assure that such factors are part of what clients can discuss in therapy. Kelly et al. (2020), for example, emphasize that the topic of race be discussed at the beginning of therapy as a way of extending permission for black families to talk about race and its impact on their lives and their work in therapy. Opening the therapy to culture and intersectionality extends beyond what therapists learn to *do*. *R*ather, learning to establish and maintain effective therapeutic alliances requires that the therapist make an ongoing commitment to the cultivation of cultural competence (Awosan et al., 2018; Kelly et al., 2014). This journey, a significant part of the development of the self of the therapist, involves developing a critical awareness that the therapist's own cultural contexts, as well as privilege, can constrain the therapist from seeing and understanding things that are real and important for their clients. The journey also requires cultural humility that engenders respect and openness to the impact of the cultural identities most important to the clients (Hook et al., 2013). Further, the therapist will need continued education about what clients are likely to experience based on their cultural contexts which will help with the process of building relationships and anticipating factors that will influence the problem-solving process. Both didactic and experiential training formats that allow for the development of critical consciousness are recommended for therapists (Awosan et al., 2018), as is an acceptance that self-reflection toward cultural humility and competence, including the understanding of power, privilege, and oppression, is a lifelong process (Hardy & Bobes, 2016).

Describing IST as a Problem-Solving Process

For some clients, the initial session is the first time they have ever been in therapy. For others, it is starting with a new therapist who may be following in the footsteps of a number of predecessors. Many clients enter therapy holding beliefs about the nature and process of therapy. Some might consider therapy to be a time to vent on the issues of the week. Some believe it is about self-actualization that will not involve the specification of goals or tasks to get there. Others expect to be given specific tools to change their current situations or symptoms. Despite clients' prior experience or preconceived notions about therapy, the IST therapist will need to explain how IST therapy works and set the tone for what clients should expect. There is no one right time in the first session to do this, but one reasonable point is after getting acquainted, orienting the clients to what will occur in the first session and covering the administrative issues. The IST therapist is transparent about the nature of "how I work." For example, the therapist might say:

Therapist: I base my work on a collaboration between myself and my clients. I focus on what they are concerned about, and I look for patterns in how their concerns develop and persist. I begin with straightforward solutions that we agree on. I call these solutions *experiments* because they either lead toward what you want to accomplish or help us learn more about what we need to know to achieve your goals. When we run into obstacles, I consider various ideas that have been developed in our field and I look for those that fit best for you. We call this approach IST, Integrative Systemic Therapy."

The clients may have some questions or there may be some conversation about the nature of therapy. Then the therapist can transition to asking the clients what they want to address in therapy. An example follows.

Therapist: There are different ways to start therapy. For me, it is very important that I understand what brings you here today because I will focus the work on your goals. I spoke with Maria briefly on the phone when she requested this appointment, but I would like to hear from each of you today. What brings you in to see me? I am going to take a back seat and ask you as a group to answer this question. I am a very curious person, though, so I may not stay silent for too long. Our conversation will create a shared sense of what there is to work on. What brings you in?"

How the system responds to this open invitation may yield information about leadership or about various members' level of concern about the presenting problem, but it is also reasonable to begin by asking the person who made the call to respond first or to begin with the parents as leaders of the family. When there are children present or when the therapist hypothesizes that generational hierarchy requires acknowledgment, it will be important to begin with the parents. The language in the example above, is appropriate for family sessions, but it can be adapted for couple sessions or individual sessions. Further, the therapist can adapt the language of the statement to fit better for both themselves and the clients.

As the conversation unfolds, the therapist is guided by the generic tasks of the IST essence diagram (see Figure 1.2 in Chapter 1) and the process specified by the IST blueprint (see Figure 1.3 in Chapter 1). The blueprint, consisting of a process of hypothesizing, planning, conversing, and reading feedback, anchors the therapist to the decision-making and decision-evaluating process of a systemic, integrative approach. The blueprint is the means by which the essence steps are accomplished, and the alliance is maintained. The essence diagram specifies tasks for the first session, including getting a good definition of the presenting problem and beginning to locate that problem in a problem sequence. It is not necessary to accomplish these tasks entirely in the initial session, but it is important to recognize that IST is designed to begin with these tasks. The pace of addressing these tasks is understandably variable as per the clients' circumstances and the therapist's level of experience. Occasionally, enough of the problem sequence emerges in the first session for the therapist to suggest an experiment with a solution sequence.

Defining the Problem

The first problem-solving task is to define the problem. IST honors the clients' presentation of the problem or concern and rests the work on a problem-centered contract (see the problem-centered guideline in Appendix B) that clarifies the purpose of therapy, focuses the work, and supports the therapeutic alliance. Sometimes the problem is readily defined, and participants agree that this is what they want to address in therapy. For example, a couple presents with concerns about the conflict and dissatisfaction associated with the intensive involvement of one partner's parents in their lives. They may not agree on a solution, but they agree on what they need to work on. Other times, clients have a narrative of distress or disappointment but do not readily state a problem to be solved. In such cases, the therapist works to distill from the narrative what the clients want to change. Often, it is helpful to invite the client to consider what might be different when their concerns have been solved. For example, "I think I understand that you don't feel as connected as you used to feel. Can you say what will be different once you are connecting? What do you think will be happening that is not happening now?"

Some clients enter therapy with a sense that they have some things to sort out or that they need a place to talk about the pressures or conflicts they are experiencing. This is sometimes the case for clients who present for individual therapy. The therapist can probe to see if the client will define a problem but should not press the client too hard in the first session to define a specific problem as this can seem judgmental or be a failure to meet the client where they are. The alliance predominance guideline of IST (see Appendix B) provides room for slowing the process down and learning more about what the client is experiencing before introducing ideas associated with change or problem-solving.

Clients will eventually identify something specific within them or in their world that is concerning to them. The therapist can merely ask, "Is that something you would like to change?" If the answer is yes, a problem is defined. Another option when clients are not specific about the problem is to enter the essence diagram at the point of identifying a problem sequence as the clients, over a series of sessions, begin to demonstrate that there are recurrent patterns that are enacted in their lives. The therapist might say, "It seems like that keeps happening. Shall we talk more about what you might like to do about it?" In this way, the therapist invites the client to collaborate in a process to address a problem sequence.

Clients often present with multiple concerns. In such a case, the therapist works carefully to define each concern and attempts to prioritize them according to the clients' preference. For example, "Of the things we have discussed, is there something that you would like to work on first?" As IST therapists often convene couples or families, there are multiple perspectives on what brings members to therapy. These perspectives may be aligned as a couple agrees they want to reduce their conflict or family members agree they need to talk about a recent loss. In some cases, though, the members of the direct client system do not agree on what to work on in therapy. With couples, this may take the form of one party wanting to save the marriage and the other interested in exploring whether they want to remain in the marriage. With a family, the different perspectives may have to do with generational differences, life cycle transitions, or disagreements about boundaries. When family members have different perspectives on why they have come to therapy, the therapist initially seeks an umbrella problem description that includes two or more perspectives. For a couple presenting with different perspectives, "I hear that you are here because one of you wants to be in the relationship and one of you wants to decide whether you want to be in the relationship. I believe this is a starting point for the therapy. Do you agree?" For a family struggling with the demands of a transition to adolescence, "I hear that you are here to solve the problems related to the difference in expectations at this stage of the family's development. As parents you are asking John to be more accountable and John, you are asking your parents not to monitor you so closely. Maybe these two things are related. This is something we can work on."

Locating a Problem in a Problem Sequence

Usually, a description of a problem is more or less formed in the minds of the clients, but they often have limited awareness of how they interact around it, that is, engage in a problem sequence. The problem sequence is a predictable, patterned, and recursive set of actions, meanings and emotions in which the problem is embedded. It is a parsimonious and first explanation of what is going on when the problem occurs. As therapy continues, constraints are identified and the systemic explanation may become significantly more complex, but the problem sequence and direct attempts to solve it are the key to discovering the complexity of the system.

A primary task for the therapist during the initial session is to provide guidance and modeling that helps the clients begin to see the problem within the context of their relationships. To accomplish this, the therapist asks Socratic (Rutter & Friedberg, 1999; Freeman, 2005; Overholser, 2018) and circular (Selvini et al., 1980, Tomm, 1987) questions about the nature of client concerns and how the members of the system are affected by them. This is true for individual clients as well as couples and families. An individual client can be asked how others react to the problem or concern and how they, in turn, respond to that reaction. The answers begin to establish how the problem is embedded in the client system's sequences, that is to say how the system contains and maintains the problem.

Locating a problem in a problem sequence is an interviewing skill that repeatedly utilizes the decision-making properties of the blueprint to formulate and ask a series of questions. The idea of what to ask about (hypothesis) leads to the formulation of a specific question (plan) which leads to asking the question (conversing) and then noticing the clients' verbal and nonverbal responses (feedback). This process is idiosyncratic and improvisational, but the questions can be guided by at least two dimensions: (1) the interpersonal dimension of how members affect and are affected by the problem and by others reacting to it, and (2) the dimension of time with an emphasis on how the problem and related events are nested and play out over time. Some clients can be coached to directly identify the sequence by thinking about what typically happens. In other cases, the conversation benefits from examining specific examples that suggest a common pattern that the therapist can interpret as a problem sequence. Sometimes clients will enact a problem sequence in session and the therapist gets to see it at work in real-time.

Here are some example questions that a therapist can ask to develop an understanding of the problem sequence. The questions are asked in the spirit of respect and curiosity with the awareness that people may feel shamed by their participation in problem sequences. The IST therapist sets a nonjudgmental course that assumes that all parties' actions are understandable and potentially modifiable.

"I understand that you want to argue less. Can you give me an example of what an argument looks like for you?"

"As you describe the argument, do you think that other arguments seem similar to it?"

"Can you tell me more about what happens in a typical argument?"
"What seems to be happening when the argument starts?"

In succession: "How does it start?" "What happens then?" "And after that?" How does it typically end?"

"Once the argument starts, are there things you do to try to stop it or improve it?"

In succession: "How are you affected by the argument?" "How are others affected by it?" "What do they do or say?"

"So, if I understand this correctly, the argument often starts when you disagree about limits for your daughter..." The therapist summarizes a description of a problem sequence and gets client feedback on whether it is accurate.

The description of the problem sequence is not expected to describe every conflict perfectly; rather, it represents what typically happens. It can be summarized for the client or even written out in circular form on a whiteboard or piece of paper: First this happens, then that, then this, etc. It can include internal reactions (i.e., thoughts and feelings) of each member that clarify what they are experiencing or trying to do in the moment. The therapist collaborates with the client system to establish a consensus on a description of the problem sequence.

Some problems might appear to involve only one person. For example, chronic pain, the trauma of a car accident, or a disappointment at work. These problems may, at first glance, appear not to have relational components, but they almost always do. For example, a client presenting with chronic pain may be a parent and have debilitating days when the ability to provide childcare is impaired. The pain exists in a relational context within which it impacts and is impacted by patterns of interaction. The conversational process in IST will lead to an interactional description of how the presenting concern is embedded in the client system. For example, a depressed man's partner repeatedly tries to cheer him up, but this discourages him further. The partner, in turn, gets frustrated and withdraws. This interactional pattern seems to worsen the depression but likely does not fully account for it as other issues of biology, personal habits, and developmental history may also be relevant. Still, given the assumptions of a systemic approach, the problem sequence is a fruitful place to start. And, it does not preclude further hypothesizing as the therapist wades into the ongoing process of assessing and intervening with the blueprint.

Sequences sometimes play out in front of the therapist during the first session. Protective sequences can be triggered by mistrust or lack of knowledge about the therapeutic process, concerns about the limits of confidentiality, fear of judgment, or fear of causing conflict or hurt feelings. For example, a couple seeks therapy for distress in their relationship, but when one of them describes some degree of unhappiness, the other one talks about the ways they are satisfied with the relationship or touches the other partner in a comforting way. The therapist may hypothesize that they are protecting themselves and the relationship. If so, the therapist can choose to comment on the relational strengths being observed and acknowledge that it is good that they can be so positive and close during the session. This can be a bridge to saying that first sessions can be uncomfortable for a variety of reasons. And from there the therapist can ask if there are any concerns about starting therapy that they would like to share. This effort acknowledges that what the clients are experiencing matters to the therapist which in turn may contribute to the establishment of the alliance.

Protective sequences may also take the form of significant resistance or avoidance in a first session. This may be associated with mandated therapy or near-mandated therapy (i.e., no legal requirement, but the client attends under significant relational or other pressure), or with some cases of complex relational trauma. In mandated therapy, clients may feel that the therapy is an intrusion or that it may expose something that will be used against them. Mandated cases are discussed in Chapter 11. In a case involving a background of complex relational trauma, the client may not feel safe in the first session. In such a situation, the IST therapist will need to slow down the process of identifying a problem sequence as it may seem intrusive or controlling to the client. Trust will need to be built and the client will need to feel that they can move at their own pace. Trauma is discussed in Chapter 9.

Obtaining Information About the Members and the Context of the Client System

In IST, assessment and intervention are inseparable and co-occurring processes that begin with the first phone call and end with the last session. This does not preclude an initial formal assessment process and, as has been discussed, assessment and management of risk are always essential. IST can accommodate comprehensive written assessments when required by an agency or preferred by the therapist, but such an assessment is not required for IST. And, the performance of such an assessment does not modify IST's commitment to continue assessment throughout therapy and to view intervention as a way to learn more about the clients and their relationships. In other words, the attempts to solve the problem will reveal much of what clients and therapists need to know about the constraints in the system. Still, at the beginning of therapy, an IST therapist requires some basic information about the client system and is interested in what the clients feel is important for the therapist to know about them as well.

Based on the initial phone call (see Chapter 2), the therapist will know the names and ages of the family members, including those who will not be joining the direct client system for the first session. This is sufficient information for the therapist to draw a very simple genogram and begin to think about the developmental stages of the members and the family. During the social (i.e., getting acquainted) and problem definition stages of the first session, the therapist will learn many important things about the client system. There will also be things the therapist will not learn until later in the therapy. To the extent that time permits in the first session, however, the IST therapist will want to learn about such things as: Work or school involvements of the participants, the cultural background of the client system, the religious or spiritual involvement of its members, current or recent medical issues, significant losses, other recent changes or stressors, other mental health providers (if any), and information about family members not present. The therapist can also gather some of this information in the second session. Lastly, the therapist can ask, "Is there anything else that you think is important for me to know?" Or, "Next time we meet I will check in with you to see if there is anything else you think is important for me to know." The information collected at the outset of therapy provides some immediate understanding of factors impacting the system and establishes a basis for hypothesizing in the early and later stages of the therapy.

Individuals, Couples, and Families in the Direct Client System

The initial session focuses on the universal and IST-specific objectives regardless of who is in the direct client system. The initial and later tasks specified in the essence diagram and the utilization of the blueprint to guide the accomplishment of these tasks comprise a universal process of IST that applies to work within the individual, couple, and family contexts of therapy. Importantly, as experienced therapists will observe, this book does not describe all there is to know about each of these contexts of therapy. Rather, it elucidates the core process of problem-solving in IST that is utilized with individuals, couples, and families. Additional books in the Routledge IST series will each focus on the special considerations for working in these contexts. Some initial considerations for the first sessions with each of these therapy contexts are discussed below.

Individuals

Clients who seek individual therapy do so for myriad reasons. As discussed in Chapter 2, the IST therapist's first hope is to convert the call for individual therapy into a relational first session attended by the caller and a partner or family member(s). Still, callers often opt to attend the first session alone. They may be struggling with one or more of a variety of contextual factors such as: They have difficulty forming and maintaining intimate relationships, they feel adrift in choosing a career path, or they are recovering from a traumatic experience. They may identify the contextual issues when they call for therapy as would be the case if they present with a relational concern, but understandably clients often use condensed descriptions or categorical language to describe the complex issues of their lives. That language may convey something about themselves (e.g., anxiety, depression, anger issues) or about another person (e.g., stubborn, mentally ill, abusive), but will rarely carry a systemic description of the problem. Even in the case of an individual attending the first session, the IST therapist looks to embed the presenting concern in a systemic context and describe it in terms of specific problem sequences. It is not sufficient to describe the symptoms or label an overall problem or condition. Rather, the therapist will want to learn about the specific patterns of action, meaning, and emotion that occur between the client and others and the specific patterns of thinking and feeling that occur within the client.

Many clients will label their presenting problem as anxiety or depression. There are evidence-based therapies designed to reduce the symptomatology of the conditions classified as anxiety or depression (Kirmayer, 2001; Hofmann et al., 2010; Normann et al., 2014; Greenberg & Watson, 2006; Watson et al., 2003). Following an assessment and plan for any risk issues and the determination that the therapist can provide the appropriate level of care, an IST therapist may incorporate one or more of these evidenced-based methods into the therapy or refer a client out for that component of the work. Prior to incorporating such methods, the therapist works with the client to describe and contextualize what the client labels as a condition (e.g., depression), so that it can be addressed more systemically. To do this, the therapist seeks to expand the presenting problem beyond the label of "depression." The first step in this process is to locate the depression within a context of living (for example, struggling to establish a career). This is accomplished with questions about what the client is discouraged or frustrated about. The second step is to construct a problem sequence that serves as the starting point to work on the systemic pattern of the problem. When individuals present with concerns about themselves, the problem sequence is almost always a hybrid sequence that includes internal sequences of meaning and emotion that are connected to external sequences of action and interaction. The interventions are chosen to fit the specific patterns of action, meaning, and emotion that comprise the client's depression.

An example of contextualizing an individual client's presenting problem is found in the case of a 20-year-old woman who presents in the first session with concerns about anxiety. She explains that she feels anxious most of the time and has trouble sleeping. She reports that she often wakes up very early and is not able to get back to sleep.

Therapist: That must be very uncomfortable for you. Have you always had this anxiety, or did it come on at some point that you can identify?

Client: I was happy as a child and in high school. The anxiety started this last Fall when I went to college. I had only been there for a month when I got a call from my dad saying that my mom had cancer.

Therapist: I'm sorry to hear that. It must be very difficult for you to be starting college and suddenly have an illness in your family.

Client: I'm so torn. I know my dad can handle my mom but part of me says I should drop out and go home to help him. My mom keeps telling me that I should stay in college. Another part of me agrees with her.

Therapist: Can you hear that debate between those two parts going on in your head?

Client: Absolutely. Logically I know I should stay, but my emotions just won't agree. Every day, the emotion pushes me to just drop out and go home.

Therapist: I'm thinking that all that second-guessing must contribute to your anxiety.

Client: Absolutely.

Therapist: Can we talk more about your mom's condition and about your conversations with your family about it?

The therapist will directly address the client's symptoms, but first will explore the interactions within the family concerning the illness as well as the client's specific patterns of thinking, feeling and acting that seem to keep the client from reducing the anxiety.

The IST therapist thinks contextually, and relationally, about the individual client, keeping in mind that intervening with an individual is intervening also in an indirect family system and that that system exists in a multisystemic context. Thus, in beginning to think about the patterns, strengths, and constraints of an individual, the therapist is mindful of the web of human experience (see Figure 1.4 in Chapter 1) that includes the levels of the system and the hypothesizing metaframeworks. Yes, hypotheses based on the mind metaframework are relevant to individual clients, but other hypothesizing metaframeworks (i.e., culture, development, organization, gender, biology, or spirituality) may be essential in understanding the client as well. For example, the 20-year-old college student's perception of her role in her mother's illness may be constrained by the family's cultural background and/or view of gender roles.

Another consideration would be the applicability of the culture hypothesizing metaframework and the social justice guideline (see Appendix B) when themes of diversity, intersectionality, and privilege emerge within the therapist's mind or are expressed directly or indirectly by the client. The therapist must remain centered and open in addressing differences and explore what the differences mean to the client and how they inform the client's view of the presenting problem and the process of discussing the patterns in which the problem is embedded.

Couples

Like individuals, couples present in myriad and complex ways. The following considerations address a few distinctions about how the therapist can think about the concerns couples bring to therapy. When couples present with problems in their relationship, the description of the problem can lead directly to the definition of a problem sequence. This is particularly true of couple conflict which, in and of itself, is a problem sequence that can be articulated through a careful conversation with the couple. Addressing what is missing in a couple's relationship requires more excavation in terms of how the couple's pattern of interactions, thoughts and feelings block communication or intimacy.

When couples present with concerns about the problems of one partner (e.g., a psychiatric condition or a physical illness), or when they present with concerns about facing a challenging circumstance (e.g., loss in the family or adjustment to retirement), they are not necessarily asking that the therapy address the patterns between them. In such cases, the therapist begins to map how the couple interacts with each other around the presenting concern, how they are each affected by it, and how each of their reactions are expressed and impact the other. Variants of the questions provided in the above section on *locating a problem in a problem sequence* can begin to unveil the context of the problem. What the partners need from each other in relation to the problem and how they might interact differently about it can emerge from this conversation. In this way, the therapist will tie the patterns of interaction to the presenting concerns and begin to make the case for seeking a solution sequence.

Families

IST's interpersonal guideline (see Appendix B) calls for as many family members as possible and appropriate to attend the initial session. This guideline grows out of the systemic underpinnings of IST and the belief that the problem sequence is more readily observable when all of the members are present. In an initial session with a family, the therapist has to devote considerable energy to introducing the family to the idea that they can benefit from working together, with the goal that by the end of the session all members are committed to a second session. The therapist must focus on the alliance with all members of the family, some of whom may be hesitant to be in the session and/or have less power and authority to speak about how they see the presenting problems. Making sure that all members, including young children, have a voice in the session is crucial.

The larger the number of members of the client system attending the session, the greater the challenge to reaching goal consensus as the adults often believe one or more of the children are misbehaving and the children and/or adolescents may have concerns about the parenting style of the adults. Finding common ground wherein all family members have bought into the goals can be challenging. For these reasons, arriving at a consensus on the presenting problem—let alone articulating the problem sequence—is sometimes not possible in the initial session with a family. Hence, it is important to get to a second session. Sharing what will happen during the second session is helpful in this regard. For example:

Therapist: It was a pleasure to meet you and learn a little about each of you and about the family. I appreciate what you all have shared today. I am starting to understand each of your ideas about what is happening in the family. Next session, I would like you to help me understand a bit more about what each of you want to accomplish so that we can find a way to describe the goal of our work that makes sense to everyone.

Conclusion

The first session is the event that launches therapy. It is designed to get a second session and to set the stage for the IST therapy that will follow. Having collaborated with the caller to decide who should attend the initial session, the therapist convenes the client(s) with the goal of defining the presenting problem, beginning to form an alliance and establishing an agreement to work together. The therapist will also try to go a step further and locate the problem in a problem sequence. However, the first session has a variety of additional objectives that include: becoming acquainted with the clients, orienting them to the first session, learning about their context, addressing administrative requirements, assessing risk, and explaining the process of therapy. Thus, the therapist in many cases may not complete the step of defining a problem sequence in the first session. Chapter 4 provides a more extensive discussion of this key essence step.

Exercises

The case scenarios below are the same as those you worked on in Chapter 2. Reflecting on your original conceptualization of the first phone calls, consider how you will proceed in the first sessions with these cases.

1   Imagine meeting with the client system. Practice, role-play or write notes about how you will open the session and begin to join with the direct client system.
2   Role-play or practice how you will orient the client(s) to the session. Role play or practice how you will describe IST therapy to them.
3   Role-play or practice constructing and asking questions to define the problem. Notice the respect, nonjudgmental attitude and curiosity in your questions and in your tone.
4   Consider how the culture and development metaframeworks might influence your approach to the session. Role-play or take notes on how issues from these metaframeworks might find expression in the session.

A family attends the first session: Mixed-sex parents (ages 47 and 45) request family therapy to discuss recent increase in conflict and acting out behavior with their middle son, who is 9 years old. They also have a 13-year-old son and a 4-year-old daughter. The parents moved to the United States 10 years ago from Uruguay. They do not have extended family members in town and report feeling isolated. The mother is contemplating moving back to Uruguay with the children. No risk factors were noted at intake.

White, mixed-sex, cisgender parents attend the first session together: They are looking to work on co-parenting skills after their recent divorce. Their marriage ended because of an affair; however, the caller is interested in rekindling their relationship. She has shared this interest with her ex-husband. He is not thinking of getting back together as a couple but states that he has an interest in co-parenting counseling. The couple would like to include their two children, ages 5 and 8, in therapy. No risk factors were reported at intake.

Same-sex partners attend the first session: The caller (white, cisgender, age: 40) asked for therapy to discuss the recent infidelity by her partner (Latina, cisgender, age 35). The couple has been together for 7 years and wants to address the trust issues in their relationship. Attempts to discuss the infidelity have not been successful. Sexual assault history in adulthood is reported by the caller outside of the current relationship. No risk factors are reported.

A mixed-sex couple (44-year-old Black cisgender man and 45-year-old Black cisgender woman) attend the first session together: He is looking to reduce anxiety and to address issues related to his father's death a decade ago. The couple has four children. He also wants to work on being more attentive to his wife and kids. He states he does not have a preference for what therapy will look like and is not sure if individual or family therapy is better for his needs. Risk factors were denied.

A 19-year-old, biracial, nonbinary person attends the first session with their parents: At the suggestion of a parent, the caller is seeking therapy for the anxiety they are experiencing. The client has difficulty linking anxiety to any specific stressor. No risk factors have been reported.

References

Awosan, C. I., Curiel, Y. S., & Rastogi, M. (2018). Cultural competency in couple and family therapy. In J. Lebow, A. Chambers, & D. Breunlin (Eds.), *Encyclopedia of couple and family therapy*. Springer. 10.1007/978-3-319-15877-8

Breunlin, D. C., Schwartz, R. C., & Mac Kune-Karrer, B. M. (1992). *Metaframeworks:Transcending the models of family therapy*. Jossey-Bass.

Fife, S. T., Whiting, J. B., Bradford, K., & Davis, S. (2013). The therapeutic pyramid: A common factors synthesis of techniques, alliance, and way of being. *Journal of Marital and Family Therapy*, *40*(1), 20–33. 10.1111/jmft.12041

Freeman, A. (2005). Socratic dialogue. In A. Freeman, S. H. Felgoise, C. M. Nezu, A. M. Nezu, & M. A. Reinecke (Eds.), *Encyclopedia of cognitive behavior therapy* (pp. 380–384). Springer.

Greenberg, L. S., & Watson, J. (2006). *Emotion-focused therapy for depression*. American Psychological Association.

Haley, J. (1976). *Problem-solving therapy*. Jossey-Bass.

Hardy, K. V., & Bobes, T. (2016). *Culturally sensitive supervision and training: Diverse perspectives and practical applications*. Routledge.

Hofmann, S., Sawyer, A., Witt, A., & Oh, D. (2010). The effect of mindfulness-based therapy on anxiety and depression: A meta-analytic review. *Journal of Consulting and Clinical Psychology*, *78*(2), 169–183. 10.1037/a0018555

Hook, J. N., Davis, D. E., Owen, J., Worthington Jr., E. L., & Utsey, S. O. (2013). Cultural humility: Measuring openness to culturally diverse clients. *Journal of Counseling Psychology*, *60*(30), 353–366. 10.1037/a0032595

Kirmayer, L. (2001). Cultural variations in the clinical presentation of depression and anxiety: Implications for diagnosis and treatment. *The Journal of Clinical Psychiatry*, *62* (13), 22–30.

Kelly, S., Bhagwat, R., Maynigo, P., & Moses, E. (2014). Couple and marital therapy: The complement and expansion provided by multicultural approaches. In F. T. L. Leong, L. Comas-Diaz, G. C. Nagayama Hall, V. C.

McLoyd, & J. E. Trimble (Eds.), *APA handbook of multicultural psychology, Vol. 2: Applications and training* (pp. 479–497). American Psychological Association. 10.1037/14187-027

Kelly, S., Jérémie-Brink, G., Chambers, A. L., & Smith-Bynum, M. A. (2020). The Black Lives Matter movement: A call to action for couple and family therapists. *Family Process, 59*(4), 1353–1957. 10.1111/famp.12614

Knobloch-Fedders, L. M., Pinsof, W. M., & Mann, B. J. (2007). Therapeutic alliance and treatment progress in couple psychotherapy. *Journal of Marital and Family Therapy, 33*(2), 245–257. 10.1111/j.1752-0606.2007.00019.x

Normann, N., van Emmerik, A., & Morina, N. (2014). The efficacy of meta-cognitive therapy for anxiety and depression: A meta-analytic review. *Depression and Anxiety, 31*(5), 402–411. 10.1002/da.22273

Overholser, J. (2018). *The socratic method of psychotherapy.* Columbia University Press.

Patterson, J., Williams, L., Edwards, T. M., Chamow, L., & Grauf-Grounds. (2018). *Essential skills in family therapy: From the first interview to termination.* Guilford.

Pinsof, W. M. (1995). *Integrative problem centered therapy: A synthesis of biological, individual and family therapies.* Basic Books.

Pinsof, W. M., & Catherall, D. R. (1986). The integrative psychotherapy alliance: Family, couple and individual therapy scales. *Journal of Marital and Family Therapy, 12*(2), 137–151. 10.1111/j.1752-0606.1986.tb01631.x

Rogers, C. R. (1965). The therapeutic relationship: Recent theory and research. *Australian Journal of Psychology, 17*(2), 95–108.

Rutter, J. G., & Friedberg, R. D. (1999). Guidelines for the effective use of Socratic dialogue in cognitive therapy. In L. Vandecreek, & T. L. Jackson (Eds.), *Innovations in clinical practice: A sourcebook* (pp. 481–490). Professional Resource Press.

Selvini, M. P., Boscolo, L., Cecchin, G., & Prata, G. (1980). Hypothesizing – circularity – neutrality: Three guidelines for the conductor of the session. *Family Process, 19*, 3–12. 10.1111/j.1545-5300.1980.00003.x

Sprenkle, D. H., Davis, S. D., & Lebow, J. L. (2009). *Common factors in couple and family therapy: The overlooked foundation for effective practice.* Guilford Press.

Sprenkle, D. H., & Blow, A. J. (2004). Common factors and our sacred models. *Journal of Marital and Family Therapy, 30*(2), 113–129.

Tomm, K. (1987). Interventive interviewing: Part II. Intending to ask lineal, circular, strategic, or reflexive questions? *Family Process, 27*, 1–15.

Watson, J. C., Gordon, L. B., Stermac, L., Kalogerakos, F., & Steckley, P. (2003). Comparing the effectiveness of process-experiential with cognitive-behavioral psychotherapy in the treatment of depression. *Journal of Consulting and Clinical Psychology, 71*, 773–781. 10.1037/0022-006X.71.4.773

Chapter 4

Strategies for Locating a Problem in a Problem Sequence

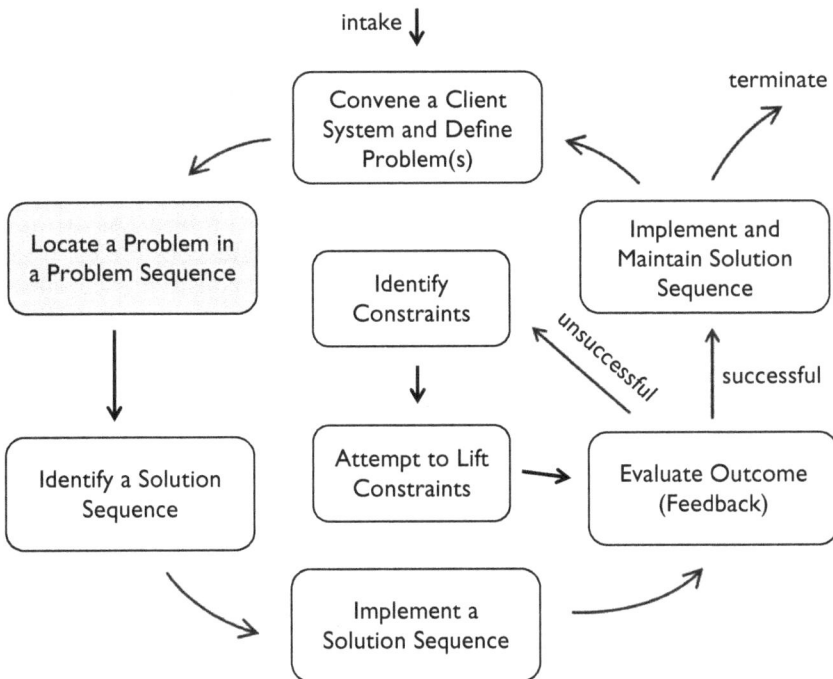

intake ↓

Convene a Client System and Define Problem(s)

terminate

Locate a Problem in a Problem Sequence

Identify Constraints

Implement and Maintain Solution Sequence

unsuccessful

successful

Identify a Solution Sequence

Attempt to Lift Constraints

Evaluate Outcome (Feedback)

Implement a Solution Sequence

IST Essence Diagram.

Objective

This chapter will show the reader how to embed the presenting concern or problem into a systemic framework. In the practice of IST, the initial description of how the problem exists within the system is known as the problem sequence. The process of collaborating with the client system to

DOI: 10.4324/9780429322273-4

uncover a problem sequence is discussed and clinical examples are provided to illustrate this process and the challenges associated with identifying problem sequences.

Introduction

Systemic practice rests on the proposition that the context within which the problem is embedded is what maintains the problem. Correspondingly, a proper alteration of the context will allow for the problem to be resolved. The context is enormously complex, but the therapist need not address all of the systemic complexity. Rather, the therapist needs to address just enough of the context to allow the problem to be solved. As the therapist begins to lead the therapy, the level of complexity required to solve the problem is unknown.

In IST, the problem sequence is a predictable, patterned, and recursive set of actions, meanings and emotions in which the problem is embedded. It is a parsimonious and first explanation of the context of the problem. The articulation of the problem sequence affords the therapist and clients the opportunity to consider an alternative, adaptive sequence (solution sequence) that would appear to solve or improve the problem. As therapy continues, it may become clear that the clients are constrained from utilizing or maintaining this solution sequence. As constraints are identified, the description of the context of the problem becomes more complex, and the therapist seeks to identify just enough of the context to allow for the solution of the problem.

IST privileges the therapeutic alliance which is built through careful attention to what the clients want to address in therapy—the presenting problem. Once the presenting problem is defined, the therapist works with the client system to locate it within a problem sequence. The problem sequence suggests an initial direction for the therapy in the form of a solution sequence. As the therapist and clients collaborate on the development of solution sequences that address the clients' goals, the therapeutic alliance is formed and strengthened.

Identifying Problem Sequences

The time it takes to articulate a problem sequence varies. Variables that come into play are the experience level of the therapist (more experience means the therapist is likely to have previously encountered similar sequences), the transparency of the client system to describe the problem sequence, the complexity of the problem sequence, and the degree of consensus among clients regarding the problem and the problem sequence. Some problem sequences emerge easily over the course of an initial session in which case the therapist may initiate the discussion of a solution sequence. Other problem sequences take several sessions to uncover. There are also cases where an additional component of the problem sequence is uncovered after one or more solution sequences have been tried.

The problem sequence is the first and most elementary understanding of how the problem is nested in the client system. Defining it is a way to jump-start therapy because it creates a focus on the pattern that surrounds the concern that brought clients to therapy and thereby gives the clients an opportunity to feel heard and valued. This focus can lead directly to a solution that will improve or solve the presenting problem or, as is more often the case, it may be the first step in a process of discovery of the systemic factors that will need to be addressed in order to accomplish the clients' goals for therapy.

A Classification Scheme for Sequences

To prevent therapists from getting bogged down in a sea of detail that reveals no sequence, IST offers a way to catalog sequences so the information provided by the clients can be more readily distilled into a problem sequence. In an earlier conceptualization of sequences, the periodicity, or length of time it took to complete one cycle of the sequence, served as an organizing principle to classify the various kinds of sequences (Breunlin & Schwartz, 1986; Taussig, 2018). Four classes of sequences with four ranges of periodicity were identified and labeled as S1, S2, S3, and S4. Sequences of shorter duration were conceptualized as nested in sequences of longer duration, and originally it was thought that each level of sequence needed to be fully articulated if it constituted part of the total problem system. With the introduction of the concepts of a problem sequence and solution sequence, it became clear that all four classes of sequences did not need to be fully articulated in order to initiate change. Further, the therapist may incorporate more than one class of sequence into the formulation of a complex problem sequence. Below is a summary of the four classes of sequences.

S1 sequences have a period of seconds to several hours. S1s can be readily observed in the here and now. They are referred to as *face-to-face sequences*. Examples of S1 sequences are the way a couple argues, problematic sexual encounters, ordeals around homework, and a battle over getting ready for school.

S2 sequences capture some aspect of the client system's daily or weekly routine. They may include aspects of the circadian rhythm. Individuals with sleep disturbances often go through episodes where they have trouble sleeping at night and resort to dealing with their exhaustion by napping during the day, which only exacerbates the difficulty sleeping at night. The length of S2 periods can range from a day to a week. For example, in a mixed-sex marriage, a husband works 12–15 hours daily while the wife is home with three children under the age of six. They are both exhausted when he finally arrives home. They have a quick dinner, and then she puts the kids to bed while he watches television. They climb into bed and barely acknowledge each other. This is a daily S2 sequence. Another example of an S2 sequence would be a divorced family in which the children spend specified days of the week with their mother and the other days with their father. This full sequence transpires over the course of a week.

S3 sequences, the periodicity of which ranges from several weeks to a year or more, consist of either ebb and flow or intermittent event sequences. Ebb and flow S3s involve a variable that varies over time, sometimes being problematic and sometimes not. For example, Seasonal Affective Disorder involves the ebb and flow of depressive feelings and thoughts that correlate with the amount of sunlight available. In the summer when there is ample sunshine the mood is positive but as the sunlight dwindles with the onset of winter, depressive symptoms increase. Another example would be libido which naturally ebbs and flows, and when this ebb and flow is out of sync for a couple, they are likely to struggle with concerns related to the frequency of sex.

S3s based on intermittent events involve circumstances that change the way the client system functions. Examples of intermittent event S3s include periodic family visits, episodes of domestic violence, binge drinking, and chronic relapsing illnesses. Each time the event occurs, the clients inevitably organize around it. Once such an S3 exists, the client system learns to anticipate it such that the precursor to it is also part of the S3. Further, there can be a period of recovery that follows the event. Thus, a couple may anxiously prepare for the visit of one partner's parents, experience the challenges of the visit itself, and then have a period of conflict about it after the parents have left. Anniversary reactions are another example of intermittent events that disrupt the lives of the people who must pass through them. The anniversary may be about the loss of a loved one or going through a divorce. For example, a Christian family endured a traumatic marital separation just before Christmas, so subsequent Christmases took on a painful anniversary reaction.

S4 sequences are transgenerational sequences. They have a period of at least two, if not more, generations. The transgenerational process can be built into the DNA of the client system, such as when a client is at higher risk for breast cancer, alcoholism, or mental illness because the illness was present in the genes of previous generations. Behavioral patterns can also transmit from one generation to the next, including repetition of such patterns as abuse, abandonment, infidelity, and suicide. Additionally, prominent attitudes, values, and coping mechanisms found in one generation are often reflected in the next generation.

The following example illustrates sequences of varying duration in a reconstituted family (i.e, stepfamily) who presented with a problem that they have great difficulty reaching a consensus regarding almost any decision. This family included a mixed-sex married couple, the wife's son, and the husband's son and daughter. Whenever there was dissent in the conversation, the father voiced his opinion passionately. The other family members had a tendency to wither in the face of his intensity and their voices were silenced. Not surprisingly, his preference for how the family should proceed, whatever the matter, was often adopted and the other members felt coerced. This interaction would be considered an S1.

This interaction typically occurred the evening the children arrived for the weekend from their respective other parent's homes. This meant they were in the midst of a transition from one household to the next, so the emotional field was inevitably heightened. This constituted a weekly S2. Furthermore, the father's former wife was often at odds with him, and the mother's former husband was upset that his son wanted to spend time with his mother. Both former spouses made negative comments about each parent from time to time which occurred on an S3 basis. Finally, the mother had been raised to never challenge her father and when she did, he would get viciously angry at her. Nowadays, she cowered in the onslaught of her husband's passionate appeals. This constituted a transgenerational transmission process known in IST as an S4.

It would be tempting for the therapist to agree with the perspective of family members who blame the father for dominating the reconstituted family. They believe the problem would easily be solved if the father would just admit that he is the source of the problem. He should just modify the way he communicates with the family. With this formulation, the problem sequence would be a simple description that does not attempt to account for systemic complexity and could be stated as: The family tries to decide something, the father speaks passionately, other members fall silent, and the matter is decided according to the father's wishes. In some cases, a simple problem sequence such as this can lead to an initial solution sequence that will either have some success or present the opportunity for learning more about other levels of sequence that constrain the initial solution sequence. In other cases, it is difficult to construct an initial solution sequence without knowing more about other classes of sequences.

An IST therapist is prepared to incorporate other classes of sequences that make the description of the problem sequence more recursive and systemic. The key question is: What maintains this problem sequence or, using the language of constraints, what keeps it from taking a more adaptive form. Using the blueprint and hypothesizing with the organization metaframework, the therapist forms two hypotheses. The first is that hierarchically, the mother/stepmother should be the one to lead the effort to reduce the father's influence. The second pertains to the reconstituted nature of the family: The family might be constrained by confused leadership as they have only been together for two years and the therapist knows it can take upwards of five years for blending to be solidified. In short, the family is evolving. The therapist would have to explore the behavioral, cognitive, and emotional implications of these hypotheses. The net result would be a more systemic and fully articulated problem sequence.

The problem sequence is the smallest nugget of the larger systemic treasure trove that comprises the family system (Russell & Breunlin, 2019). This nugget allows the clients and therapist to agree upon a goal and to focus on selecting and implementing solution sequences (often framed as experiments) to reach that goal. In this sense, the problem sequence is a point of entry into the system. If the solution sequence works, the therapist does not have to look further into the systemic nature of the clients' system. If multiple constraints keep the solution sequence from working, then the therapist keeps elaborating and expanding the systemic frame until enough of it is understood to address the therapy with sufficient comprehensiveness (Russell & Breunlin, 2019).

Method

Holding a Systemic Frame

Holding a systemic frame means continually hypothesizing and conversing in relational and contextual terms about the relevant behaviors, cognitions, and emotions that together comprise the experience of the client system. It is this systemic frame that enables the therapist and clients to piece together the problem sequence. Holding a systemic frame does not come naturally to most people, including therapists, because we all grow up being taught to view the world in linear terms. For every action, there is a reaction, and it is just the action that causes the reaction. Therapists must embrace a frame that events are far more complex than this simple action-reaction model. Once a systemic frame is embraced, it still takes patience and effort to see the systemic underpinnings of phenomena in the world and particularly in the world of relationships.

When clients are first asked why they have sought therapy, the therapist joins with them and collaborates to define a workable problem. A problem is workable when the clients can impact it. For example, if a client reports having schizoaffective disorder, that diagnosis is not something the client system can solve; however, if the therapist works with the client and they agree that poor mood regulation is disrupting the client's relationships, the problem called mood regulation is a workable problem in that members of the client system can work on improving mood regulation. A workable, interactive solution has also been called a workable reality (Minuchin & Fishman, 1981; Churven, 1988). A workable reality is essentially an explanation of a strategy for a solution sequence. The process of identifying solution sequences will be discussed in detail in Chapter 5.

IST therapists are attuned to the language of process. The adage is: think process, not content. Often clients initially describe the problem simply or categorically as if it existed in isolation from its context. For example, "Our son is doing poorly in school," or "We have been told that our daughter has an eating disorder." With this starting point, the therapist must contextualize the problem in order to uncover the problem sequence.

Sometimes clients' description of the problem includes a description of an interactional process. When this happens, the therapist has a head start defining the problem sequence. For example, "Our son is doing poorly in school, and we have nightly battles where we try to get him to do his homework," or "Our daughter has been diagnosed with an eating disorder and we are exhausted because every night at dinner we have a battle with her over food." In these two examples, the therapist is given at least part of the problem sequence. Sometimes the problem is presented relationally, in which case the problem and the problem sequence partially overlap. For example, "I feel like the only thing keeping my partner in the relationship is sex. He is constantly wanting it," or "We have a problem with communication. When we fight it almost always gets ugly." In these instances, the therapist fleshes out the problem sequence by asking the clients to elaborate thoroughly on their interaction.

Locating a Problem in a Problem Sequence

The process of identifying a problem sequence involves a conversation or set of conversations that unfold in a unique manner based on specific client and therapist factors. Although these are distinctive conversations, there is a commonality to the kinds of questions that the therapist can ask to accomplish this process. Here are some example questions:

Therapist (about a specific incident):	Tell me what happened in as much detail as you can.
Therapist (for greater detail):	And what happened next?
Therapist (for greater detail):	What did you feel then?
Therapist (generalizing):	Do things like this happen from time to time? If so, how often?
Therapist (generalizing):	How does it typically go? Can you describe it in general terms?
Therapist (for greater detail):	How does it typically start?
Therapist (for greater detail):	What happens next? And after that? How does it end?

Therapist (for detail of mind):	I imagine you have some important thoughts and strong feelings along the way. Can you talk about that?
Therapist (for detail of mind):	At what point in the sequence do you begin to feel that?
Therapist:	How does that feeling influence what you do?
Therapist (for outcome):	What is it like for you once the sequence has ended?
Therapist (for precipitant):	Is there something that causes the sequence to begin?
Therapist (reaching consensus):	So, let me see if I can summarize what you have described, and we can see if it fits for you.

The clients' responses to the inquiry will send the conversation in a variety of directions. The questions provided here demonstrate in a general way the initial understanding the therapist seeks about how the system works with respect to the presenting problem. For families attending therapy to work on the problems of identified patients, such as depression, anxiety or a behavior disorder, the therapist can ask about attempted solutions to the problem (Watzlawick et al., 1974). For example, "What do each of you do to try to help or change this?" An analysis of how the family is responding to the problem and how they try to manage it or themselves often begins to reveal a problem sequence.

Protecting Alliances

The alliance priority guideline states that the alliance takes priority over the therapist's plans for therapy (see Appendix B). Most often this guideline applies to decision-making regarding solution sequences or the removal of constraints; however, it must also be considered when identifying the problem sequence. It is one thing to state a problem, for example, "we don't get along." But it makes clients far more vulnerable to share the specific details of not getting along. To do that requires a level of disclosure about self or others that uncovers thoughts, feelings, and sometimes actions heretofore not revealed or fully understood by other family members. Revelations of this sort can create embarrassment, require defense mechanisms, and/or create a rupture in the alliance. The therapist must monitor and support the alliances while in the process of articulating the problem sequence.

For example, Lori and Sami, white cisgender women in a same-sex marriage, report a problem sequence that occurs when they discuss a challenging issue. The conversation is manageable until Lori starts pressing Sami to see her point of view. The more Lori does so, the more Sami gets defensive or seeks to withdraw. Lori then escalates to the point where she is yelling at Sami, at which time Sami disengages and accuses Lori of being a bully. To the therapist, it sounds like the problem sequence includes what may be bullying on Lori's part, but simply labeling it as such may rupture the alliance. The therapist knows there will be a need to address Lori's escalation and what fuels it but thinks that the description of the sequence may already be embarrassing to Lori. The therapist decides to seek an agreement that the sequence does recur, that it is a problem, and that the couple will work together to change it so that they can complete important conversations. The therapist will search for a way to understand each of their needs, emotions and meanings that occur in the conflict, and will look for a way to supportively address Lori's escalation as understandable given how she experiences the conflicts, but counter-productive and possibly damaging to the relationship.

Managing Multiple Points of View

Two people who have participated in the same interaction will rarely remember it in exactly the same way. Therapists should make it clear that respecting multiple perspectives is part of the process of therapy. Moreover, listening and trying to understand the perspective of another family member is not tantamount to giving up one's own perspective. Here, the IST pillar on epistemology is evoked through the concept of progressive knowing. When a couple, for example, reaches a point where each can say to the other: "I understand your perspective about the way you treated me, but I would like to share what it was like for me," they can have a conversation that involves a healthier give and take.

Some components of the problem sequence involve the thoughts and feelings held by the clients about the problem. Sometimes clients have shared these feelings but often they are held privately. The therapist must gently coax the clients to be transparent about their privately held thoughts and feelings. To do so, the therapist must establish an agreement with all clients in the direct system that the therapy is a safe space, and that no retaliation will follow in the wake of honest exchanges.

Vagueness

To arrive at a workable problem sequence, the clients must be able to access information about their relevant actions, meanings, and emotions. For any number of reasons, clients sometimes struggle to produce this information, resulting in vagueness surrounding the presenting problem. The therapist can slow the process down and be very concrete about defining the problem and locating it in a problem sequence. Some clients have difficulty generalizing from incidents to patterns. In some cases, it may take many descriptions of specific events to assist clients in finding the pattern. A whiteboard can be used to depict the sequence in a circle. Heightened emotion can constrain the process, so calming the emotion before describing the sequence can be helpful. Lastly, vagueness can exist when clients fear being put on the spot or blamed. For these clients, it is important to create a greater sense of emotional safety. With a sense of safety, a calming of emotion, and careful attention to detail, reflection on pattern can be increased and clients can see internal sequences of mind and/or external sequences of interaction. For example, one partner in a couple who often gets angry over apparently minor issues would come to see and be able to say to the other partner: "Yes, when I start to think that some of the things you do mean that you don't love me, I get hurt feelings and then I get angry and say something harsh."

Two or More Stories Offered

If two or more clients are providing discrepant versions of a problem sequence surrounding a given problem, the therapist is challenged to create a consensus about the problem sequence that both can accept. This may require a more broadly stated description of the sequence or an inclusion of the disagreement within it. Extreme examples of this are akin to each client watching different videotapes of the same events. These discrepancies and how the members deal with them can, themselves, be framed as a problem sequence. Participants may need to learn how to find some truth in the other's observations or learn to talk differently together about them.

Attitudinal Tools for Identifying a Problem Sequence

Attitudinal tools reflect how the therapist views the nature of the therapeutic endeavor. Three attitudinal tools drive the search for a problem sequence: curiosity, creativity, and courage.

Curiosity

IST therapists are tinkerers who are passionate about figuring out how something works; in this case, how a problem sequence is embedded in a client system. They succeed because they have massive amounts of curiosity. The presenting problem serves as the entree into the client system. For some therapists, when a client starts therapy and reports feeling depressed, a diagnosis of depression could be made, and treatment would follow a manualized therapy designed to treat depression. Instead, IST therapists are curious about the impact of the depression on the client's life and the impact of the client's life circumstances on the depression. They are always in search of clues as to how the problem shows up in the clients' daily lives. The who, what, when, where, and why must be meticulously fleshed out for the problem sequence to emerge. Although clients enact their problem sequence frequently and often daily, they seldom fully formulate and describe it without assistance from the therapist. The therapist's curiosity is focused on: "I wonder how the problem sequence transacts for these clients?"

The conversation could include the following kinds of questions: "Please tell me what it feels like when you have mood changes that make you think you might be depressed?" "Is the depression better and worse throughout the day or over the course of the week?" "Did something happen in your life about the time the depression started or worsened?" "Is there anything you do that makes the depressive symptoms lighten or deepen for you?" "Is there anyone in your life to whom you talk about your symptoms?" "How do you think your partner is affected by the depression?" "How are you affected by your partner's reactions?" It is relentless but respectful curiosity that fuels the therapist's push to understand the problem sequence.

Creativity

A popular pastime for children before the age of cell phones and the internet was a piece of paper on which were a set of dots that were numbered. The child's task was to draw a line between two dots with consecutive numbers (e.g., 8–9, etc.). When the dots had all been connected, a picture (e.g., an animal) would appear. Identifying the problem sequence is analogous to connecting the dots, except there are no numbers associated with the dots. The therapist must use creativity to hypothesize how the dots are connected. Through a trial-and-error process of asking questions, the problem sequence (the picture) emerges. There are infinite variations of how problem sequences exist in client systems. They are analogous to snowflakes. There will always be some common elements, but in the end, every problem sequence is unique. The creativity of the therapist is instrumental in finding that uniqueness.

Clients live in their problem sequences, but they are not always aware of how their interactions constitute a repeating pattern. For example, in the case of a white, cisgender, mixed-sex, married couple, the husband, during arguments, regularly accused his wife of being like her mother. The wife always reacted with strong anger to this statement. In this example, the creativity of the therapist might lead to the hypothesis: What might the connection be between the accusation that the wife is just like her mother and the strength of her reaction to it? With this hypothesis in mind, the therapist would formulate a question (planning per the blueprint) and advance the conversation by asking it. For example (to the wife): "I get that you are offended when your husband compares you to your mother, and you may just want him to stop doing that, but your reaction to it seems stronger than I would expect. I wonder if you can identify anything that might make that comparison so difficult for you?" In this case, uncovering the connection to her mother's abusive behavior and carefully defining its impact had the effect of helping the husband see the importance of discontinuing the practice of comparing his wife to her mother.

Courage

Therapists are always challenged with the decision to make the unspoken spoken or, for the moment, to leave it unsaid. For therapists to make the unspoken spoken requires courage for two related reasons. First, any spoken observation about the problem sequence puts the party most involved in it on the spot. Second, the observation is also about the relationships among the clients and can be taken as critical of the relationship and/or other people in it.

When deciding whether to offer an observation, the therapist weighs the importance of the observation against the risk that it might damage the alliance. If the risk of a substantial tear in the alliance is great, the clinical activity (e.g., question, statement, or suggestion), will be modified, postponed, or abandoned, depending on its perceived importance in the process of therapy. The exceptions to this rule would include matters of safety which always require direct and immediate attention, and critical points in therapy at which the integrity or effectiveness of the therapy will be compromised by not directly broaching an issue. In these situations, courage is summoned, and the therapist speaks directly, though respectfully. In other situations, therapists temper their courage with concern for the alliance. If they conclude that the potential alliance tear is repairable, and that there is an opportunity to advance the definition of the problem sequence, they will need to summon the courage to directly broach the issue.

For example, during their third session a multi-ethnic, cisgender, mixed-sex couple began to engage in a conflict. The conflictual sequence escalated quickly, and both spouses first complained, then criticized, and finally the husband began to speak to the wife with what the therapist coded as contempt, saying: "What have you ever done with your life? You never finish anything." The therapist knew from Gottman's (1993) research that contempt is corrosive to a relationship and its presence is highly correlated with the demise of relationships. Thus, the therapist knew it was imperative to identify contempt as a major component of the problem sequence.

Considering the alliance, the therapist sensed that the husband might take offence, and might also conclude that the therapist is siding with his wife. Although the therapist felt the first two sessions went well, the alliance was in an early stage of development, so the conversing component of the blueprint became critically important here as the therapist summoned courage and sought a way to minimize the stress on the nascent alliance. There are many alternatives for doing this. Below is one scenario.

Husband:	What have you ever done with your life? You never finish anything.
Therapist (to wife):	How did it make you feel when your husband said that to you?
Wife:	It felt awful.
Therapist (to husband):	We are working on trying to improve your conflict style. Your wife just told you that the way you spoke to her made her feel awful. Can you ask her why it felt awful to her?
Husband:	(to wife) Sure. So, what was so bad about what I just said to you?
Wife:	(to husband) You just sounded so disgusted. It made me feel like you see me as a complete idiot.
Therapist:	That was a good short exchange. You both took a risk. *(To husband)* Your wife sounded hurt by your words. How does that make you feel?
Husband:	I think she's way overreacting.
Therapist:	Well, maybe, but another word very similar to disgust is contempt. *(To wife)* Does that word also describe what it sounded like?
Wife:	Yes.
Therapist:	When things get heated in a conflict, we sometimes say things we don't mean, but when we say something to our partner that sends a message that we don't value who they are, it can be a sign of contempt. Some excellent research on couple interaction has shown that contempt in a relationship is hurtful and puts a couple at higher risk for the relationship to fail.

In this way, the therapist begins to address the damaging nature of what the husband said, connects it to established knowledge about relationships, and defines a part of the problem sequence that needs to change. As the alliance develops, the therapist can afford to speak more directly to both parties.

The Therapeutic Conversation

The problem sequence emerges from the therapeutic conversation in one of three ways. First, the most straightforward way is for the problem, itself, to be a problem sequence. For example, a quite common presenting problem is difficulty with communication. Communication, itself, can be thought of as a set of sequences, so when the clients describe their communication problems, the therapist is careful to help them name the components that make their communication problematic. For example:

Natasha:　No matter what we talk about, we seem to disagree and almost immediately we are upset with each other.

Therapist:　I see. Almost any topic can create a disagreement.

Max:　That's pretty much it.

Therapist:　Let's see if we can understand more precisely what happens when these arguments escalate. Let's start at the beginning. What is generally going on when you start one of these conversations?

Natasha:　Well, that's part of it. We both work and by the time we get the kids to bed, there isn't much time for us, so we are always trying to squeeze a conversation in when we are both exhausted.

Therapist:　That sounds like it will be a key factor for us to consider. So, conflicts often happen in the evening when you are exhausted. Maybe you can describe the pattern they take. Or it could be good to start with the story of a recent conflict, if you like.

Many problems presented for therapy, for example, "doing poorly in school," do not, in and of themselves, describe or refer to a sequence. The second way for the problem sequence to begin to emerge in a therapeutic conversation is when clients provide interactional context for the presenting problem. For example:

Mother:　Our son is doing very poorly in school. His grades have been dropping, and we can't seem to motivate him to do his work. We talk to him about it every day, and he says he will try harder, but there is no follow-through.

Therapist (to son):　Do you agree with your mom that school isn't going as well as it once did?

Son:　School is a waste of time.

Therapist:　Your mom says they try to encourage you. What does it feel like to you when they do?

Son:　They tell me I should be like my brother. He's a genius and a total nerd. I could never be like that.

Here the comparison of the son to his brother constitutes an interaction that is likely to be part of a problem sequence. The therapist uses contextual information as springboards from which to track the sequences. In this case, there will be sequences related to schoolwork and sequences related to conversations with parent(s) about schoolwork.

Third, in some instances problem sequences only emerge through extensive questioning by the therapist. This is sometimes the case with clients, who seek individual therapy and initially describe the presenting problem in a de-contextual way. A problem sequence exists but it can only be described from the perspective of the individual client. Some of these clients focus on their internal experience and less on descriptions of interactional patterns. In such a case, the therapist can work to co-create a problem sequence that consists of the internal sequence of meanings and emotions. For example, clients whose presenting problem is anxiety are guided by the therapist's questions to organize their thoughts, feelings and actions into a problem sequence that explains how they experience their anxiety. Some examples of questions are: "What kinds of things bring anxiety to you?" "When is anxiety the strongest?" "Does your anxiety ebb and flow throughout the day?" "Are you more anxious when you are by yourself or around other people?" "What do you say to yourself when the anxiety begins to increase?" "What do you do then?" With sufficient, compassionate inquiry, the context of the anxiety–its problem sequence–will emerge.

As is sometimes more apparent in individual therapy, people have two types of interlocking problem sequences: Internal sequences and interactional sequences. Interaction patterns evoke thoughts and feelings which, in turn, impact and are part of what maintain the interaction patterns. The therapist must establish that both are important in the understanding and resolution of the problem. To accomplish this, the therapist can work with the client to establish and understand the impact the internal problem sequence has on other people in the client's life; hence, the problem takes an interpersonal as well as a personal toll.

For example, a white cisgender gay man sought therapy after he had been given a diagnosis of borderline personality disorder. He shared that he had a significant abuse history and had been depressed and anxious for most of his adult life. His goals were to find meaning in life and to be more at peace with himself. When asked if he were in a relationship, he became more somber and said that he had been living with a man for a year who had recently told him that he did not think he could tolerate the instability of their relationship much longer. The client agreed the relationship was in trouble. With guidance from the therapist, he pieced together a problem sequence. He said that frequently his partner would say something to him that may be innocuous but made him feel denigrated. He would then immediately become angry, and the partner would try to explain why he said what he said, but the surge of anger was too powerful, and the client would tell the partner to leave him alone. Dismayed, the partner would try to pursue the client, sometimes into the next room until the client disengaged and slammed the door. The partner would disengage and stew over the hurt of being so misunderstood. When asked how he would feel should his partner break off the relationship, the client said he would be devastated. In this example, an internal sequence and an interpersonal sequence were interlocked in such a way that each amplified the other, thus threatening both the emotional wellbeing of the client and his relationship.

Operational Tools

Working collaboratively with a client system to co-construct a problem sequence requires careful attention to the use of the blueprint, particularly the hypothesizing, conversing and reading feedback components. The planning component of the blueprint increases in prominence when alliance issues need to be directly addressed or work on the essence diagram shifts to creating a solution sequence.

Identifying the problem sequence commits therapists to think about the small part of the total system that enables the therapist to set a goal and give a task, two crucial components of alliance formation. This is done in total recognition that the problem sequence is embedded in a client system that is far more complex, and that some of the complexity will likely have to be accessed at a later point in therapy.

Using the blueprint to construct a problem sequence harnesses the recursive nature of its components: Hypothesizing, conversing, reading feedback, and planning. In the discussion to follow, for heuristic purposes only, each component is discussed separately.

Hypothesizing

Hypothesizing is an endeavor by which information (feedback) offered by clients is given meaning. The parts of a problem sequence are not isolated actions, meanings, and emotions that are strung together in a sequence. Rather, each action, meaning, and/or emotion exists in the context of other actions, meanings, and emotions. Although the primary task is to piece together a problem sequence, each part of the problem sequence can evoke hypotheses about the client system. The level of therapist experience comes into play here. Beginning therapists should focus more on just getting the actions, meanings and/or emotions into a problem sequence. With experience and deeper knowledge of the hypothesizing metaframeworks, the process of constructing the sequence will trigger hypothesizing that enriches its salience. An example related to hypothesizing is presented below. Take a moment and ask yourself what your hypothesis would be and compare it to a possible IST hypothesis.

A parent complaining that a 7-year-old son with attention deficit hyper-activity disorder (ADHD) won't start getting ready for bed: He knows he must get off all screens and take his bath, but when I call up the stairs to tell him to start taking off his clothes, he just ignores me.

Your hypothesis:

One IST hypothesis: Best practice for parenting a child with ADHD begins with the premise that these children have difficulty paying attention; therefore, to get the message from parent to child, it is important to be standing face-to-face with the child. When giving a command, therefore, it will exacerbate the problem for the mother to call up the stairs believing that her son hears and follows her command. This hypothesis informs the description of the problem sequence.

Conversing

Conversing in IST is an active and engaged process. As discussed earlier in this chapter, the clients often are not aware of how their internal and interactional problem sequences work so therapists must assist them in the construction of such sequences. The causality pillar (see Chapter 1) comes into play as IST therapists adopt the construct of recursiveness that holds that for any two variables in the sequence the relationship between them is mutually influencing rather than causal.

IST therapists model this recursiveness through their use of language. One of the most effective ways to do this is through circular questioning (Selvini-Palazzoli et al., 1980). A circular question is constructed whenever two variables (e.g., an action and a meaning) are juxtaposed and presented as a question. For example, "When he says that to you, how does it make you feel?" The answer to the question constitutes a partial arc of the whole problem sequence. When all of the partial arcs are assembled, they constitute the problem sequence.

A problem sequence describes the relationship among actions, meanings, and emotions in a client system. These domains of action, meaning, and emotion can be juxtaposed in the formulation of questions as illustrated in the following examples:

Action/action: When she yells at you, what do you do?

Meaning/meaning: If you told her, you no longer believed in her, would that change the way she looks at the relationship?

Emotion/emotion: When you feel that fear welling up inside of her, how does that affect your sadness?

Action/meaning: When he says he'll be home in an hour and then is three hours late, what does that mean to you?

Action/emotion: When you find out that he has smoked weed, how does that make you feel?

Meaning/action: When you tell yourself that your son is lazy, what do you do?

Emotion/action: When you feel her sadness overwhelming you, what do you do or say?

Meaning/emotion: When you tell yourself she must be having an affair, how does that make you feel?

Emotion/meaning: Your daughter says she is very angry at the teacher. How do you understand what that means to her?

Feedback

Feedback is the driver of the blueprint. Whatever feedback the clients provide about their interpersonal and intrapersonal system serves as the source of information for hypothesizing, planning and conversing, all of which lead to the construction of a problem sequence. Feedback includes everything that happens verbally and nonverbally during a session and everything the clients report about their lives outside of the session. Several moments of feedback are presented below. The reader is invited to decide what that feedback means and compare it to the IST hypothesis.

EXAMPLE 1

Client (on the phone making an appointment to be seen in individual therapy): Oh, I can't schedule an appointment next week because I will have the kids.

Your hypothesis:

One IST hypothesis: The language "I will have the kids" suggests the client is likely divorced and shares custody with the children(s)' other parent. I wonder if there is an S2 pattern of children moving between households during the week that is relevant to the problem sequence?

EXAMPLE 2

A gay couple seeking therapy for communication problems come into the therapy room for their first session and elect to sit on the sofa side by side, one putting a hand on the knee of the other.

Your hypothesis:

One *IST hypothesis:* The partners seem comfortable, close, and willing to show this aspect of their relationship to their new therapist. This seems like a strength for them.

EXAMPLE 3

A mixed-sex, cisgender, married couple in their early 40s is arguing about the husband's periodic nights out with his friends and the wife's complaint that he does not let her know when he is going to be home.

Wife: You act like you can do whatever you want. I can't do that. Who would watch the kids?

Your hypothesis:

One *IST hypothesis:* This is an intermittent event (S3) in which the husband's night out destabilizes the relationship and contributes to the intensity of the arguments.

EXAMPLE 4

A mother, father, and a 15-year-old daughter are discussing the father's complaint that his relationship with his daughter is contentious and distant.

Father	When I knock and come into your room to tell you
(to daughter):	something, you just grunt and tell me to get out without any response.
Daughter:	You are such a bore. Why should I want to talk to you?
Father:	Don't talk to me that way.
Mother:	That's the problem. You can't get anywhere with her so long as you do nothing but criticize her.

Your hypothesis:

One IST hypothesis: The mother defends the daughter which suggests that she may have a cross-generational coalition with her. Perhaps the daughter strengthens her voice when the father criticizes her as she knows she will be protected by the mother.

Case Example

The following example illustrates how the problem sequence serves as one of the key components of the essence diagram.

Juanita, a Latina, cisgender, heterosexual woman in her late 40s, contacted an IST therapist requesting to work on her relationship with her 76-year-old mother, Stella (Estrella). Juanita mentioned that her relationship with her mother had always been strained, and now that her mother was at an age where she might need the daughter's involvement in her life, she felt she should improve their relationship. The mother lived alone in another city, having been divorced decades earlier.

Hypothesizing that the care of an elderly parent is best managed as a collaboration among the parent's children, the therapist asked Juanita whether she had any siblings. Juanita said she had a sister named Eva who was two years younger. When the therapist asked Juanita whether she thought Eva would be part of a plan to help the mother, she replied that Eva's relationship with Stella was very strained and the two hardly ever spoke to each other. When the therapist asked Juanita whether she intended to ask her sister to share the responsibilities that would eventually arrive, Juanita replied that Eva had fixed opinions about their mother, and it would require too much work to get her on board. To get the therapy started, the therapist decided to try to first build an alliance with Juanita and to leave Stella and Eva in the indirect client system until a later time.

When the therapist reflected on the initial phone call with Juanita, the broad strokes of a problem sequence emerged. The mother and her two daughters had but sparse communication, and there seemed to be some underlying tensions among them, particularly between Stella and Eva. Although Stella was currently in fairly good health, Juanita was concerned that sometime in the coming years her mother would need someone more involved in her life. She reported that there had been no conversations about her mother's future.

When Juanita attended the first session, she provided additional background information. She revealed that the parents had divorced when the children were very young, and that Stella had been the one to leave the home post-divorce. Juanita seemed more reconciled to this than Eva, the latter having spent years of therapy understanding Stella's departure as an attachment disruption to which she attributed her mental health struggles. Juanita felt that Eva tolerated her mother but had never forgiven her for leaving her children. She said that her conversations with Eva about their mother inevitably ended in an intense argument; hence, they rarely broached any topic that touched on Stella.

At this point in the conversation, the therapist hypothesized that the target problem sequence was between the sisters. It involved avoidance and conflict escalation whenever the two women discussed Stella. The therapist could coach Juanita to change that problem sequence or bring Eva into the direct system and deal with the problem sequence in a session. The latter was chosen.

The therapist provided Juanita with a rationale that explained why, in the long run, Eva needed to be involved. Juanita eventually reached out to Eva and talked with her about attending a session. Eva was surprisingly receptive to attending a session. She shared with Juanita that it pained her greatly that Stella drove such a wedge between them. In the next chapter, the concept and use of solution sequences will be presented. In this instance, a solution sequence was drawn from the action planning metaframework and involved a straightforward challenge to the avoidance component of the problem sequence by having both sisters in session. That would give the therapist direct access to the second component of this problem sequence—conflict escalation ending in polarization and disengagement.

Juanita and Eva attended the next several sessions. Eva made it clear that she was very reluctant to engage with Stella. She felt that Stella had never apologized for abandoning the sisters and that throughout her adult life had continued to show a selfish side to Eva. Juanita countered that, despite all that had happened, she loved Stella and felt sorry for the life of challenge and loneliness that awaited their aging mother. Eva felt that Juanita owed her mother nothing, and Juanita felt Eva was hiding behind her hurt and unwilling to do her fair share. Unlike their private conversations about Stella, the therapist was able to keep the conversations civil, so the polarization did not occur, and over time both sisters better understood the perspective of the other. Eva was able to say she knew it would not be fair for the burden of the mother's care to fall solely on Juanita, but it was also clear that she believed Stella would never change and feared wading too deep into a relationship with Stella that could threaten her mental health.

In the next session, Juanita revealed that Stella was aware of Eva's view of her and would complain to Juanita about it. Juanita stated that she felt stuck in the middle. Eva hadn't been aware of this triangulation. At first, Eva was angry that Juanita talked behind her back, but Eva quickly softened with the recognition that it would be difficult to avoid such conversations with their mother. This pattern of triangulation further complicated the problem sequence.

When the therapist mused about involving Stella in the therapy, Juanita was guarded but ready to hear more, and Eva immediately said that nothing good could come of it. Recognizing that the therapist's alliance with Eva was at risk, care was taken not to rupture the alliance. By the end of the session, Eva had agreed for the therapist to speak to Stella and said she would trust the therapist's judgment on whether a session with the mother could be helpful.

When Stella did attend a session, the three women seemed uncomfortable and interacted in an awkward manner. It was clear that they avoided certain topics about their current relationships and made no mention of the early history. It was also clear to the therapist that Stella presented more favorably than Eva's internalized representation of her. This representation may have been galvanized by years of Eva's therapy that characterized Stella in a deficit-oriented way. This too played a role in maintaining the problem sequence and constraining alternative sequences.

The first meeting was sufficiently successful to continue working with the mother and daughters. The following topics were broached. First, since the daughters were very young at the time of the divorce, they had no personal knowledge of it and had always accepted their father's narrative of it that had Stella abandoning her children. This narrative plays a role in the problem sequence as it predisposed the daughters, particularly Eva, to hold anger toward Stella. Stella's narrative included details the daughters did not know; hence, it helped them soften toward their mother. This narrative approach supported the development of new patterns of interaction, the solution sequences.

As the mother and daughters felt safer in the sessions, Eva was able to say that she felt her mother always acted and spoke in a self-centered manner when they interacted. Stella was shocked by this revelation. It took a lot of work to unpack this issue, but in the end, Stella committed to pay more attention to her daughter and gave Eva permission to call her on it when Eva thought it was happening. These interventions were examples of solution sequences.

Juanita also raised the problem sequence involving Stella's penchant to learn about Eva by asking Juanita about her. Disentangling this triangulation proved challenging because Eva was still reluctant to engage her mother in a dyadic conversation. She finally relented when Stella committed to not always direct topics back to herself.

The final problem was the daughters' concerns that Stella's needs would be met as she continued to age. At first, Stella protested that she was in good health and didn't need any assistance from her daughters. The therapist offered the distinction between "young old age" when an aging individual is in good physical and mental health and "old old age" when an illness or injury partially or totally incapacitates the individual (Duvall, 1957). Stella was currently in the stage of "young old age." Experts on aging encourage families to discuss and plan for "old old age" while the aging parent is still of sound mind and body. Stella saw the logic of this, and the women discussed what needed to be done. They prepared a list and then discussed how best to execute it. It included issues like power of attorney, medical power of attorney, whether Stella would move to an assisted living facility, and what circumstances might trigger that. Eva showed reluctance to step forward to take responsibility for items on the list, but this was a far better situation than the original problem sequence where it was just assumed that Juanita would do it all. Enough of a relationship had been built between Eva and Stella to enable them to discuss how to proceed. Juanita suggested Eva select items that she could handle with consistent but minimal back and forth with Stella and all agreed. Within several sessions, the list had been addressed and it was clear that the women felt both closer to each other and successful in their progress.

Conclusion

There is an old expression: "Well begun is half done." While it is very tempting to slip into a case and begin the work without obtaining a full understanding of the problem sequence, the price paid for doing so can have a negative impact on the outcome of the case. Taking time to identify a problem sequence will have long-term benefits as the case unfolds. The problem sequence will serve as a reference point for the case. It will serve as the basis for your first interventions in support of a solution sequence and if the solution sequence fails, as it often does, the next step will be to locate the constraints that kept it from being successful.

Exercises

1   Think of a problem that you struggle with. Note the recurrent nature of it. Using the knowledge you gained by studying this chapter, seek to discover the specific sequence of action, meaning and emotion that you exhibit in relation to this problem. Write down each step of your problem sequence.

2   Consider a recent session you conducted. Jot down the main theme of the session. Identify how you were handling the session. Reflect on whether the process of the session included a focus on a problem sequence (even if you called it something different). Describe this sequence in writing. Review it and ask yourself what might be missing from the sequence. Write this down. Reflect on what you would have to do to fill in the gaps of the sequence. Be sure to consider whether the client(s) who attended the session could provide the answers. Reflect on any new ways of looking at the case that may have come out of this exercise.

3   Think about a case you have. Describe your focus for the case. Think of a problem sequence that could be part of the case. Write down the problem sequence based on what you know. Review it and ask yourself how complete it is. What additional information would you need to gather to complete a workable problem sequence?

4   Record several of your sessions with the intent of identifying problem sequences that occur in session or are described in session. From one recording to the next, is your ability to articulate the problem sequence with your clients improving? Review the *attitudinal* and *operational tools* described in this chapter. Check to see if you are using them. If you are not using them, ask yourself what is keeping you from doing so. Pick one tool and focus on it during your next recording.

References

Breunlin, D. C., & Schwartz, R. C. (1986). Sequences: Toward a common denominator of family therapy. *Family Process, 25*(1), 67–87. 10.1111/j.1545-5300.1986.00067.x

Churven, P. (1988). Marital therapy my way: Creating a workable reality. *Australian and New Zealand Journal of Family Therapy, 9*(4), 223–225. 10.1002/j.1467-8438.1988.tb01269.x

Duvall, E. M. (1957). *Family development*. J. P. Lippincott.

Gottman, J. M. (1993). The roles of conflict engagement, escalation, and avoidance in marital interaction: A longitudinal view of five types of couples. *Journal of Consulting and Clinical Psychology, 61*(1), 6–15. 10.1037/0022-006X.61.1.6

Minuchin, S., & Fishman, H. C. (1981). *Family therapy techniques*. Harvard University Press.

Russell, W., & Breunlin, D. (2019). Transcending therapy models and managing complexity: Suggestions from integrative systemic therapy. *Family Process, 58*(3), 641–655. 10.1111/famp.12482

Selvini-Palazzoli, M., Cecchin, G., Prata, G., & Boscolo, L. (1980). Hypothesizing, circularity, and neutrality: Three guidelines for the conductor of the session. *Family Process, 19*, 3–12. 10.1111/j.1545-5300.1980.00003.x

Taussig, D. (2018). Sequences in couple and family therapy. In J. L. Lebow, A. L. Chambers, & D. C. Breunlin (Eds.), *Encyclopedia of couple and family therapy*. Springer, Cham. 10.1007/978-3-319-15877-8_915-1

Watzlawick, P., Weakland, J. H., & Fisch, R. (1974). *Change: Principles of problem formation and problem resolution*. Norton.

Chapter 5

Identifying a Solution Sequence

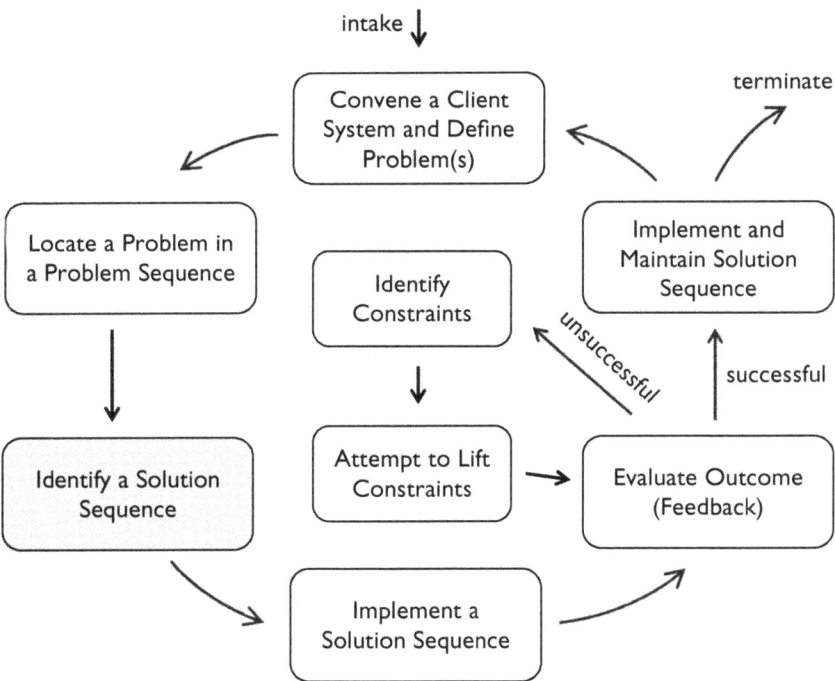

intake ↓

Convene a Client System and Define Problem(s)

terminate

Locate a Problem in a Problem Sequence

Identify Constraints

Implement and Maintain Solution Sequence

unsuccessful

successful

Identify a Solution Sequence

Attempt to Lift Constraints

Evaluate Outcome (Feedback)

Implement a Solution Sequence

IST Essence Diagram.

Objective

This chapter will discuss and demonstrate how to collaboratively identify a solution sequence. A solution sequence is an alternative, adaptive sequence that replaces a problem sequence and contributes to the improvement or resolution of the presenting problem. Various hypothesizing metaframeworks may inform the selection of a solution sequence. Particular attention needs to

DOI: 10.4324/9780429322273-5

be paid to assuring that the solution sequence fits the developmental levels and cultural context of the clients. The role of IST's culture metaframework in the selection of a solution sequence will be elaborated.

Introduction

The identification of a solution sequence is an essential step in the IST process. The solution sequence is developed based on the problem sequence, and its implementation leads either to problem resolution or to the identification of constraints. In and of itself the solution sequence may be quite simply formulated, but it can be the means of discovering great complexity within the system. As clients seek relief from a problem sequence, identifying and implementing a solution sequence provides a point of entry to the factors that will need to be addressed and resolved. The solution sequence will typically involve a change in action or interaction, as clients agree to try something new. Although the focus is on the realm of doing, the therapist will need to work within the realm of meaning and language to establish a rationale for the solution sequence and connect it to what the clients want to get out of therapy. The therapist will also need to be attuned to clients' emotional reactions to establish and maintain a therapeutic alliance. Thus, changes in patterns of action require attention to meaning and emotion. Further, many solution sequences include a modification of an internal sequence of mind that is linked to the external pattern of action or interaction. Importantly, a solution sequence will need to fit with the context of the clients' lives. Since at this stage in the process the therapist is not uncovering all of that context, the therapist solicits feedback from the clients to see whether a solution fits for them.

IST therapists often describe solution sequences as experiments that lead either toward problem resolution or to the identification of constraints in the system. This experimentation is a collaborative effort that helps the therapist and clients learn more about how to proceed with problem-solving. Success with the solution sequence advances problem solving, but the failure of a solution sequence also advances problem-solving by virtue of what can be learned about the constraints that will need to be addressed in therapy. Thus, the therapist can project a respectful, collaborative, win-win attitude about the experiments that clients agree to try. It is great when initial solutions work, but immediate change is not the only way forward.

Solution sequences will be more relevant and appealing to clients when they see the relationship between the solution and the carefully described problem sequence. As per Chapter 4, the therapist helps the clients see that there is a pattern to their problems and that change in that pattern is required to solve the problem. By identifying problem sequences, the therapist can illustrate how members of the family or other system recursively influence each other as they act and interact in relation to the presenting problem. Sequences have elements of action, meaning and emotion, each recursively contextualizing the others. As previously stated, initial solution sequences typically involve changes in action supported by a rationale (meaning) and attunement to the clients (emotion). At times, though, due to the nature of the problem presented or a strong client preference, an action strategy will not be the best first step. Alternatively, the meaning/emotion planning metaframework is a source of strategies for solution sequences. For example, a client grieving the loss of their partner clearly did not want to do something early in the therapy. The therapist respected this and began the work in the realm of meaning and emotion. Other grieving clients may be more open to doing something such as reaching out to family or friends, attending church services, taking a nature walk, lighting a candle each night, or visiting the grave of a loved one.

A solution sequence, when successfully performed and maintained, may be sufficient to solve the presenting problem. More often, there will be more than one problem sequence associated with a particular presenting problem and there may be more than one problem. So, the meaning of the success with a solution sequence is contextualized in the larger patterns related to the clients' concerns. For example, a 44-year-old white cisgender single gay man presents with depression. Risk issues are assessed and ruled out and the therapist explores the patterns in the client's life. There does not seem to be a clear precipitant to the depression, but a problem sequence of isolation is identified: the client thinks about connecting with someone, feels shame about being seen as depressed, and decides not to make the contact. The therapist works to empower the client to modify the internal avoidance and reach out to a friend of his (solution sequence). The client does so and feels good about it. The therapist works to help the client maintain this gain, but also begins to address another problem sequence that involves inactivity. Sharing the research on behavioral activation (Kanter et al., 2010), the therapist helps the client establish a new pattern of activity and begins to modify how time is spent (solution sequence). The client does get involved with some activities and feels better doing so. The therapist works to help the client maintain the new activities. The client shares his disappointment concerning his romantic life and the therapist helps him explore a problem sequence of self-defeating thinking which they agree to examine with special attention to a particularly painful break-up that had occurred 2 years before the initiation of the therapy. If one or more of the solution sequences are unsuccessful, the therapist will hypothesize about constraints. For example, there may be a biological constraint that governs mood and can be addressed by a biobehavioral intervention such as exercise or psychotropic medication. In this case, there was a set of problem sequences that comprised what the client (and others) called depression. Improving the depression required progressively implementing solution sequences to address the problem sequences that were identified.

Method

Experiments

As therapy is a collaborative process, the therapist explains how IST works and invites the clients to join the effort which will be designed to address the issue(s) they want to work on in therapy. In IST, this process is best described by talking briefly about the process of defining the problem and the patterns that surround it, experimenting with solutions, and identifying and working with the things that get in the way of solutions. As the therapist begins to discuss a solution sequence, it is important to return to the concept of experimenting and emphasize that experiments tried in session or between sessions will provide the opportunity to find a solution or identify constraints. The therapist advances a spirit of collaboration by emphasizing that clients will have the opportunity to ask questions and give feedback at each step in the process.

In keeping with IST's strength guideline, the therapist believes that client systems can help generate solutions, so the therapist asks clients to work from the problem sequence in considering a solution sequence. The therapist might say:

Therapist: It seems that you have been working hard to manage this (the problem they are presenting), but it has been challenging. Last week we put together a description of a pattern that occurs. It repeats itself and seems to be closely related to what brought you into therapy. Have you had any thoughts about changing that pattern or doing something different that might help with the situation?

In couple or family sessions, if one person suggests a solution sequence or an element of one, the therapist would ask what the other members think about the suggestion. If there is a consensus that it is a good idea, the clients would be asked if they would like to try it. Ideas from the clients are often excellent starting points for a solution sequence. For example, a family of five described a pattern of disconnection. The oldest daughter came up with the solution sequence of a weekly, "old-fashioned Sunday dinner." The parents chuckled at the old-fashioned part wondering where their daughter had heard about this, but they liked the idea, and the two other children were open to trying it. The therapist supported it as a worthy experiment and the family discussed in session how it would work. This quite simple solution sequence was reasonable in that it might be a vehicle for connection. The therapist praised the family for developing the solution and shared the idea that the advantage of the experiment was that they would either make it work or if that proved difficult, there was a lot to learn from trying. The dinner did not work out on a weekly basis, but it was a concrete way to begin to explore the circumstances and history that constrained them from connecting. A few years later, the family contacted the therapist to work on a new issue. In a light moment of reuniting with the therapist, they reported that now and again they still had an "old fashioned Sunday dinner," a ritual that had become part of the narrative of the family and a metaphor for what they had worked on in therapy.

Solution sequences can also be suggested by the therapist. Sometimes these are based on common sense solutions that provide a good initial experiment. Oftentimes, they are based on formal strategies and interventions drawn from one of the planning metaframeworks. An example of how the therapist can communicate a potential solution sequence is as follows, "I have been giving a lot of thought to the way you are contending with (the issue of concern) and I wanted to share my thoughts with you." The therapist's thoughts will include a justification for how the solution fits the problem sequence. That justification is a connection to the problem sequence that is described in terms of common sense, therapist experience, best practices, or research. It states why the therapist thinks it is a good solution to try. This justification has elsewhere been described as a *workable reality,* a shared conception of the problem that suggests a way to solve it (Minuchin & Fishman, 1981; Churven, 1988). A workable reality gives a description of what clients can do to solve the problem.

Any of the hypothesizing metaframeworks may come into play when considering a solution sequence. The development and culture metaframeworks are especially important to consider. What the therapist suggests will need to be consistent with the developmental levels of participants which is especially important when children are involved. For example, an 8-year-old child should not be asked to do things that require deductive reasoning, abstract thinking, or systematic planning that are associated with the later, formal operations stage of cognitive development. Therapists who have professional experience with children or who are parents themselves will understand some of the factors to consider. Other therapists will need to review their studies in human development and consult their supervisors for guidance on what can be expected of children at various ages.

In formulating a solution sequence, the therapist will need to consider the clients' cultural contexts of membership (intersectionality) and worldview as well as the contextual factors in the clients' lives. Attunement, respect, and curiosity are essential elements of conversation that the therapist uses to make sure the developing solution and experiment do not leave the clients feeling misunderstood or disrespected. Offering a solution that disregards the family's value system or the real-life constraints they face may result in a rupture of the therapeutic alliance, which can lead to premature termination and further discouragement. The following case example illustrates the introduction of a solution sequence that negatively impacts therapy. In this case, a couple is struggling with whether they will get married.

Therapist: I hear that your main worry about getting married is not knowing if you will enjoy each other in the same way once you are under the same roof, and I hear there is a pattern of conflict that begins when you approach topics related to moving things forward in your relationship. Do I understand this correctly?

After confirmation of the hypothesis, the therapist goes on to say:

Therapist: It seems like a solution here is simply to move in together for a trial period without giving up your own separate apartments just yet to see how it feels to live under the same roof before marriage.

In this example, the therapist identified the problem sequence and received confirmation that it was accurate. However, the therapist abruptly suggested a solution without sufficient consideration of how it would fit with the clients' belief system, cultural context, the indirect client system, and socioeconomic factors. It is preferable to slow things down and begin with what the clients can offer about how to contend with the dilemma, including the options they have considered. In this way, the therapist will learn more about their worldview with respect to the dilemma and will be in a better position to tentatively propose a solution sequence and seek client feedback on it. If it does not seem contraindicated by what the clients are sharing about their worldview or circumstances, the therapist might decide to say something like:

Therapist: I am not sure how this idea will fit for you but some couples who face this dilemma decide to move in together for a period to see how they do together. I would be interested in your thoughts about this approach.

The importance of guiding a conversation with a genuine interest in a client's meaning system, emotional experience, and actual circumstances cannot be overstated.

Strategies

In some cases, the therapist will propose more formal strategies or interventions to construct a solution sequence. With consideration of contexts of membership and client circumstances, the therapist can look to IST strategies (see Appendix A) when addressing a problem sequence. Strategies are general plans that can be accomplished in a variety of ways. A strategy can be accomplished by various interventions that are borrowed from existing models of therapy. For instance, in the case of a client with a phobic problem sequence, the therapist may propose a strategy of exposure with the idea that being exposed, in prescribed ways, to what is feared can reduce the fear. There are a variety of ways to provide therapeutic exposure, including progressive exposure and prolonged exposure. Exposure can be done in-vivo, via imagination (imaginal exposure), or via virtual reality. In IST, the specific ways of doing exposure therapy are classified as interventions that can be chosen in support of the general strategy of exposure. In selecting the intervention, the therapist is guided by the nature of the problem sequence, relevant research findings, and client feedback.

Another example of a strategy would be to access primary emotion (Greenberg & Safran, 1989) as a means of addressing conflictual sequences in a couple system. The therapist could choose specific interventions from the emotion-focused (Goldman & Greenberg, 2015; Greenberg, 2011) or emotionally focused therapy (Johnson, 2015) models to fulfill this strategy and help the couple modify the problem sequences that have contributed to the conflict. A final example of a strategy is seen in a case of a blended family seeking therapy for interpersonal conflict. The therapist might recommend a strategy of designating the biological parent as the one primarily responsible for setting expectations for the adolescent children. This strategy for a solution sequence may draw on structural family therapy interventions such as marking boundaries.

The collaborative process of identifying a solution sequence is a complex, moment-by-moment conversational process that is guided by the IST blueprint (hypothesizing, planning, conversing, and reading feedback). The therapist attends carefully to the clients' verbal and non-verbal feedback and the interactions between and among clients in conjoint sessions. The therapist leads this process with a planful approach to *when* and *how* questions are interjected during the clients' recounting of a narrative. As such, the therapist can identify the ways emotions and meanings are a part of the clients' experiences and have become part of the problem sequence or serve as a constraint to solution sequences. Observing and tracking problem sequences with an eye on emotions and cognitions facilitates the therapist's understanding of how the system works in relation to the problem and suggests how it might be changed to solve the presenting concerns.

Enactments

Interactions observed in sessions are a wonderful source of information about sequences. Problem sequences often make themselves known to the therapist as clients talk together during a session. For example, one parent might be talking to a child and suddenly the other parent interrupts and takes over the conversation. The therapist sees this interaction and hypothesizes that it is a recurrent pattern that may be related to the presenting problem, in other words a problem sequence. Clients may spontaneously talk together in session, but the therapist can also ask them to do so. In an enactment (Minuchin & Fishman, 1981; Nichols & Colapinto, 2017) the therapist asks the clients to talk directly with each other. This is done either for the purpose of seeing how clients interact or for working with them to modify their sequences of interaction.

The therapist begins to set up an enactment by deciding what needs to be the topic. The therapist then gives a clear rationale for why it is suggested. For example, "I am noticing that it seems challenging for the two of you to stay on a topic you are discussing. Could you talk to each other about something specific and let's see how that goes?" Sometimes the enactment is developed based on the clients' description of an interaction that takes place outside of the session. For example, a parent might describe how the bedtime routine misfires every night. The therapist can conduct an enactment by asking the clients to show in the session what they have just described to the therapist. In another example, a parent might report that she cannot get her child to start doing homework. The therapist might say: "Can you show me here and now how that conversation goes?" The therapist would ask the parent to talk to the child the way she would at home and the child would be asked to respond as if at home. The enactment provides a concrete way of examining the problem sequence and discussing a solution sequence.

An enactment can serve as a stimulus to experimentation with a solution sequence. This happens when the therapist sees the enactment unfolding as a problem sequence and suggests that the clients try to do something different. In the example above where one parent interrupts the other parent, the therapist, if the alliance is solid, might say: "Let's see how the conversation progresses if Lois (the mother), you let your daughter and her father talk this through without you providing input." If the mother stays out of the conversation and the father and daughter communicate better, the therapist has part of a solution sequence on which to build. If the mother continues to interrupt, a constraint question is warranted: "I wonder what keeps you from being able to let your husband and daughter sort this out themselves?"

In the case of individual therapy, the enactment might occur between therapist and client or even between the client and a part of themselves. The latter could involve an empty chair exercise in which the client addresses a part of themselves that is imagined to be in the empty chair. This can also involve the client moving to the other chair to answer back from the part. This is an example of a skill a therapist can learn and incorporate into their practice. The point here is that role-playing with a therapist or talking with a part of self can produce significant new patterns that comprise an effective solution sequence the client can utilize in their lives outside of the session.

When an in-session enactment evolves into a solution sequence, it is important to allow time in the session to discuss the change that has taken place and to compliment everyone for their participation. For example, in the enactment described above, the therapist might say: "Great work. We see that father and daughter can successfully discuss an issue. And Lois, you were able to trust them to have a good discussion." The therapist will often extend the solution sequence to a between-session experiment in which the clients practice what they accomplished in the session. The main intent here is to generalize the solution sequence to the natural environment of the home. This can help build confidence in the therapeutic process and strengthen the therapeutic alliance.

Cultural Considerations

Cultural factors may influence the range of solution sequences that are appropriate for the clients that seek therapy. Historically, some therapy models made generalized and overarching normative assumptions about mental health and relationships that did not account for clients' varying experiences and cultural backgrounds. One of the advantages of IST is that it is not based on normative assumptions about health. Rather, it is based on collaborating with clients to solve the issues for which they come to therapy. For example, a common mental health value in the United States is for people to access and express their primary emotions. The therapist who is thinking of incorporating this as a part of a solution sequence will need to determine whether this is a fitting strategy for a client who is from another cultural background.

Therapists can also make the mistake of incorporating a simplistic understanding of the client's culture into a solution sequence. For example, a therapist hypothesizing about a client's pattern of isolation and loneliness may propose a sequence based on a fixed idea about their culture.

Therapist: I have met many people from your cultural background and one thing I have found to be true among them has been that they have strong ties to their families. What would you think about spending more time at your mother's house since she lives so close? This way neither of you would be alone as much.

Such a proposal should not be made on the basis of the therapist's assumptions about a cultural context. It would only be suggested if it fits with a set of shared understandings that have been carefully developed between the therapist and client. Therapists must take a more exploratory approach to culture such that they neither make assumptions about it nor dismiss its importance.

Assumptions about cultural contexts can lead the therapist to introduce a solution sequence that is unfitting and even triggering for the clients. This exchange, in turn, can lead to the rupture of the therapeutic alliance (Watson & Greenberg, 2000), without which even the best solution sequence will not be successful. It is critical for therapists to be cognizant of the emotional toll that a rupture in the alliance can have. It can lead to a client needing to explain to yet another person the impact of being misunderstood and othered.

Client-Therapist Differences

For an IST therapist, considering culture in identifying solution sequences begins with the acknowledgment of the importance of person-of-the-therapist (Aponte & Kissil, 2016) training in IST (Pinsof et al., 2018; Hardy & Bobes, 2017; He et al., 2021), which includes a focus on developing the facility to recognize and acknowledge the differences that exist between therapists and their clients. Acknowledging and conversing about differences facilitate the search for solutions that fit the client system. A generalized example of how to state the importance of difference in the search for solution sequences follows:

Therapist: I'm glad that you feel that I have a good understanding about the problem you bring to therapy. I think that's a good start. The next step is to begin to think about solutions. I acknowledge and respect that my clients' traditions and backgrounds are different than mine because I don't want to assume that what might occur to me as a solution will necessarily fit for you. So, as we work together to identify solutions, let's make sure we make room to talk about how your values, background and current-day experience impact the solutions we select. I'm interested in any thoughts you have about this.

This type of statement is worth making to any client system that is encountered, as there is always difference, even when there is a set of similarities (e.g., white therapist and white client, both cisgender, straight, and 30-something in age). Directly addressing specific differences between therapist and client (e.g., race, ethnicity, gender identity, sexual orientation, ability/disability) is another important step that will inform the search for solutions and support the alliance. Care should be taken not to underestimate or overestimate the importance of the difference as either can be insulting or embarrassing for the client. It is the meaning of the difference for the client that matters.

The alliance depends on the client having the feeling that their views and experiences matter to the therapist and matter in the problem-solving process. Additionally, addressing differences can reduce the clients' hesitancy to talk about problems or solutions that seem to carry implications for the therapist by virtue of the therapist's membership in a cultural context. For example, by inviting a client to consider her thoughts about the impact of the therapist's disability on the therapy, the therapist was able to help the client communicate her discomfort in describing a problem sequence related to her body dysmorphic issues in the presence of a therapist who uses a wheelchair.

In another example, a daughter's resentment of her mother constrained the search for a solution sequence. The therapist wondered about the place of racial and ethnic differences in the therapy system and decided to explicitly address the differences between her ethnicity and race and that of the mother and daughter. The discussion that followed led to the daughter admitting that she resented her mother for making comments throughout her life about her skin color being darker than others in the family. After further exploration of how the issue of colorism had influenced her feelings about her mother, the daughter revealed that she had been hesitant to talk about it in therapy because the therapist seemed to be darker-skinned, and the daughter did not want to raise the issue due to fears of offending the therapist. As a result of this conversation, an essential source of resentment was discovered and subsequently worked through such that the mother and daughter were able to improve their communication and the daughter reported becoming progressively more confident in her own identity and place in the family.

Client-Therapist Similarities

A perceived similarity between the therapist and the client system sometimes leads to an assumption of sameness. If the therapist and the client system share membership in a cultural context or are from similar ethnic backgrounds, both the therapist and the client system may be at risk for assumptions that constrain the exploration of possible solution sequences. In one instance, a young cisgender, straight man sought therapy with a therapist who was from the same ethnic background. The client felt ashamed to talk about his sexual problems with the therapist due to the topic of sex being taboo in their shared cultural background. Given this, the therapy did not address the client's sexual concern, and thus the problem and solution sequences identified were unrelated to one of the client's most pressing issues. It is important for therapists to explicitly point out that while they may have similar cultural backgrounds, some of their experiences may be very different. This sets the expectation early on that both therapist and client may bring different and valuable ideas to the table.

Therapeutic Alliance

The therapist needs to solicit and monitor client feedback on whether there is an alliance with respect to the goals and specific tasks of therapy. Alliance on these dimensions will help develop and strengthen the third dimension of the alliance, the bonds. The therapist strengthens the alliance by soliciting and respecting the client system's views of possible solutions and monitoring their readiness to accept and implement a solution sequence proposed by the therapist. Thus, the questions that therapists ask themselves at this step of the essence (identifying solution sequences) are crucial to the alliance and the course of therapy: What tone am I taking? How is the tone being interpreted? Do the clients agree with the description of the problem sequence? Is the suggested solution sequence fitting with the client systems' cultural and contextual factors? Are the clients on board with it? Am I rushing them? These types of questions are considered in relation to feedback that includes verbal and nonverbal responses of clients. When in doubt—and doubt is encouraged here—the therapist can ask a client for feedback with the intent that it can be used to protect the alliance and thereby enhance the probability that solutions can be agreed upon and tried.

Case Example

The following case example illustrates how the solution sequence serves as a device for anchoring and tracking the progress of therapy. It demonstrates how IST affords a wide range of strategies and interventions to make the solution sequence work. The example also illustrates the key role of the hypothesizing and planning metaframeworks in creating effective solution sequences.

Gloria, a 24-year-old, cisgender, straight Columbian woman, came to the United States with her mother, Maria, when she was four years old. Maria had fled an abusive marriage and an unsupportive family of origin.

In the United States, Maria became a successful businessperson and at the peak of her career owned three businesses. She never remarried. By the time Gloria was in middle school, Maria moved the family to a suburb with the idea of providing Gloria with a good education. Gloria graduated with a degree in political science and was in a graduate program at the time she entered therapy.

The precipitant for therapy for Gloria was the onset of a major depression accompanied by a suicide attempt and a brief hospitalization followed by two weeks in a partial hospitalization program. When she was discharged from the hospital, she was prescribed an antidepressant medication that she continued to take. Gloria reported that both programs were traumatizing and unhelpful and she vowed not to repeat them. She was referred to outpatient therapy with a woman therapist of Brazilian descent who practiced IST. When the therapist first met with Gloria, they worked on a written contract regarding Gloria's continued suicidal ideation. The therapist believed the risks of suicide were manageable with the contract and twice-weekly outpatient therapy.

Gloria was still enrolled in her graduate program when she started therapy, but needed to decide whether to make up the work lost during her hospitalization, drop out, or take Family Medical Leave. With the help of her therapist, she elected the latter; hence, she stopped attending classes. The therapist identified her routine at home, an S2 sequence, to be one of the prominent problem sequences. Once she no longer attended classes, she stayed at home and became increasingly reclusive. She admitted to daily suicidal ideation without a plan or intent and spoke to no one including her mother, with whom she reported she had a poor relationship.

The therapist hypothesized that Gloria's sequences of rumination and immobilization exacerbated her depression; therefore, using the action planning metaframework, the strategy of behavioral activation was chosen. The therapist briefly summarized the research on behavioral activation and framed the solution sequence of activation as an experiment. Gloria agreed to work on simple tasks such as taking a shower, cleaning her room and preparing a meal. She also agreed to walking, which was an activity she had enjoyed in the past. Gloria enacted the solution sequences and soon reported feeling a bit less depressed but still had recurring suicidal ideation without intent.

One persistent complaint was the relationship between Gloria and Maria. Gloria found it frustrating to talk with her mother as she did not feel her mother could carry on a conversation on topics that interested Gloria. Further, Gloria said that her mother always pushes her to do more than she can do. The therapist proposed that Maria join them for a session to discuss how the two women could improve their relationship. Bringing Maria into the direct client system and improving communication might reduce Gloria's isolation and help her depression. The therapist was surprised when Gloria said she didn't want to meet with her mother. The therapist pressed gently, but Gloria was adamant; consequently, the therapist evoked the alliance priority guideline and backed off. Instead, she asked Gloria for permission to call Maria. Gloria agreed and provided formal written permission for the call to occur.

When the therapist and Maria talked, they connected around their shared heritage with South America. The mother worried about Gloria, but clearly did not fully grasp the severity of her depression nor the risk associated with her suicidal ideation. Maria thought Gloria had made a mistake in dropping out of her graduate program. She admitted that when she did see Gloria, she persistently pushed her to do things. The therapist hypothesized that the mother's belief system that led her to push Gloria to do things made Gloria feel guilty about her level of productivity. The therapist used the meaning/emotion planning metaframework and chose the strategy of altering beliefs in the hope that Maria would back off and stop making statements that resulted in Gloria feeling guilty. To alter beliefs, the therapist chose the intervention of externalizing the problem of depression. The therapist carefully discussed the power of depression to sap the energy of a person and stressed that Gloria's behavior was not a sign of weakness or laziness. The therapist stressed that Maria could best help Gloria manage depression by honoring her current, limited capacity to do things. Maria agreed to try this solution sequence.

As Maria backed off from pushing Gloria to do things, Gloria reported being more interested in talking with her mother. Gloria began to discuss how she was becoming increasingly ambivalent about her chosen field of political science. The therapist realized that the one activity that might have ended Gloria's reclusiveness—going back to study—was now threatened, so the therapist decided to explore the constraints that had emerged that kept Gloria from wanting to become a political scientist. The exploration then turned to what career alternatives might exist. Gloria had few interests. The therapist suggested that some testing might provide information. A basic occupational inventory served as a good starting point. Gloria appreciated the results, but they did not open any obvious directions. The therapist continued to track Gloria's suicidality and used a progress instrument to gain additional feedback. Gloria's scoring on relevant items pertaining to depression and suicidality had significantly improved.

In one session, the therapist mentioned having gotten a puppy. Gloria asked many questions about the puppy and reminisced about once having a dog. In the next session, Gloria started talking about getting a dog. Using the mind metaframework (M3), the therapist hypothesized that Gloria had developed a twinning transference with her (Kohut, 1984), which suggested a deepening of the alliance. Although the therapist was not practicing Kohut's self-psychology with Gloria, she did recognize that twinning was an experience that allowed the client to feel understood and valued.

Gloria's interest in getting a dog increased. The therapist wondered if getting and caring for a dog might be an additional solution sequence for Gloria. The conversation shifted to discussing the process of obtaining a dog. Gloria was becoming very motivated. She obtained permission from her condominium board to have a therapy animal. Maria was equally excited, and they began to have daily conversations about a dog. The idea of a dog also brought Gloria a new perspective on her life. She said: "If I commit to a dog, I have to commit to be there for it, so I guess I have to let go of suicide as a solution to my depression." Her scores on the progress instrument went into the normal range and she reported adopting a future orientation to life for the first time in a long time. Eventually, Gloria found the dog of her choosing and devoted herself to being an excellent owner. Her depression lifted. She left the field of political science, obtained a job, and began to explore with energy and excitement the direction she would take in life.

This case example illustrates how the quest for solution sequences is tied to reading client feedback and adapting therapy to the needs of the client. The example of getting the dog illustrates how serendipity is often involved in producing change. The therapist's openness to these moments is made possible by the integrative and systemic nature of IST, something that is often not possible with a rigid adherence to one model of therapy.

Conclusion

Identifying a solution sequence is a key step in the problem-solving process. The construction of a solution sequence is designed to address the carefully identified problem sequence and provides a vector for the therapy that will lead to improvement in the problem or an opportunity to learn more about what factors in the system constrain problem-solving. With this win-win approach in mind, IST therapists frequently refer to the solution as an experiment. The solution sequence may be proposed by the clients or by the therapist. It may be based on common sense or an established therapeutic intervention. It may primarily involve a change in what people do or it may have a significant cognitive or emotional component. It is important that the clients feel the solution fits for them and that they do not feel pressured, judged, or shamed by its proposal. In formulating a solution sequence, the therapist in concert with the clients will need to consider the client's cultural background, intersectionality, and any social justice issues that may pertain.

Exercise

Identifying a solution sequence: Case illustration and questions to consider

Nima is a 16-year-old cisgender male, who identifies as biracial and lives in a suburban neighborhood with his parents and two older brothers. He was admitted for the second time in 16 months to a partial hospitalization program for symptoms of depression and anxiety. Nima admitted himself to the hospital because he was afraid of the suicidal thoughts (with plans) that he was having which led him to ask for help. His parents adhered to his request and brought him to the hospital. He was hospitalized for one week and discharged with a plan for outpatient therapy.

The referral for outpatient therapy came with significant background information on Nima and his family. He is described as the "good child," showing little conflict with other members of his family. Nima grew up in a family where his father's alcoholism played a significant role within the family. As a result of the alcoholism, his parents divorced when Nima was three years old, and neither his mother, an African American woman, nor his father, an Armenian immigrant, ever remarried. Although Nima's father was not part of his ongoing daily life until the age of ten, Nima reports having a close relationship with his father and denies holding him at fault for his absence during the early part of his development. The family (which included Nima and his two brothers, mother, maternal grandmother, and maternal grandfather) all lived together. Nima indicated his maternal grandfather had played the role of his father but passed away two years ago. Since then, Nima's parents reconciled and the father, now sober, has moved back into the home. Although he has reported having a good relationship with his parents, Nima has expressed that within the last year his relationship with both of his parents seemed more distant, and he admits to keeping more to himself with fewer interactions with his family than previously experienced.

Within the social and educational domains, Nima finds himself struggling and feeling discouraged, as evidenced by his withdrawal from friends, ending a one-year relationship, and failing several of his Junior-year classes. Nima also reported a spinal cord injury several years ago which led to having to take pain medication for a month following surgery. Although Nima has the mobility to complete daily tasks, the injury kept him from participating in high school sports in which he had previously shown interest. Nima's parents present with the concern that Nima is isolated and inactive, and they do not know how to help him or connect with him. They are very concerned about his suicidal thoughts, though he has provided them (and hospital staff) with reassurance about his safety. Nima indicates a strong desire to understand himself better and a willingness to adhere to treatment, however, he does not identify specifically what he wants to work on in therapy.

Now that you have been introduced to Nima, consider (or discuss) the following.

1　Who would you convene for therapy? Why?
2　What is your initial hypothesis about a problem sequence in Nima's current situation? List some initial questions you would ask to clarify the problem sequence. Consider what you need to ask to clarify a problem sequence.
3　How will you converse with the client system about cultural or contextual factors that may influence the choice of solution sequences? Write down some questions you might ask.
4　What strategies for a solution sequence come to mind for this case? Pick one and formulate how you will present it.
5　How do you feel when you think about working with this case? How might your internal reactions (person-of-the-therapist factors) influence your inclination to move forward or refrain from introducing a solution sequence?

References

Aponte, H. J., & Kissil, K. (Eds.) (2016). *The person of the therapist training model: Mastering the use of self*. Routledge.

Churven, P. (1988). Marital therapy my way: Creating a workable reality. *Australian and New Zealand Journal of Family Therapy*, 9(4), 223–225. 10.1002/j.1467-8438.1988.tb01269.x

Goldman, R., & Greenberg, L. (2015). *Case formulation in emotion-focused therapy: co-creating clinical maps for change* (Ist ed.). American Psychological Association.

Greenberg, L. S. (2011). *Emotion-focused therapy: Theory and practice*. American Psychological Association.

Greenberg, L. S., & Safran J. D. (1989). Emotion in psychotherapy. *American Psychologist*, 44(1), 19–29.

Hardy, K. V., & Bobes, T. (Eds.). (2017). *Promoting cultural sensitivity in supervision: A manual for practitioners*. Routledge.

He, Y., Hardy, N., & Russell, W. P. (2021). Integrative systemic supervision: Promoting supervisees' theoretical integration in systemic therapy. *Family Process*, 61, 58–75. https://doi.org/10.1111/famp.12667

Johnson, S. M. (2015). Emotionally focused couple therapy. In A. Gurman, J. Lebow, & D. K. Snyder (Eds.), *Clinical handbook of couple therapy* (5th ed., pp. 97–128). Guilford.

Kanter, J., Manos, R., Bowe, W., Baruch, D., Busch, A., & Rusch, L. (2010). What is behavioral activation? A review of the empirical literature. *Clinical Psychology Review*, 30(6), 608–620. 10.1016/j.cpr.2010.04.001

Kohut, H. (1984). *How does analysis cure?* The University of Chicago Press. 10.72 08/chicago/9780226006147.001.0001

Minuchin, S., & Fishman, H. C. (1981). *Family therapy techniques.* Harvard University Press.

Nichols, M. P., & Colapinto, J. (2017). Enactment in structural family therapy. In J. L. Lebow, A. L. Chambers, & D. C. Breunlin (Eds.), *Encyclopedia of couple and family therapy.* Springer. 10.1007/978-3-319-15877-8_969-1

Pinsof, W., Breunlin, D., Russell, W., Lebow, J., Rampage, C., & Chambers, A. (2018). *Integrative systemic therapy: Metaframeworks for problem solving with individuals, couples, and families* (1st ed.). American Psychological Association. 10.1037/0000055-000

Watson, J. C., & Greenberg, L. S. (2000). Alliance ruptures and repairs. *Journal of Clinical Psychology, 56,* 175–186.

Chapter 6

Implementing a Solution Sequence

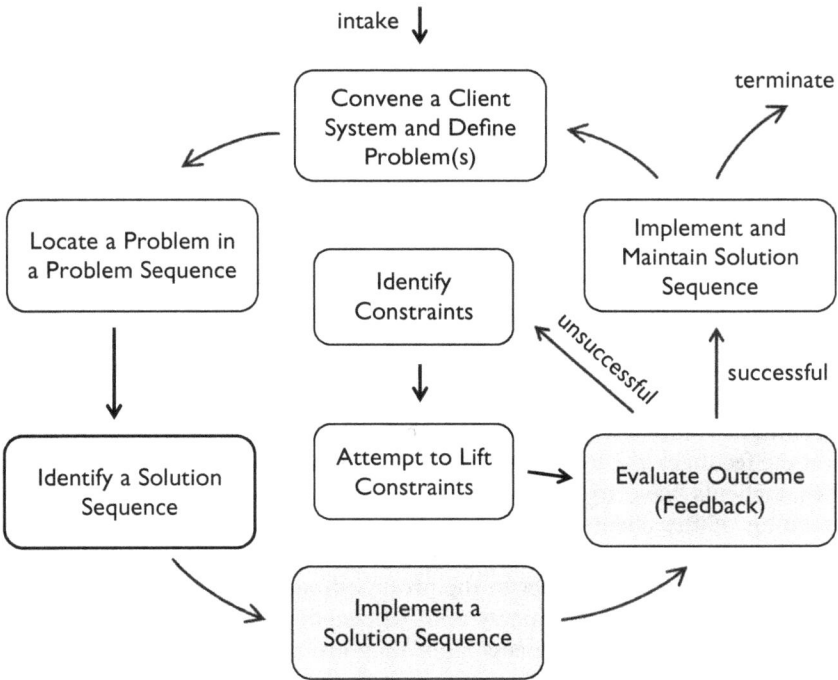

intake ↓

Convene a Client System and Define Problem(s)

terminate

Locate a Problem in a Problem Sequence

Implement and Maintain Solution Sequence

Identify Constraints

unsuccessful

successful

Identify a Solution Sequence

Attempt to Lift Constraints

Evaluate Outcome (Feedback)

Implement a Solution Sequence

IST Essence Diagram.

Objective

This chapter will discuss the four components of solution implementation. To successfully implement a solution sequence, therapists must collaborate with clients to establish a shared understanding of their readiness to try a solution and, if they are inclined to try it, consolidate the plan, establish their commitment to it, and review the results of their

DOI: 10.4324/9780429322273-6

attempts at it. Solution sequences are typically described as experiments for clients to try. Experiments with new sequences when successfully enacted can produce movement toward problem resolution. When the experiment is not attempted, or when the clients have difficulty sustaining their effort or maintaining the solution, then the therapist and clients can learn from the experiment as they explore the factors that constrained its performance.

Introduction

The principles discussed in this chapter can be applied to both in-session and between-session experiments with solution sequences. In-session experiments (enactments), discussed in Chapter 5 can often be initiated less formally. The therapist provides an explanation for what is to be done and why and solicits an agreement from the clients that they will try it. The preparation for an in-session experiment is less intensive because the therapist is present to guide the process. If a client system conveys ambivalence or resistance to an in-session experiment, however, the therapist is wise to take more time to carefully discuss the purpose of the experiment and its specific requirements and explore the clients' readiness for it and their commitment to do it.

Following an in-session experiment, the therapist follows up on what it was like for the clients and may ask questions about what it means to them to have done it. In-session experiments can also be the basis for the suggestion that the clients "try this at home." In other words, the therapist can discuss with the clients whether they would be open to trying the solution sequence during the time between sessions. Depending on the feedback the therapist observes from the enactment itself and from what clients have to say about it afterward, as well as the therapist's reading of the clients' comfort with the idea of trying it at home, the therapist will decide how much time to spend on readiness and commitment issues with respect to the proposed between-session experiment.

Between-session experiments tend to benefit from a fuller articulation of the implementation process since they are not guided directly by the therapist in session. The description of methodology in the method section of this chapter is the more fully articulated version. Implementation of a solution sequence consists of four components: *Readiness, refinement, commitment,* and *follow-up.* The therapist needs to assess client readiness to do the experiment, refine the experiment with client feedback, solicit a commitment from the client to do it, and follow up in the next session on both the clients' level of success in doing the experiment and the impact of it.

Method

Readiness

To accept suggestions or implement solutions, clients need to achieve a level of readiness. Therapists often wonder if clients are sufficiently motivated to put significant effort into the therapy. In IST it is preferable, especially in the early phases of therapy, to wonder less about an overall assessment of whether the clients want to work hard in therapy or are ready to make a meaningful change, and more about whether clients are ready and willing to work on specific problems and experiment with specific solution sequences. In this way, the therapist meets clients where they are at and encourages them to consider the prospect of experiments that may impact the specific issues they bring to therapy. Admittedly, some of these issues may involve major life changes, but IST begins with more targeted experimentation.

For example, James and Grace, a white, cisgender, heterosexual couple in their 50s with two independent adult children, presented with concerns about their conflict. In the second session, the couple and therapist defined a problem sequence that involved James stopping with friends for drinks after work/Grace complaining about it when he arrived home/ James arguing back or withdrawing/Grace feeling helpless and frustrated. Rather than feeling the immediate need to determine whether James is an alcoholic or assessing how willing he is to come to terms with his drinking, the therapist explores the place of the drinking in the problem sequence. This involves asking James about the nature of his drinking, as well as what he intends to do about Grace's concerns. In this case, the conversation led James to agree that the drinking was an issue in the relationship, but he affirmed that he did not have concerns about his drinking and did not intend to quit. Grace shared that her father was an alcoholic and that, in her view, James would eventually need to achieve abstinence. They agreed that finding a new pattern for the drinking sequence that they could both live with for now would help them in their relationship. The therapist helped the couple negotiate an experiment that involved Grace accepting that James would stop after work with friends for a drink once per week. They agreed that he would do so as per agreement with Grace, he would drink moderately, and Grace would not criticize him if he stayed within those bounds.

Readiness for this solution sequence was enhanced by three factors. First, what they agreed to do was related to what brought them to therapy. Second, the therapist did not ask them to do something they were not ready to do. Third, rather than having to be ready for a permanent commitment, they just had to be ready to perform the experiment until the next session. In the Transtheoretical Model of Change

(Prochaska & DiClemente, 1984), the stage of contemplating change precedes making the change (preparation and action stages). The couple was contemplating how to modify patterns in their relationship, but James was clearly not contemplating abstinence at that time. Later in the therapy, if the drinking continued to constrain the relational patterns, the therapist could use motivational interviewing (Miller & Rollnick, 2012) to invite James to move into the contemplation stage and begin to look at his drinking in a different light.

Enhancing readiness can begin with earlier steps in the essence diagram, such as locating the problem in a problem sequence and identifying a solution sequence. Being careful to fully define the problem sequence often enhances readiness and motivation as clients gain awareness and acceptance that what they are doing clearly is not working for them. The therapist takes a curious, non-judgmental stance with respect for how clients are trying to manage or solve the problem (Therapist: "I see what you are saying. Can you tell me more about how you respond to these situations?"). Often, as their hard work and intentions are clarified, so is the fact that what they are doing is not working (Therapist: "I see how hard you are working to improve this situation." and "I hear you saying that you don't feel that what you are doing is working as well as you would like it to."). In such cases, clients can begin to look objectively at current patterns and begin to experience themselves as ready to try something new (Therapist: "Would you be open to talking about other options for managing this?"). Once this shift in client experience occurs, the therapist and clients can discuss solution sequences. As the therapy moves to the task of implementing a solution sequence, the therapist has the prior work to draw on (Therapist: "I remember you saying that you very much wanted to find a new way forward with this. Do you feel ready to try this way forward?").

Once a solution sequence is discussed, a variety of questions can be asked to assess and possibly enhance readiness to try the solution sequence. For example, "On a 1–10 scale, how ready do you feel to try this?" or "What do you think it will be like to try this?" In this way, the therapist invites the clients to imagine doing the experiment in their real lives and not just think about it abstractly. It also communicates clearly to clients that the therapist understands that the things they agree to do will need to fit for them and their circumstances.

In family therapy, sometimes a family member will not seem committed to a solution sequence. The therapist needs to acknowledge this ambivalence and ask the client about their concerns. Examples of statements or questions the therapist can pose include: "I am not sure you are on board with this suggestion." Or "I would be interested in hearing your concerns about this." Or "It may be that we are missing something important here. Are you concerned about what will happen if you try this?"

Or "I think it is important to hear more about what you want to see happen." If an agreement is not reached among all members, and the parental subsystem wants to forge ahead, the therapist can ask what the impact on each member will be to have one or more members not be on board. The therapist can also raise the possibility of limiting an ambivalent person's role in the experiment to see if an agreement can be reached in that way. Sometimes in family therapy, especially with families with young children, the parents (or parent) will need to decide about a course of action whether or not a child is fully on board.

The therapist is also wise to ask clients if they think there is anything that will keep them from performing the experiment. The therapist can ask, "As you think about doing this, do you think there is anything that would get in your way?" In this way, constraining factors can be identified and planned for in advance of implementation. Another dimension to explore is whether the clients see a risk of a negative consequence. Especially when the therapist senses resistance or ambivalence about the solution, the therapist can ask something like, "Do you see any risks or downsides to trying this?" Or "Do you think anything stressful or hurtful could come from trying the experiment?" As with inquiry about any step in the essence diagram, questions can be formulated to address the perceived relational impact of what is being proposed. Given a level of task-ambivalence in a family context, a more extensive round of questions can help the family members address whether they anticipate that the proposed solution would have an impact on any of the other members or their relationships. These circular questions were formulated and classified by Tomm (1985, 1987) and provide an important supplemental learning opportunity for an IST therapist.

A final element of readiness is addressed by the win-win nature of experimenting with solution sequences. The therapist and clients win if the solution improves things, and they win if it does not. The therapist might say something like, "Remember, this is a win-win situation. We will learn something about what it will take to get where you want to go whether or not this experiment accomplishes what we intend." Maintaining the language of experimenting in addressing readiness carries a what-do-you-have-to-lose implication. Further, it can reduce the sense of shame clients anticipate feeling if they are not successful with the solution sequence. The reduced risk of feeling ashamed may, in turn, support readiness.

Refinement

For many solution sequences, it is important to be specific about who is agreeing to do what and when. This means that as the therapist establishes a shared readiness with the clients to do the experiment, it is important to discuss and negotiate the details about how it will work. For example, in the case of James and Grace, it would not be sufficient to conclude the conversation with the idea that James would not stop at the bar as often. Rather, it is preferred to establish what each party will do differently. The therapist might say, "Let's talk a bit more about how this will work." Or, "I think we have a general idea of what you will be doing, so let's talk more specifically about how this will actually play out."

In the case of James and Grace, the therapist can ask specific questions about who will do what and when. "Let's talk about what you will be expecting of each other and yourselves as you try this experiment over the next week." The therapist can also ask them to talk to each other about this by saying, "Talk together about how this is going to work this week." Using a variety of questions and statements, the therapist can prompt for specifics. "As this is an experiment, what can you live with, Grace, in terms of how often James stops at the bar and how long James should be delayed in getting home?" "James, can you live with stopping once per week for a couple of hours?" "James, you feel strongly that you can manage your drinking. How long would you propose to stay at the bar and about how much would you anticipate drinking?" "Let's talk about your needs in terms of communication about these events. Do you agree that the days be specified in advance?" "Grace, what do you feel should happen when James returns?" The therapist can also make recommendations. "I think it would be a good idea not to discuss your relationship or the success or failure of the experiment on an evening when James stops at the bar. What do you think of that idea?"

Developing specificity about what is expected is helpful in three ways. First, the clients know exactly what they are going to try to do and can focus on that. Second, it increases the likelihood of success as certain issues have been anticipated and negotiated. Third, it brings difficulties in the implementation of the plan into sharper focus and facilitates later discussion of where things went off course and, importantly, what circumstances, actions, thinking or emotions may have constrained the clients. With Grace and James, the specificity in expectations will allow for an accumulation of shared observations of James' success or failure in managing his drinking. The outcomes will be there for all to see. The need for abstinence or treatment of the drinking problem can be assessed by whether a person can sufficiently control their drinking.

Sometimes a general idea for a solution sequence is agreed upon near the end of a session. In such a case the therapist and clients need to agree to either try it or wait until the next session to further clarify the task. If the therapist hypothesizes that the lack of specificity for the experiment may risk unnecessary frustration or disappointment, then the therapist can ask the clients not to try it yet. For example, "I am sorry to say that we are running out of time today. I think we are on a good track, but I don't recommend you try this yet. Let's talk next week and get more specific about how this will work. Is that okay with you?" Other times, the solution sequence seems uncomplicated, and the clients are ready to try it. In such cases, it can be worthwhile to encourage them to enact the plan. For example, a couple decides they want to establish a date night and does not feel there are any risks associated with it. The therapist can say something like, "It seems like you agree and feel ready to do this. I hope you enjoy it. I look forward to following up with you."

Some solution sequences require significant preparation and refinement. For example, when Grace and James are discussing James' drinking or other issues they disagree on, they often get into a pattern of escalating conflict. The therapist introduces the idea that they would benefit from taking a time-out when conversations become too conflictual and that they calm themselves before resuming the conversation. With the initial agreement of the couple, the therapist selects an established time-out procedure to address the problem sequence of their conflict. This procedure is of sufficient complexity to require that the couple be taught what to do, practice it, and anticipate challenges they may have with it. Further, the time-out intervention needs to be tailored to their life situation. For example, how will they know to ask for a time-out? What will they notice that they feel in themselves or see in the other person that will be the measure of when to implement the time-out? Guided by the therapist, the couple needs to agree on how long a time-out will last, what they need to do during it, and what mindset they need to bring when the conversation resumes. It can take the better part of an entire session to work through the details of this procedure, but if it can interrupt damaging conflict sequences, it is well worth the investment of time.

Commitment

Given a level of readiness and a further refinement of what is involved with a solution sequence, the therapist next addresses the issue of commitment. "Okay, I think we are pretty clear on what each of you will be doing. Do you both feel ready?" Also, it is often helpful to ask something like, "Do you have any last-minute questions or reservations about doing this?" If there is a question or reservation, it is better to learn about it and address it before they experiment with the solution sequence. If they do not ask questions or share a reservation, this may indicate that the clients are deepening their commitment. It is important to address reservations because as the task has become more refined, the clients may begin to feel differently about it. For example, the general idea of a time-out is not the same as the actual procedure for a time-out. The specificity might make it seem more real or suggest a downside of adopting the procedure (e.g., "I can't wait that long to talk about these things. I'm afraid that if we stop talking, we will never get to the bottom of the issue."). In continued service to the therapeutic alliance, it is important to acknowledge such feelings and offer reassurance that they will be addressed. It is helpful to remind clients that they are not expected to adopt the solution sequence permanently. Rather, they are agreeing to experiment with it until the next session. The therapist can say something like, "Remember that this is just until the next session and it is win-win in that we either find that this experiment works, or we learn more about something we need to know to find what works."

The therapist discovered a reservation in the case of Grace and James. As the therapist discussed with James the parameters of his plan to spend time at the bar after work, Grace seemed to stiffen in her chair. The therapist asked if the conversation was having an impact on her. Grace shared her worry that James would take the designated weekly stop at the bar as a license to get drunk. The therapist honored Grace's fears and asked James to respond. James was initially defensive, but with the encouragement of the therapist was able to see this less as a criticism and more as a reasonable fear for which he could offer help. He agreed to not over-drink and to arrange a ride-share home. The therapist emphasized that this was a first step toward finding a pattern they could both accept.

Follow up

The purposes of the follow-up are to maintain the focus of therapy, establish a sense of accountability, and ascertain the outcome of the experiment. The outcome of the experiment is feedback for the therapist that suggests whether to continue the direction of the experiment, identify what prevented the clients from performing it, or begin to reconceptualize the solution sequence.

In the session following the one in which clients commit to trying a solution sequence, the therapist asks about it. "Tell me, how did the experiment go?" or "Did you have a chance to try the experiment we talked about last week?" This typically would occur early in the session, but sometimes events have occurred that the clients need to address prior to the follow-up. When this is the case, the therapist will need to be careful to allow time for the follow-up. Occasionally, much of the session will be taken up with an urgent matter. In such a case, the therapist can acknowledge that they will discuss the experiment during the next session. The therapist's focus on the solution sequence conveys that there is continuity from session to session and reinforces the idea that some of the work is done between sessions.

Throughout the follow-up, it is essential that the therapist maintain a curious, nonjudgmental stance. People ordinarily are sensitive about whether they did well enough with the experiment, and the therapeutic alliance can be damaged if the therapist comes across as judgmental or harsh in tone. This is especially true early in therapy before the alliance has formed, or with clients who are particularly sensitive to judgment or vulnerable to strong feelings of shame. For these reasons, the therapist is respectfully curious when it comes to the experience the clients had with the experiment. What it was like for them is an important source of feedback. The therapist might ask, "What was it like to do this experiment?" This question explores the experience the clients had with the experiment, which may need to be addressed in order to move forward with the alliance and problem-solving. If they found the solution experiment frustrating, or if they feel ashamed about not doing it, their emotions may color their view of therapy. The nature of the clients' experience with the experiment can be explored before or after a more careful review of what the clients actually did and what came of it.

If clients felt good or encouraged by the experiment, this would be a green light for continuing their efforts. The therapist might ask, "Do you feel it is worth continuing this experiment?" If they say "yes," then there can be a discussion about whether it can be improved upon in some way. If clients continue the experiment week to week, and it continues to be effective, then the therapist leads a discussion about whether the problem has been addressed sufficiently in which case they may be moving toward termination or on to another problem.

Clients sometimes report that they did not try the experiment. Or, they may report trying it but not continuing with it. In these cases, the therapist does not know if the experiment would be helpful or not, nor can the therapist assume that the clients were resistant. As a part of gathering feedback on their experience, the therapist can ask if there seemed to be something wrong with the plan for the experiment. "When we talked about doing this, we might have missed something. Do you think that the plan was not right for you in some way?" or "I (we) could be off base with this experiment. What do you think?" The therapist can also ask if the plan poses a risk or could have unwanted effects for the clients or others that need to be considered: "I was wondering if you felt the plan could cause a problem for you or anyone else in the family." An example of this is a depressed man who agrees with the need to exercise to improve his mood but worries that doing so would reduce his time with his family.

Sometimes clients report that they did not fully understand the plan. In such cases, the therapist takes responsibility for not being clear. The therapist can say something like, "My mistake, I did not describe the experiment carefully enough. Are you open to giving this another try? I can explain it better." In some cases, clients may have internalized the experiment as an idea or a suggestion and not necessarily something they were committing to try. This is a sign for the therapist to more explicitly address the commitment phase of the experiment. Client resistance need not be interpreted until or unless the failure to do the experiment shows itself to be a pattern. There are many reasons that clients do not do experiments between sessions. The therapist seeks to understand this from the clients' perspective.

In describing the implementation of the experiment (solution sequence), many clients will give less detail than the therapist needs. In most cases, therefore, the therapist will want to explore exactly what was done and compare that to the established plan. The therapist might say something like, "I appreciate that you took this task on. I think it will be helpful for me to understand in detail exactly what happened. Can I ask you some questions about it?" The therapist will want to track whether the clients did the experiment when it was called for (by schedule or circumstance), the extent to which the clients did what was expected at those times, and what resulted from the attempts. Example questions include: "So, tell me how often you tried it?" "How would you describe exactly what you did?" "Were you able to continue the experiment at other times?"

In the case of James and Grace, the solution sequence of a once-weekly, safe visit to the bar after work was agreed upon. Part of the decision was that within the parameters established for the week, James would communicate directly and truthfully, negotiate the day he would stop at the bar, utilize a ride-share, and drink moderately. Grace agreed not to register concerns about James' drinking. Two weeks later, during their next session, the therapist asked, "So, how did the experiment go?" Grace replied, "Not so well" and looked at James. James sheepishly stated, "I F-ed up. I did it right the first week, but not this last week." He went on to say that he had stopped at the bar twice that week. The therapist stated, "I am interested in what this experiment was like for each of you." Grace shared that she felt betrayed and was concerned that James could not control his drinking. James shared that he felt "bad" but did not think it was as "big a deal" as Grace did. The therapist stated that the experiment was already bringing information that would be useful in the therapy. The therapist planned to explore what kept James from fulfilling the terms of the experiment (constraint identification), but first, it was important to understand in detail what had occurred.

The therapist asked a series of questions. "So, let's look at the first week first." The therapist asked a series of questions: "Tell me how you came to agree on the day that the visit to the bar would occur." "How late did you stay at the bar, James?" "Did you feel impaired?" "Grace, how were you feeling when James was at the bar?" "Did the two of you discuss the drinking when you returned home?" "How did you get along together the next day?" "Did this pattern feel workable to you, Grace? "How about you, James?" It was established that despite some initial anxiety for

Grace, this pattern seemed workable to both of them. Comparable questions were asked about the second week which revealed that James did have some concern about how much he drank on one occasion. The therapist acknowledged the feelings they expressed, including how difficult this was for Grace and that it was painful for James to see the impact of his actions on her. The next step would be to explore what constrained James from fully following through with his commitment during that second week. This step in the essence diagram, identifying constraints, is discussed in detail in the next chapter.

Grace and James' therapist knew that clients' failure to perform a designated solution sequence can carry a wealth of information about the system. The therapist may discover an uncomplicated pattern of constraint, or they may find that there are multiple and/or challenging constraints. The therapist need not make a judgment about the degree of constraint (simple or complex) at this stage of the process. The work with solution sequences is meant to allow for successive identification of factors that prevent problem-solving. It could be that James can get a much better handle on his drinking through determination, additional coping mechanisms, and a modification of patterns of interaction with Grace. Alternatively, James may be constrained by an alcohol dependency or addiction process, the pull of which will require significant additional intervention. The therapist and clients can experience and discover together which of these scenarios is closer to the truth about James' drinking.

Hypothesizing and Planning

Hypotheses based on the various hypothesizing metaframeworks (see Chapter 1) present important considerations for the formulation and implementation of solution sequences. These hypotheses govern the range of appropriate solutions. An obvious example would be that the therapist will need to avoid solution sequences that are not developmentally appropriate for the children in the family. Similarly, the way the family is organized, or their religious beliefs may influence how the solution is formulated. Importantly, the therapist will need to consider the culture hypothesizing metaframework for every solution sequence.

Culture

IST is a collaborative, client system-centered approach. Rather than specifying norms or values that clients "should" adopt, it encourages the therapist to collaborate with clients to find solutions that fit their needs and patterns. It allows therapists to join the family, couple, or individual where they are and conduct therapy with respect for clients' identities and values.

IST's culture hypothesizing metaframework presents a set of concepts that can guide the therapist in identifying and implementing culturally considerate solution sequences. Understanding clients and their families in terms of this metaframework's contexts, including race, ethnicity, socioeconomic status, education, gender identity, and sexual orientation, allows for the examination of the meaning and implications of intersectionality (Crenshaw, 1989), including the disadvantages and injustices that accrue from membership and the intersection of memberships. The therapist needs to be mindful of intersectionality and its effects when identifying and implementing a solution sequence.

Some questions a therapist should consider are: Is what I am about to propose inconsistent with anything I have come to understand about the clients' values or circumstances? How will I introduce the idea so that clients see that I am soliciting their reactions to it? Am I asking clients to do something that requires access to resources that they do not have? What do I need to ask them to know if aspects of the solution sequence are doable for them? Am I being collaborative enough with them to reduce the power dynamic and assure that they feel fully on board with the experiment? Is my privilege getting in the way of understanding the challenges of implementing this plan?

For example, Angela, a 43-year-old, African American, straight, cisgender woman and single parent of three adult children, sought therapy for advice on how to handle her 20-year-old son who had a psychiatric history and seemed to be having a relapse. He refused to attend the therapy session. Angela reported that his behavior was becoming increasingly strange, and he was intimidating to her at times. As he became more delusional, she was unable to communicate with him. Angela was afraid and confused about what to do.

The therapist, a white, straight, cisgender woman, felt it was important to address Angela's safety as well as a plan for hospitalizing the son, if necessary. The therapist began to think about the role the police could play. Then, the therapist wondered, given the incidence of injury and death of black citizens at the hands of police, how Angela would feel about involving them. It occurred to the therapist that the mention of the police might be unsettling for her. The therapist realized that her own privilege allowed her to see the police as a resource; however, given a traumatic personal or community history with law enforcement, some people are understandably reluctant to involve the police in their lives.

The therapist did not assume that the idea of calling the police would be a trigger for Angela, but she also did not assume Angela would see them as a resource or feel safe about that option either. Rather than go right to the suggestion of police assistance, the therapist gathered information about what would help the client feel safe and what thoughts she had about getting her son the help that she felt he needed. As the conversation progressed, the therapist asked, "Can you say what you think about whether the police could be helpful?" This tentative, open question led to a conversation in which the risks and benefits of police involvement were discussed, and Angela defined the circumstances under which she would seek their help. As the therapist learned about Angela's readiness to call the police under certain circumstances, she steered the conversation to refining a plan for that if it was needed. The plan included what she would say in the call to the police and how she would try to meet them when they arrived. The plan also included contacting her employee assistance coordinator to get help selecting a hospital for her son.

The therapist encouraged Angela to bring her two other adult children into the next session to explore ways they could work with their mother to help their brother. Before the next session, Angela called the therapist to let her know that things had gotten worse and that she had called the police. The police had brought her son to the emergency room, and he had been hospitalized. The therapist supported Angela in her further contacts with the hospital and met several more times with her to define the circumstances under which her son could live in the home. Among Angela's requirements were that he remain under the care of a psychiatrist and a therapist and be compliant with the medication that would be prescribed.

As illustrated in this case, being helpful to clients requires attention to cultural and contextual factors that influence their lives. Therapists need to continually work at developing cultural competence and pay special attention to issues of inequality and social justice that impact their clients' lives.

Therapeutic Alliance

In IST, establishing and maintaining the therapeutic alliance is given priority over the planning guidelines (see Appendix B) and the therapist's ideas about intervention. The essence step of implementing a solution sequence carries risks for the alliance. The first risk has to do with conversations that pertain to the clients' readiness to experiment with a solution. The therapist needs to be respectful of the clients when discussing readiness so that the clients do not feel judged. Tone and language choice are key. The therapist can also check in with the client about the process. "I am asking you a lot of questions. Are you feeling okay about that?" Or, "I want to make sure that we don't ask you to try something that does not seem right for you."

Another challenge to the alliance can come in the commitment-related conversation. It is sometimes important for the therapist to encourage or even strongly encourage clients to try an experiment. This process can present risks of the client feeling pressured or controlled. Thus, in the process of collaborating on implementing a solution sequence, it is important for the therapist to seek feedback on the effects of the encouragement. The therapist might say, "Am I pushing this too hard?" Or "I am thinking this will be an opportunity for you. Do you think I am off base?"

The implementation step that may be most fraught with challenges for the alliance is the follow-up. Clients will naturally be sensitive about how their involvement in the therapy will be judged. When things with the experiment don't go as planned, they may feel a sense of failure. Their response in therapy might be apologetic, avoidant, or defensive. The therapist's tone and nonverbal communication in the follow-up are as important as what is said. When an alliance has been developed over time and is strong, the therapist is in a better position to be more direct about the expectations related to what the client agreed to do; however, in the early phases of therapy, or when the alliance becomes challenged later in therapy, the therapist needs to be especially careful with word choice and tone when following up on an experiment such that respect and acceptance are communicated.

Feedback is invaluable to the process of following up on a solution sequence. The therapist can make note of the client's body language, tone of voice, and the information they report. The therapist reads the feedback and either adjusts the approach or asks the clients directly about it. In the case of James and Grace, "James, you seem uncomfortable with the discussion of your drinking this week. Would you say that is accurate?" It is important to ask the clients about what they are experiencing in the discussions concerning the follow-up. The therapist can say something like, "How do you feel about this conversation?" Or "I am asking a lot of questions. Am I making this conversation uncomfortable for you?" If clients do say it is uncomfortable, the therapist can ask what is uncomfortable or what would feel better for them. Though clients often deny discomfort, it still may be worth reassuring them that the purpose of the inquiry is to learn about the details of what they did in order to help them better. Therapists develop their own styles of reacting to these situations, and those styles may vary from client to client and situation to situation, but the spirit of the communication is that the clients are respected, that the therapist sees their significant strengths, and that the therapist is there to help them do the things that will make a difference in their lives.

Alliances within the family can be split with respect to implementation as one member of a couple or family may demonstrate less commitment than others to an experiment. It is important for the therapist to establish clarity on who is on board and what the ambivalent members are thinking about the task at hand. One way to discuss this is in terms of the reasons a member has for not committing to the experiment. In a family system, the other family members may decide to embark on the experiment without the member who feels resistant to it, but the therapist is wise to delay the implementation until there has been further discussion of it. The therapist needs to consider that the reluctant family member may be scapegoated, or that the alliance between family members and the therapist could be affected. For this reason, the therapist will want to provide a calming and positive approach to what is ultimately a family decision. The therapist can hear the reluctant party out, validate their concerns and attempt to help them become comfortable to try the solution. Family members in alliance with the reluctant person can also help them get on board. When an agreement is not reached, further discussion can be had at the next session.

Options to consider in the case of family disagreement on the experiment include the following. First, the therapist may discourage the family from doing the experiment until all are on board. Second, the therapist can say that all members have good reasons for being for or against the experiment and frame their reasons as protective of or in the best interests of the family. Third, the therapist may ask the reluctant member what solution they would suggest. Fourth, the therapist can carefully explore the constraints of the reluctant member and may even talk individually with that member about their concerns. Fifth, the therapist may ask the resistant member to do a different task or to become an observer of the experiment. Sixth, the therapist may ask the resistant member or the whole family to consider other solution sequences with which to experiment. Seventh, the therapist may propose a new solution sequence. One or more of these strategies might be utilized as the therapist seeks to maintain the alliance with all members and move toward a solution sequence.

In the case of couples who disagree on whether to commit to an experiment, the process is somewhat more straightforward since it clearly takes two to proceed. The therapist can explore the concerns of the reluctant partner and acknowledge that their concerns are important and can say that the viewpoint and experience of both partners have important value in the relationship. For example, the therapist might say that a partner who initiates difficult discussions is holding up the value of resolving their conflicts, and the partner who avoids difficult discussions is holding up the value of protecting the relationship from the hurt that can result when they try to resolve conflicts. The therapist can also hypothesize about what may be constraining the reluctant partner and ask questions that relate to various hypotheses. For example, "I hear that you may be reluctant to talk with your partner about a plan for the holiday. I wonder if you are worried that a conversation between the two of you may compromise your wish to be loyal to your family-of-origin's holiday tradition?"

Absent an agreement between partners, it may be best for the therapy to move on to other solutions. Before moving on, however, it is wise for the therapist to ask the couple if the difference in their feelings about the experiment reminds them of other conversations that they have. If it does, the therapist has the opportunity through further questioning to uncover an additional problem sequence that may constrain any number of solution sequences. In other words, the disagreement they have on whether to experiment with a solution sequence may itself be an example of a sequence that limits the functioning of the relationship.

Conclusion

The implementation of a solution sequence is sometimes more straightforward than at other times. The implementation consists of four components: Readiness, refinement, commitment, and follow-up. The therapist needs to assess the clients' readiness to do the experiment, refine the experiment with client feedback, solicit a commitment from the clients to do the task, and follow up in the next session on both the clients' level of success in doing the experiment and the impact of it. Special attention to each of the components of implementation is required when clients are unclear on what the experiment with the solution sequence will look like, or when one or more members express ambivalence about the solution sequence.

Exercises

1   Recall a time when you were working with one or more people in a team effort. Consider a course of action you wanted the group to undertake. Did you feel effective in the conversation? Do you think you could have been more effective? Imagine applying one of the four components of implementing a solution sequence (readiness, refinement, commitment, or follow-up) in that conversation. Write down specific questions you might ask or statements you might make in the conversation to address the component you are imagining. Then see if there is another component of implementing a solution that you can apply. Write down the questions you would ask and the statements you might make in exploring this solution-implementation.

2   Develop a few questions you can ask for each of the components of implementing the solution. Practice saying these questions in a manner that is nonjudgmental and respectful. Make a video recording of yourself saying the questions one by one. Or, say the questions while looking in the mirror and observe your facial expressions. See and hear yourself. Do you seem sufficiently interested and respectful? Imagine using these questions with a particular client.

3   Think of one of your current clinical cases. Identify something clients had agreed to do between sessions and remember the conversation about it as well as the outcome of the between-session experiment. If available, review recordings of the session in which the plan was made and review the conversation carefully. Think of how you might have enhanced the conversations by consciously utilizing the four elements of implementing a solution sequence. Write down some specific questions to ask and statements to make for each of the four components. Recall things clients have said that could be considered feedback concerning one of the solution-implementing components.

4   Consider one of your current cases as an opportunity to enhance your skills in implementing a solution sequence. Once the solution sequence is identified, work through each component of implementation as thoroughly as you can. Take a few notes on what you did and how you did it. When you have progressed through the follow-up component, reflect on how you did and whether you would do anything differently.

References

Crenshaw, K. (1989). Demarginalizing the intersection of race and sex: A black feminist critique of antidiscrimination doctrine, feminist theory and antiracist politics. *University of Chicago Legal Forum, 1989*, 139–167.

Miller, W. R., & Rollnick, S. M. (2012). *Motivational interviewing: Helping people change*. Guilford Press.

Prochaska, J. O., & DiClemente, C. C. (1984). *The transtheoretical approach: Crossing traditional boundaries of therapy*. Dow/Jones Irwin.

Tomm, K. (1985). Circular interviewing: A multifaceted clinical tool. In D. Campbell & R. Draper (Eds.). *Applications of systemic family therapy: The Milan approach method* (pp. 33–45). Norton.

Tomm, K. (1987). Interventive interviewing: Part II: Intending to ask lineal, circular, strategic, or reflexive questions? *Family Process, 27*, 1–15.

Chapter 7

Identifying Constraints

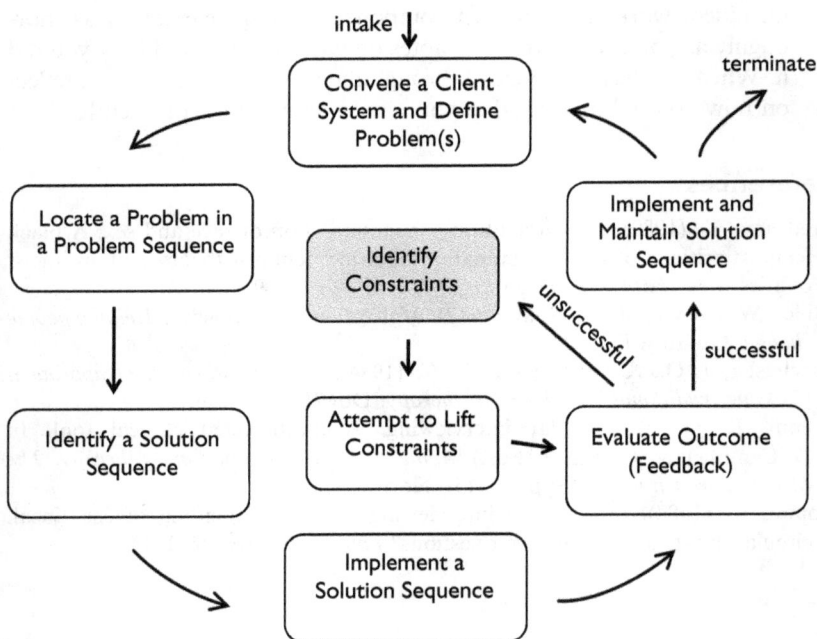

intake

Convene a Client System and Define Problem(s)

terminate

Locate a Problem in a Problem Sequence

Identify Constraints

Implement and Maintain Solution Sequence

unsuccessful

successful

Identify a Solution Sequence

Attempt to Lift Constraints

Evaluate Outcome (Feedback)

Implement a Solution Sequence

IST Essence Diagram.

Objective

As clients experiment with solution sequences, they often find themselves constrained from implementing them. This chapter illuminates the process through which constraints are identified and described. This process enables the therapist and client to agree that the constraint is present and interferes with implementing the solution sequence. The web of human

DOI: 10.4324/9780429322273-7

experience including the biopsychosocial levels of the system and the seven hypothesizing metaframeworks is used to consider where constraints can be located and what they might consist of. Examples of constraints from within each of the hypothesizing metaframeworks are provided.

Introduction

Early in the history of family therapy, what came to be known as the theory of constraints was an important proposition for systems theorists. First described by Gregory Bateson (1972) as *negative explanation*, the proposition was that a system is distressed because something is preventing it from performing in an adaptive way. Australian family therapist Michael White was one of the first family therapists to codify the use of negative explanation in clinical practice. He used the word restraint rather than constraint (White, 1986). In *Metaframeworks: Transcending the Models of Family Therapy* (Breunlin et al., 1992), the word "constraint" was used rather than restraint, because it was more prevalent than restraint in the United States where the Metaframeworks approach originated. As the Metaframeworks approach evolved into IST, the language of constraints was preserved.

As the many models of psychotherapy developed and evolved, the systemic theory of constraints was not a particularly dominant feature of them. Further, the language of direct, linear causation that seems to be embedded in mainstream thought in the United States and perhaps some other countries, does not view causation primarily through the lens of systemic constraints. Thus, therapists drawn to the integrative and systemic nature of IST need to make a conceptual leap to embrace constraint theory. This chapter is designed to help make that leap for newcomers to IST and to strengthen it for existing systemic practitioners. Having made the leap, the journey is just begun. IST therapists spend a lifetime developing and maintaining their constraint-identification abilities.

Method

Constraints are identified in two ways. First, clients identify constraints either spontaneously or in response to the therapist's questions and comments. Second, the therapist hypothesizes about what constrains the clients and presents the hypotheses to them. In both cases, the language of constraints is an important means of identifying systemic factors in a manner that is accepting and respectful of clients. Adopting the language of constraints requires practice, but it is not hard to master once the commitment to it is made.

Constraint Questions

The first means of identifying constraints draws on the clients' knowledge of themselves and their situation. In this case, the identification of a constraint begins with a version of the *constraint question*. The question takes the form of a stem followed by a description of the solution sequence. The most common stems of the constraint question are: "What keeps you from...?", "What stops you from...?", "What gets in the way of...?", and "What blocks you from...?".

A classic example of the application of constraint theory in couples therapy can be found in the case of a partner who complains that the other partner frequently lies. The therapist's question to the untruthful partner might be, "Why do you lie to your partner?" The corresponding constraint question would be, "What keeps you from telling the truth?" Constraint questions are delivered empathically and do not have an accusatory tone. The partner accused of lying can respond in myriad ways. One example is the following: "You know what? Sometimes my friends want to go for a drink after work. If I call home and tell the truth, I'll be told 'no, come home now!' Then I can't go out with my friends without a fight. So, I call and say, 'I'm held up at the office.' I know I'm not being straight, but I don't want to fight about it."

Although this is a tense moment, the groundwork is laid for the clients to see the lying as something that negatively impacts their relationship. The constraint-oriented interview also signals that the therapist is interested not in judgment or shaming, but in finding solutions.

Practicing Constraint Questions

Below are several issues common to therapy. Consider each one. Ask yourself how you would normally ask a question about the issue and then construct a constraint question as an alternative. Examples of corresponding constraint questions are provided just below the set of issues.

> Refusing to attend school.
> Relapsing with alcohol use.
> Feeling emotionally numb.
> Not addressing a critical issue in a relationship.

IST Examples of constraint questions:

> What keeps you from going to school?
> What's getting in the way of you staying sober?
> What do you think keeps you from experiencing your feelings?
> What stops you from bringing the issue up with your partner?

Proposing Hypotheses about Constraints

The second way constraints are identified is by means of a therapist's hypothesis. Clients may have difficulty identifying certain constraints. In such cases, therapists can propose hypotheses about what they think may be holding the clients back. The therapist observes patterns and uses knowledge about hypothesizing metaframeworks to consider what may constrain the clients. For example, a single mother and her two children attended therapy. The work took a focus on bringing more structure and leadership to family life. The mother saw the need to be firmer with the children in certain circumstances, but the initial solution sequences for limit-setting were not successful as the mother found it difficult to hold the line. The therapist understood from a prior conversation that the mother had been physically abused by her own mother. Given this childhood experience, the therapist hypothesized that the mother may have an aversion to remaining firm with her children.

Therapist: You have been working hard on the limit setting and it seems that it is so difficult to hold firm. I wonder, given your own childhood, if holding firm is scary for you.

Client: Maybe. I feel relieved when I give in. Resentful, but relieved.

Introducing a hypothesis typically is preceded by a contextualizing statement that states why the therapist is suggesting the hypothesis. The therapist may also begin the contextualizing statement with, "I had an idea and I wanted to share it with you." The hypothesis can be presented tentatively, with language such as "I wonder if…" or "I think perhaps…" Under some circumstances, it may be more assertively stated "I think that…" or "I really want you to give some thought to…" (the idea just shared). Whether generated by the client or therapist, the identification of a constraint is a collaborative process, and both will need to agree that it is a factor in order to proceed to the step of lifting or addressing it.

The Nature of Constraints

By now the reader may imagine that a client system could present with an unlimited number of constraints. While this is theoretically possible, IST has two built-in safeguards to keep therapists from being inundated with constraints. The first safeguard grows out of the problem-centered contract of IST. IST does not seek to uncover all constraints. Rather it seeks to uncover the constraints that interfere with solving the problem the clients wish to solve. When the client system fails to implement the solution sequence that was formulated to solve the problem (the experiment), the therapist asks the question: "What kept you from doing this (the solution sequence)?" The answer to this question usually uncovers at least one (and sometimes several) constraints. At that moment, the therapist focuses therapy on a constraint that interferes with a particular solution to a specified problem. The other constraints might eventually be important targets of the therapy, however, so the therapist makes a mental note of them and acknowledges to the clients that they can be addressed later in therapy. For example, a woman attending a first session shares that her mother died a few years ago. During the final years of the mother's life, the client had served an important caretaker function. The woman does not think this issue has an impact on her presenting problem. The therapist would empathize with the client about the journey of caretaking and loss and indicate that they can return to this issue, if it is something she decides to focus on in therapy.

The second safeguard is IST's use of the web of human experience (see Figure 1.4 in Chapter 1). The web provides levels of the biopsychosocial system to support the search for *where* constraints occur and hypothesizing metaframeworks to inform hypothesizing about *what* factors constrain the client system. A partner in a couple system found taking a time-out virtually intolerable. The therapist and clients came to an understanding that there was a constraint of mind (feeling abandoned) operating at the individual and the relationship levels of the biopsychosocial system. This description of a constraint specified both the *what* and the *where* of it.

In Figure 1.4 (Chapter 1), each of the concentric circles represents one of five levels: the person, the relationships (dyads and triads), the family or families, the community, the society, and the global context. One might question how the broadest levels, global context, society and community, can have a direct impact on the practice of psychotherapy, but IST believes they do. For example, at the global and societal level, the pandemic of 2020 overwhelmed many people and either exacerbated their existing anxiety or depression or served as a precipitating cause of these conditions. During the pandemic, at the level of community, Black and Latinx people were disproportionately impacted by COVID-19, including higher rates of illness (CDC, 2021), hospitalization (CDC, 2020) and death (CDC, 2021). Moving to the next level of the multi-level system, the family is the incubator of relational and individual development. Families organize themselves in ways that facilitate or constrain attachment, communication, autonomy, and problem-solving. The next level down, the dyad/triad level, recognizes that a family consists of subsystems that constitute relationships within the family. Several of the most important relational subsystems are the couple subsystem, the parental subsystem, the sibling subsystem, and various parent-child subsystems. Subsystems can also form around interests, for example, the artistic siblings and the athletic siblings. Finally, there is the level of the individual, which includes biological and psychological dimensions.

The levels of the biopsychosocial system point to *where* constraints exist. The IST therapist must also identify *what* the constraints are. The hypothesizing metaframeworks serve as a template for constraint identification. Reviewing the various models of therapy, the authors abstracted seven primary domains of human experience that permeate the field of psychotherapy: mind, organization, development, culture, gender, biology, and spirituality. Each of these is a framework of frameworks or a metaframework within which theory and research findings explain various aspects of that domain of experience. The domains give therapists the ability to read client feedback and code its relevance to the problem sequence through the theoretical lens of one of the hypothesizing metaframeworks without having to first enter through the theoretical lens of a therapy model. Eliminating this step is one example of the advantages of an integrative perspective. Below is a summary of the information contained in each of the hypothesizing metaframeworks. The material is intended to be representative of a particular metaframework but not exhaustive. Moreover, as new knowledge emerges, it can be added to a metaframework. For example, with advances in the understanding of the human genome, genetics has become an important consideration in the treatment of both physical illness and psychiatric problems (Kendler, 2013; McGuffin & Murray, 2013; Miller et al., 2006). Thus, genetics has become a part of the biology hypothesizing metaframework.

Mind

The metaframework of the mind captures the mental process of clients. It has long been the heart and soul of psychotherapy. Many psychotherapies look no further than the mind and propose elegant theories explaining how mental processes regulate the lives of clients for better and for worse. Mental processes encompass both meanings and emotions. Meanings include cognitions (perceptions, thoughts, ideas), beliefs, stories, narratives, and memories. Emotions include feelings and affective states. Mental processes can be conscious or unconscious. Mind is ubiquitous, occurring during waking hours and at night in the form of dreams that can sometimes be remembered and sometimes be terrifying. Any aspect of the above can serve as a constraint. For example, a white, cisgender, mixed-sex, married couple in their early 50s enters therapy with the presenting problem of an unsatisfactory sex life. Exploration of the problem sequence reveals that they have never had a substantive conversation about their sex life. The therapist asks them to experiment with a simple solution sequence to spend 15 minutes talking about sex. They agree but arrive at the next session not having had the conversation. The therapist asks them what kept them from having the conversation. The wife responds that it made her feel "dirty" just thinking about having the conversation so she could not bring herself to initiate it. The husband responds that he had imagined that the conversation would include making requests for what he preferred to do in bed, and he believes that asking for that would be a form of entitlement. Believing this, he did not initiate the conversation. Each of them was constrained by a matter of mind.

Constraints of mind are always present when a solution sequence fails. Nevertheless, systemic therapy postulates that the mind metaframework itself frequently does not provide the necessary and sufficient explanation for the failure of the solution sequence to be implemented successfully. Constraints of mind are most often nestled in constraints associated with other metaframeworks. For example, an immigrant Muslim family consisting of cisgender, mixed-sex parents, three daughters, 25, 19 and 15, and two sons, 17 and 12, seek therapy for the intense arguments that are primarily initiated by the mother. Her anger is usually an expression of her frustration that one of the children has violated a norm that she feels they should be following. Her screaming is met with retaliatory screaming from the accused child and before long, other family members join the fray by taking sides. Using a concept developed by Gottman (1993), the therapist establishes that their arguments currently begin with a "hard start-up" and that it would be good to make an effort to replace it with a "soft start-up." In the next session, the mother was still using a hard start-up and several severe arguments had occurred. The therapist asked a constraint question: "What kept the soft start-up from working?" The mother replied that it was her duty to prepare her children for the world, and she would have to do it her way. The emotional chaos that inevitably followed such outbursts was a necessary price to pay.

Working only with constraints of mind, the therapist could hypothesize that the mother held rigid beliefs that kept her from seeing the value of a soft start-up. In addition, one could hypothesize that she was prone to become emotionally dysregulated whenever she acted on these beliefs. To contribute her part to the solution sequence, therefore, she would have to become more flexible in her beliefs and develop control of her emotions so she could use a soft start-up. If this were the only intervention, it would result in blaming the mother.

The view of the family shifts dramatically when a systemic view is taken. This view is facilitated by examination of other hypothesizing metaframeworks. The first is organization. Though this is a traditional patriarchal Muslim family, the mother holds sway over domestic matters. The father is mild-mannered and often out of town, as his job involves travel. His voice is not a factor in the arguments, and he does not seem to have the inclination or ability to influence his wife's approach to the conflicts. Another hypothesizing metaframework is culture. As with many immigrant families, the rate of acculturation among family members is uneven, with children tending to acculturate more readily (Chun & Akutsu, 2003). In this case, most of the arguments are saturated in issues of acculturation with the adolescents wanting to act in accordance with their conception of how teenagers and young adults act in the United States, and the mother wanting them to practice the beliefs and actions consistent with their culture of origin. The family is not effectively addressing the cultural divide in the household. It seems that work on soft start-ups or mechanisms of mind, if necessary, will need to follow a frank discussion of the acculturation-related constraint. Hopefully, the parents can become more understanding of the American aspects of the children, and the children more accepting of the mother's role in preserving aspects of their traditional way of life.

Since we all experience the world through our minds, it is tempting to assume that attention to the mind should be the primary focus of therapy. A systemic view of therapy, however, seeks to capture a much broader spectrum of how context contributes to problem formation and maintenance. It is important, therefore, that therapy be able to view the mind at an adequate level of complexity, but not give it so much attention that other aspects of the system are obscured. IST allows constraints of mind to be identified and addressed without maximizing their relevance until it becomes clear that it is essential to do so.

IST employs a framework that uses three increasingly complex ways to view the mind. The three levels are labeled M1, M2, and M3. The guideline for deciding which level to use is to begin with the least complex level (M1) and to go to the next levels only when the description of the constraint of mind requires more complexity. This reduces the risk of focusing more deeply on mind than required and allows the therapist to hypothesize with mind more readily in conjunction with other hypothesizing metaframeworks.

The M1 level of mind simply describes sequences of meaning and emotion without evoking a complex psychological theory to explain them. An M1 analysis may include a cognition or emotion, a sequence of meaning and emotions, or a complex narrative. In the case of the couple who was constrained from talking about sex (above), the constraints reported by the partners (talking about it feels "dirty" and asking for something is "entitlement") are described at the M1 level as they could be discussed and potentially modified without regard to a psychological theory of the mind. In the case of the family discussed above, the description of the mother's view of her role in preparing the children for the world is an M1 analysis. Her view is part of a larger narrative which can also be described at the M1 level of analysis.

When M1 constraints of mind will not lift, the therapist searches for explanations for this resistance. This may call for a more complex view of the mental process. When this is the case, the shift occurs as the therapist becomes more familiar with the clients' mental processes and recognizes the patterns involved. At the M2 level of analysis, IST therapists utilize theories that describe how components of the mind are organized and fit together. Examples of such M2 models are internal family systems (IFS; Schwartz, 2013) and object relations (Kernberg, 1976). For example, a woman presents with a concern that her husband resists closeness, which is something that she desperately wants. Interviewing her on her experience with this problem revealed an M1 analysis that included her process of noticing the distance, then feeling deflated which leads to resentment, and then judging her husband as "cold and uncaring." The husband initially states that he is a doer kind of guy who shows his love for his wife by being a good provider and helping around the house. He eventually buys into her request for greater closeness, but solution sequences designed to help the couple make a connection repeatedly fail. Moving on to an M2 analysis, the therapist draws on Internal Family Systems (IFS; Schwartz, 2013). Using this approach, the therapist suggests that a part of the husband can turn toward closeness but in such a tentative way that it feels disingenuous to his wife. The husband acknowledges this, and the therapist invites the couple to get to know that part better. What is then learned is that closeness for the husband is associated with an exiled part of him that lurks in the shadows of his mind and is fearful of coming forward because the closeness can result in too much hurt. He revealed that his mother died when he was just four years old. This is an M2 analysis in that it utilizes a theory of how the human mind is organized, namely the Internal Family Systems approach.

Sometimes a client seems to lack the resiliency needed to address constraints and implement solution sequences. Gradually, the therapist realizes that the client's failures are experienced as defeats, which seem to be discouraging for the client and damaging to the therapeutic alliance. This realization, along with the failure of interventions targeting the M1 and M2 levels of mind, is a reason to consider an M3 hypothesis. The M3 level examines the structure of the self which may be deemed too vulnerable to implement and maintain the solution sequence (Kohut, 1977, 1984). Strengthening the self so that it can do the work of therapy becomes a goal. In the case of a family or couple case, the client needing this work is typically referred for individual therapy. An M3 analysis of mind is occasionally indicated from the outset of therapy when compelling information or client feedback support a hypothesis of a significantly vulnerable self. Constraints to the flexibility and stability of self (M3) have traditionally been addressed by self-psychology (Kohut 1977, 1984), which is a long-term intensive therapy, and more recently by the behavioral and relational approach of functional analytic psychotherapy which does not hypothesize a self, but directly targets the interpersonal behaviors associated with M3 constraints (Kohlenberg & Tsai, 2007). However, if the client is self-harming, strongly reactive to criticism or rejection, or satisfies the diagnostic description of borderline personality disorder, IST would suggest a dialectical behavior therapy program (DBT; Linehan, 2014) be tried first as it has emerged as a preferred treatment for these issues.

Organization

The organization hypothesizing metaframework grows out of IST's ontological pillar that embraces systems theory and the sequential organization pillar that asserts that systems are organized through sequential patterning. Sequences are a temporal description, but if one were to take a metaphorical photo of the pattern, the result would be a visual rendering of the system's organization that shows how it works as a whole. The family therapy theorists closely associated with the organization metaframework are Minuchin (Minuchin, 1974; Minuchin & Fishman, 1981), Haley (1976, 1981), and Madanes (1981). Structural Family Therapy (Minuchin, 1974; Minuchin & Fishman, 1981; Fishman, 1993, 2013) has been the most prominent family therapy model grounded in the principles and practices of organizational theory. The IST authors preferred to name the metaframework "organization" rather than "structure" in order to provide latitude for a variety of concepts and theories related to systemic organization to live within the metaframework. The organization metaframework is closely related to the culture metaframework. When some aspect of organization is being considered as a possible constraint, it is vital to embed the organizational issue within the cultural norms of the client system. A form of organization that might be considered appropriate in one culture might be considered inappropriate in another culture.

One key organizational concept addresses how decisions are made in the family. Minuchin referred to the "who's in charge?" question with the structural concept of *hierarchy*. IST has replaced this concept with *leadership,* which represents a broader set of functions including: Allocating resources and responsibilities; mediating conflicts among members; seeing to the needs of members; encouraging the growth of each member; providing firm, fair limits; and representing the system in interaction with other systems (Breunlin et al., 1997). Leadership pertains at each level of the multi-level biopsychosocial system.

The ways leaders lead can be constraining to the system. For example, a single parent and children live with the children's grandparents. Family members all bring significant strengths to the table, but the children are struggling in school. The mother tells the children to start their homework right after school and before she arrives home from work. She needs to count on her mother (the grandmother) to facilitate that homework plan. Since the presenting problem is difficulty with school work, this homework routine would constitute a solution sequence. When the children do not perform this sequence, the therapist asks a constraint question: "What kept you from starting your homework?" One of the children replies that grandma said they could play outside for a while after school. If this is a recurrent sequence, it would signal an organizational constraint to the leadership of the family that would have to be lifted for the solution sequence to be implemented successfully.

Another key concept of the organization metaframework is boundaries—those metaphorical fences that regulate the flow of communication and resources across subsystems of the client system. The boundaries should be clear so that the right amount of communication takes place and adequate resources get shared. If the boundaries are too permeable, too much communication occurs. For example, a daughter might talk to her mother daily and reveal information about the daughter's marriage that is better kept within the boundary of the marriage. If the boundaries are too rigid, too few resources are shared, and too little communication occurs. For example, in a post-divorce decree involving mixed-sex parents and a 17-year-old daughter, the daughter elects to live with her father, which angers the mother who then cuts off communication with her, therefore creating a rigid boundary. A year later, the father meets a woman who soon moves in with him and his daughter. The woman argues frequently with the daughter and finally tells the father that she does not want the daughter to live at the house. By doing so, she is insisting on rigid boundaries that create an organizational constraint for the father, who must now choose between his daughter and his partner.

In another example, a couple who have almost no contact time together are asked to spend 30 minutes per day doing something together. They agree but in the next session they report that they had only spent time together once. When asked a constraint question, the wife reported that their daughter, who lives next door, frequently and without prior arrangement drops her children off for childcare. The therapist wonders if a diffuse boundary with the daughter's family is a constraint for the couple.

Development

The development metaframework contains the theories and concepts pertaining to the development of the various biopsychosocial levels of the system. The levels included are the person, relationship, family, community, and society. This is a vast territory of knowledge that encompasses myriad contributions from the literatures on life-span development, psychology of the person, family therapy, couples therapy, psychiatry, social work, counseling, sociology, and anthropology. From this store of information and theories, however, the therapist only focuses on the aspect of development that constrains a given solution sequence. When some aspect of development is construed as a constraint, it is vital to embed the developmental issue within the cultural norms of the client system. Behavior that might be considered age-appropriate in one culture might be considered immature or too mature in another culture.

At the level of the person, any of the stages of lifespan development are potentially relevant to a case. At each stage of individual development, a person is expected to be *on time* and meet developmental milestones. This constitutes age-appropriate behavioral, cognitive, emotional, and social competence. When a person exhibits either too little or too much competence for a given age, the result can be a constraint for the client system. Even more constraining are those situations where the person sometimes acts too mature and sometimes too immature. This situation results in a developmental oscillation where it becomes difficult for all members of the client system to know what is to be expected (Breunlin, 1988, 1989).

There are biological, psychological, and social components to development. Attachment theory posits that normal social and emotional development is dependent on the child's early attachment experience with at least one primary caretaker (Bowlby, 1979). Disruptions in early attachment can lead to attachment styles that can constrain problem-solving. Identification of these types of constraints may require focus on the attachment issues themselves before the presenting problems can be adequately addressed. Attachment-based family therapy (Diamond et al., 2014) is attachment-informed, but unlike individual psychodynamic therapy, it seeks to directly improve the attachment between parents and their children.

Theorists who have studied couples believe that couples also develop. Wynne (1984), for example, argued that couples go through five stages of relational development: attachment, caregiving, communicating, problem-solving, and mutuality. What Wynne meant by mutuality was the ability of the couple to change the fundamental rules that govern the relationship. For example, if one spouse of a dual-career couple is offered a job in another city, can the couple come to an agreement on how to deal with the job offer that would impact the other spouse's career and necessitate a move to another city? Wynne's model is epigenetic, meaning that one stage must be mastered before a subsequent stage can be. For example, a cis-gender, mixed-sex, married couple at mid-life initiates therapy to decide whether the wife, who had stayed home to raise the children, should return to the workforce. They have a history of non-productive arguing that involves mutual recriminations. They also report that problem solving has always been difficult for them. They could not agree on how to save money or how to help their children choose a university. For the wife to return to the workforce, the couple will need to alter the fundamental rules of their relationship. Since they have not mastered the stages of communication and problem solving, it is unreasonable to assume that they can renegotiate their rules without significant help from the therapist. They are constrained by their relational development. Wynne's theory suggests the development of the ability to change rules in their relationship (mutuality) without the intervention of a therapist will require them to work first on developing better communication and problem-solving skills.

Family development has typically been understood through the lens of the family life cycle (Duvall, 1957; McGoldrick et al., 2016). The family life cycle has been updated to reflect more current trends in family life and attend more comprehensively to a multicultural perspective (McGoldrick et al., 2016). In the life cycle view, families pass through predictable stages that are punctuated by transitions that separate one stage from the next. During a stage, certain processes and competencies are progressively mastered. In a transition, new processes and competencies are introduced. The family must reorganize for this to happen. For example, the transition to adolescence is often fraught with turmoil because the parent(s) and adolescent become engaged in battles over age-appropriate levels of autonomy. Too much or too little autonomy can result in conflict between the parents and an oscillation for the adolescent, both of which are constraining for a solution sequence.

Because of an absence of universal norms and values in multicultural societies, societal development can be difficult to articulate, but there is ample evidence to suggest that societies do develop. How this happens can have a major impact on the individual, relational, and family levels of the system. Consider the development of the rights of sexual minorities in the United States. As time has passed, the stigma associated with same-sex relationships and partnerships weakened and gay and lesbian people and their relationships started to appear in the media. Advocacy advanced the cause and, eventually, same-sex marriage was legalized. The way gay and lesbian relationships are nested in society has changed over time. Although this illustrates how a culture can develop, it in no way suggests that safety, equity, and inclusion for sexual and gender minorities have been sufficiently established and protected. This is an ongoing struggle.

In a rapidly evolving society, normative development for all age groups is not easily determined; hence, family members and the parents serving as leaders often cannot reach a consensus on what to expect. This can trigger conflict and constrain parent-child harmony. Questions include, at what age should a child be given a mobile device and how much screen time should an adolescent be allowed?

As society evolves, the conception of the life cycle itself continues to develop. Emerging adulthood is a new stage that extends to the age of mid-20s. During this stage, unlike their parents who typically were expected to be living independently and supporting themselves after high school or college, an increasing number of young adults are living with one or both parents (Burn & Szoeke, 2016; Otters & Hollander, 2015).

At the other end of the life span, the increase in life expectancy and improvements in healthcare have baby boomers working into their retirement years (Simon-Rusinowitz et al., 1998). Clients live in the context of evolving developmental expectations.

Culture

In recent decades, there has been a growing body of literature focusing on the importance of adopting a multicultural perspective for the practice of systemic therapy. The literature has addressed the need to step away from both universalist practices and the ethnic-focused approaches to therapy, and instead develop multiculturally-informed practices (Rastogi & Thomas, 2009; Krause, 2012; Falicov, 2015;) and incorporate an understanding of intersectionality into the work (Hernandez et al., 2005; Seedall et al., 2014). Furthermore, many scholars (McDowell, 2005; McGoldrick & Hardy, 2008; Rastogi & Thomas, 2009; Esmiol et al., 2012; Falicov, 2015; Kelly et al., 2020) have highlighted the need to acknowledge and navigate power structures present in communities and society, emphasizing the need to focus on oppression, privilege, and social justice in the lives of clients and therapists. In recent years, scholars have suggested moving away from U.S. and Eurocentric considerations to a broader framework that recognizes global influences. This would allow consideration of the larger context and interventions tailored to the needs of families and communities around the world (Bischoff et al., 2016; Patterson et al., 2017; Rastogi, 2020).

IST's culture metaframework supports the incorporation of a multicultural perspective, intersectionality, and social justice into an ongoing practice. It is built on the premise that clients' identities and experiences are shaped by their *contexts of membership*, that is the various groups with which they identify or in which they participate. Context of membership is similar to the concept of *intersectionality* (Crenshaw, 1989; Cole, 2009; Watts-Jones, 2010) that analyzes multiple aspects of social identity along with the patterns of inequity, oppression, and privilege associated with them.

Individuals belong to many contexts of membership. These contexts can be defined by economics, education, ethnicity, race, religion, gender, sexual orientation, age, majority/minority status, regional background, etc. (Breunlin et al., 1997). Sometimes people are aware of their contexts of membership and how participation in those contexts impacts their lives, and sometimes they are oblivious to it. For example, a white person who was raised in a wealthy family in a predominantly white, affluent community may not be aware of the tremendous privilege afforded them simply by virtue of being a member of that context.

The identity formed through intersectionality defines and limits how people behave, think, and feel at each moment of their lives. For example, a German American man who is an engineer celebrates his precision and problem-solving prowess and does not comprehend his wife's appeal to just listen to her feelings during a conversation. A solution sequence that asks him not to try to solve what he sees as his wife's problem, but to listen and understand her feelings, is not successful as he is unable to resist problem-solving. The therapist respects the man's intent but wonders if membership in the cultural context of his profession or conceptions of gender formed in his culture of origin may be constraints. The exploration of his intersectionality in relation to the proposed solution sequence brings further awareness to his problem-solving tendency and facilitates conversation in which the therapist helps him understand how it is in the best interest of marital harmony for him to learn to override his problem-solving penchant and just listen and empathize with his wife's feelings. If the man accepts this formulation, the therapist can create an enactment in session in which the man is coached to listen carefully and then share his understanding of what is being said.

IST employs the principle of *goodness of fit* between the inter-sectionalities of people, whatever the relationship might be. Opposites may initially attract, and partners with differences can find their own *fit*, but memberships in differing cultural contexts can be challenging for partners. When the *goodness of fit* is limited, the respective disconnects of each partner's contexts of membership can be constraining. For example, an interracial couple met and fell in love. The dyadic relationship contained their racial differences and produced minimal distress. The context of their relationship expanded when the couple decided to introduce each other to their respective families. If both families were accepting of the relationship, they would have a better chance to remain stable and satisfied. If one family disapproved, the couple would have to absorb the challenge. Fortunately, they reported that their relationship was accepted and supported by their respective families. The relationship thrived and they decided to have children, which led them to consider where they would like to raise a family. They looked for a community where their relationship would be celebrated and their biracial child would find acceptance and opportunity. Fit is a multi-level systemic phenomenon.

To work effectively with the cultural metaframework, therapists need to develop an understanding of the constraining influence of their own cultural contexts of membership and an openness to understanding the implications of the client system's cultural contexts of membership. Included in this effort is the devotion of attention to learning about non-dominant cultural contexts and their impact on clients, including the existence and effects of oppression. This work on developing cultural competency is required both for advancing therapeutic alliances and hypothesizing about the problem-solving process, including identifying constraints related to cultural contexts of membership (intersectionality).

Gender

Gender is intricately linked to culture and could potentially be subsumed within the culture metaframework; however, gender-related strengths and constraints are important in most cases and can be so impactful in a client system that the IST authors (Breunlin et al., 2011; Pinsof et al., 2018) decided to heighten awareness of gender as a factor in therapy by designating gender as a metaframework. Feminist family therapist, Rachel Hare-Mustin (Hare-Mustin, 1978) first highlighted the importance of gender to therapy. Goldner (1988) later argued that gender should be treated at the same level of importance as a hierarchy. More recently the need for affirmative practice with transgender and nonbinary clients has been emphasized (McGeorge et al., 2021; Singh & Dickey, 2017). IST emphasizes the importance of understanding the experience clients have and the meanings they develop with respect to their gender identity, gendered roles (if any) and the way gender may factor into equity, power, and influence in their relationships. Constraints related to gender develop in relation to the way partners or family members interact and fit together in their system and/or in relation to oppression within the community or at the societal level of the system.

Gender Identity

Beliefs about gender have been evolving, but not uniformly across societies and communities. There may be regional and local differences in terms of prevailing attitudes, and families live and function in the context of their communities. Importantly, families also vary in the way gender is construed. For example, transgender and gender-nonconforming clients may have been shamed or shunned by family members. Transgender people have higher rates of depression and suicide and are more likely to be subjected to violence (Budge et al., 2013; Stotzer, 2009; Toomey et al., 2018). External sources of oppression are seen within IST as constraints to safety, opportunity, connection, and peace of mind. The importance of an informed and affirmative approach to transgender and gender nonconforming clients cannot be overemphasized. McGeorge et al. (2021) highlight the negative effects of cissexism and propose a model for becoming an affirmative therapist for transgender and nonbinary clients.

Although mainstream society in the United States may have made some initial strides in promoting equity for sexual and gender minorities, the society is still constructed in the interests of a binary understanding of gender and a primarily heterosexual orientation. The persistence of oppression for individuals and groups with non-binary and non-hetero orientations is still prevalent at the family, community, and societal levels. Sexual and gender minorities do not enjoy the same privilege as cisgender, straight individuals, nor can they necessarily feel as comfortable as they navigate their communities and the larger society. Therapists working with gender-diverse and sexually diverse clients, therefore, must possess the requisite knowledge, expertise, and compassion to form strong alliances and understand the challenges these clients face.

Gender Roles

Gender roles can constrain in a variety of ways. For example, a cisgender man, who in childhood was scolded by his father for crying, years later may struggle to express his vulnerability. A cisgender woman socialized as a young girl to privilege the continuity of the relationship over her own needs or opinions may struggle to maintain assertiveness in a conversation with her partner about expectations and needs in the relationship. Despite the significant changes in gender roles that have occurred over the last 50-plus years within the United States and other countries, many families, to a greater or lesser extent, maintain certain gender role traditions. Cisgender and gender minority clients in both mixed-sex and same-sex partnerships may struggle with current-day contexts of those traditions and/or with the implications of early gender socialization.

When couples must deal with loss, developmental changes, illness, or disability, their beliefs about gender or their experience with gender roles in their family of origin may constrain the implementation of solution sequences. For instance, a partner's shame about erectile dysfunction led to sexual avoidance and emotional alienation between the partners, rather than a frank discussion about the sources of the dysfunction and possible emotional, behavioral and/or pharmacological alternatives. Solutions were constrained by the powerful lesson the partner learned in childhood that men did not talk about what was "wrong with them."

Gender and Relational Equity

Power disparities are present in all relationships, including traditional and nontraditional mixed-sex relationships. More traditional relationships, however, are often laden with the vestiges of patriarchy and, therefore, are more prone to have constraints related to power that are grounded in gendered beliefs and expectations. Although many mixed-sex couples aspire to a relationship characterized by equality, gendered influences can create significant imbalances that can play out in such issues as access to money, availability of free time, distribution of childcare and housework, and decision-making. Schwartz (1994) first described the phenomenon of *near peers,* who are couples who state that they aspire to an egalitarian peerage, but who are to some extent living more traditional roles which constrain the balancing of power. Housework and childcare distribution are sometimes markers for the extent to which a couple has achieved a "partnership of equals" (Pinsof et al., 2018). Although there is some evidence that more couples in the United States share housework than in past generations (Carlson et al., 2016), most couples seem to take a more conventional approach to labor division, and household labor contributions remain unequal (U.S. Bureau of Labor Statistics, 2019; Daminger, 2020), with about half of respondents in one study reporting that women do most of the routine housework (Carlson et al., 2016). A similar disparity is found in childcare as mothers on average spend almost twice the time as fathers caring for and helping children (Bureau of Labor Statistics, 2020). The disparity in household labor and childcare surely must have increased during the pandemic as children were home for remote learning and an alarming 80% of the 1.1 million people who exited the workforce through September of 2020 were women (U.S. Bureau of Labor Statistics, 2019).

With the arrival of a first child, couples face decisions about childcare and income generation. The couple's responsibilities increase exponentially, and degrees of freedom are reduced correspondingly. Whatever decisions are made with respect to roles, gendered inequity can result if a woman's share of the housework or childcare begins to constrain equity in access to money, resources, free time, or decision-making. Research on the satisfaction of partners strongly supports egalitarian partnerships (Rampage, 2002; Carlson et al., 2016). A sense of fairness (Carlson et al., 2016) contributes to satisfaction and induces flexibility in problem-solving. Couple therapy often facilitates a journey toward gender equity in terms of the benefits, burdens, and responsibilities of family life. For some couples, this journey is relatively uncomplicated, but for other couples, steeped in the lore of a traditional relationship, the journey can be challenging in part because such substantial changes, especially later in life, are harder to make, and the past can be steeped in resentments that are not easily forgiven. Sometimes the journey ends in divorce, the rate of which for couples who are over 50 years old has doubled in less than 30 years (Lin et al., 2018; Brown & Lin, 2012). Even in divorce, however, couples can work to modify problem sequences or accept intractable constraints with the goal of improving adaptation for themselves and their children.

Biology

Biology pervades all client systems, yet therapists may miss its significance for therapy, particularly how biological constraints can block the implementation of a solution sequence. They may consider it to be the province of medicine and thus cleave it from their view of the client system. Mind/body dualism also leads us to split off the mind from the body. Still, there are very few client systems where there are no biological constraints. Of course, as with all constraints, a biological constraint becomes relevant in therapy when it impedes the problem-solving process.

Illness and Injury

Constraints associated with illness have a profound impact on not just the person with the illness but also on other members of the client system. For example, adult children providing care for their parents with Alzheimer's spend endless hours providing the care while also attending to both their jobs and their family life. The quality of their partnerships or other adult relationships suffers as does the parenting of their own children. People in this situation have been referred to as the "sandwich generation," that is, caught between the needs of their aging parents and that of their adolescent children.

If a child in a family has a chronic illness, the parents must provide the level of support needed to maintain the child's health and support optimal development. Since the children who are well usually receive less attention, the consequence is that sometimes one or more of them feel neglected or even abandoned. For example, a 15-year-old boy's grades show a gradual decline. The parents first try to structure his homework time, but the grades continue to deteriorate. In a family therapy session, the therapist asked the student what keeps him from using the homework tools his parents have provided. He finally opens up and says he is on his own because his parents must spend so much of their time attending to the illness of his younger sister. When the parents acknowledge his experience and begin to have a more hands-on approach to helping with his homework, his grades begin to improve.

Most therapists are not physicians, so they cannot prescribe treatments for medical issues. But the ability of a therapist to recognize the negative impact of biology on the client system sometimes provides the client system with the first message that a biological constraint must be addressed. Many individuals neglect their physical health. They forego their annual physicals for years and ignore symptoms of illnesses such as diabetes, often out of fear of what the symptoms might mean. For example, a client complained of being fatigued, discouraged, and unmotivated. The therapist could attribute these symptoms to depression and/or lifestyle issues such as insufficient sleep. But fatigue can also be a symptom of an underlying illness. The therapist explored with the client the importance of ruling out physical causes of the fatigue. The client saw the doctor, underwent testing, and returned to the next session with the report that she had been diagnosed with lymphoma. The referral led to early diagnosis and treatment which was beneficial for the client's health.

Therapists can also intervene in the interactional processes surrounding health issues. Individuals in partnerships may know little or nothing about each other's health. When one of them goes to the doctor, any health-related issues that arise are not shared with their partner. At some point in the aging process, the partners will need each other's help and care. Therapists can change this pattern by emphasizing the importance of sharing health information throughout the life cycle.

Illnesses can be acute, chronic, or recurrent (Rolland, 1994, 2019), and each form of illness presents unique constraints. The timing of an acute illness can abruptly interrupt attempts to implement a solution sequence. For example, a father has a heart attack just when he is trying to get more engaged with his estranged children. Chronic illness drains the energy of both the ill family member and the members providing care. Respite is one tool to consider in these situations. Finally, a recurrent illness has exacerbations that constitute S3s that can interrupt the progress clients have made to implement adaptive patterns of interaction and functioning. The effect of this ebb and flow sequence may be unknown to the therapist at the beginning of therapy and only appear as a constraint when the illness recurs and impacts the progress of the therapy.

In dealing with illness, therapists can draw on the principles of Medical Family Therapy (Doherty et al., 1994; McDaniel et al., 2014) which takes a systemic approach that supports collaboration among providers, clear communication and partnership between patient families and providers, and assistance to families coping with the impact of illness on their lives and relationships. A central tenet of this approach is that psychosocial problems have biological features and medical problems have psychosocial features (McDaniel et al., 1992). This fits with IST's concept of the multi-level biopsychosocial system within which all problems in living are embedded.

Like illness, injury can be the reason a client initiates therapy or it can create constraints that can keep a client from achieving their goals in therapy. Sometimes it is an old injury, for instance from a car accident, that has created residues of PTSD or permanent disability. At other times, it is a recent injury that limits the mobility of a client and/or forces the client to have an operation such as a knee or back surgery that impacts both the mobility and morale of the client.

Neurobiological Constraints

The brain obviously plays a significant role in human behavior. Neurobiological patterns are associated with presenting problems and constraints such as anxiety, depression, and relational distress. In IST, unless a compelling hypothesis overrides this, the therapist begins to address these factors by proposing changes in patterns of action or by seeking to modify meanings (cognitions, beliefs, or narratives) and/or emotional process. Exercise, mindfulness, distress tolerance, or a new view of a situation can impact the neurobiological aspects of behavior and experience. Interpersonal neurobiological constraints have been identified in the relationships of couples (Fishbane, 2007, 2013). Automatic emotional reactions accompanied by physiological arousal can significantly constrain their interaction patterns. Fortunately, partners can work in therapy to pause, calm themselves, reappraise situations, and seek to attune to their partner.

Neurobiological constraints that respond to psychotropic medication are an aspect of biology often encountered by therapists. These neurobiological factors, often bearing psychiatric diagnoses, are viewed in IST not as the cause of the problem, but as one of the constraints keeping the problem from being solved. Medication can be viewed as one of the solution sequences. For example, a 50-year-old cisgender woman sought therapy for depression. It soon became clear that her depression was derivative of her isolation that stemmed from the demands on her time to care for her elderly mother. The woman had an older brother who rarely participated in the mother's care. The therapist hypothesized that a possible solution sequence would be for the two siblings to share the mother's care. When asked if the client had spoken to the brother in the hopes of achieving a more equitable balance of caregiving, she said she could not talk to her brother about it. The conversation occurred as follows.

Therapist: I think your life, and probably your depression, would improve if you and your brother shared the caregiving duties more equitably. What do you think would happen if you did talk to him?

Client: I can feel myself almost having a panic attack just thinking about that conversation.

Therapist: Do you get that panicky feeling talking to people besides your brother?

Client: Yes, if the subject is at all controversial, I get very anxious.

Therapist: So, can we think about this anxiety as a constraint that keeps you from having difficult conversations, and that includes the conversation with your brother?

Client: Yes, you could say that.

The therapist proceeded to discuss social anxiety and gave the woman a screening test for anxiety. She scored high. After five sessions of working behaviorally on the elevated level of anxiety, the therapist suggested that the woman schedule an appointment with a psychiatrist for a medication evaluation. The psychiatrist prescribed an antidepressant medication, and the therapist used some strategies borrowed from cognitive behavior therapy to strengthen the woman's assertiveness. Not long thereafter, the woman did talk with her brother and the conversation was constructive, resulting in the two siblings making plans to share in the mother's care.

Additional Biological Issues

Other biological issues include addictions, aging, hormones, and genetics (Rolland & Williams, 2005). Many clients are challenged by substance dependence or addictions that constrain their ability to participate in so-lution sequences. Often, the addiction itself is the presenting problem. When addiction is part of the problem sequence but not the presenting problem, there is often controversy among clients about the severity and impact of substance use on the problem sequence. In this instance, the therapist must be mindful of not damaging alliances when factoring sub-stance use into the solution sequence. For example, a young man living in his parents' basement and struggling to launch smokes cannabis daily. If the solution sequence includes getting a job, cannabis use might be a constraint. The parents contend that cannabis use is a major constraint, but their son disagrees. Here, the therapist may need to evoke the stages of change model (Prochaska & DiClemente, 1984) and view the young man in a pre-contemplative stage of change. At this point, the therapy may shift to some individual sessions with him to provide him with the opportunity to contemplate the impact of his usage and explore other factors that may be keeping him from getting a job.

Aging is a biological and psychological process. Life-span development often emphasizes the latter, but IST therapists are also interested in the biological aspects of aging. For example, a white, cisgender, mixed-sex couple in their late 50s present with concerns about diminished sexual interest. Both would like to improve their sex life but admit that part of the problem sequence is their pattern of avoiding sexual activity. The experiment with a solution sequence involves sensate focus exercises twice a week. When they return, they have not done the exercise. When asked what kept them from doing the exercise, they report that they have never even discussed sex, so the exercise seemed too scary to them. The solution sequence shifts to helping them talk about sex. When they try, it becomes clear that this communication constraint also contains a knowledge gap between them. The woman, who is post-menopausal, has never even told her partner that she has gone through menopause and avoids sex because of post-menopausal vaginal dryness. The male partner also confesses that he is afraid he will not get an erection so he, too, avoids sex. When these issues of aging are acknowledged and discussed, the couple agrees to return to the sensate focus exercises.

Therapists frequently overlook the crucial role of hormones in the lives of their clients. A suboptimal level of hormones (too little or too much) impacts physical health and one's sense of wellbeing. This can occur during times of transition such as adolescence, pregnancy, menopause, andropause, illness, and moving into later stages of life. Therapists do not prescribe or advise about issues related to hormones, but can suggest that clients talk with their doctor about addressing possible hormonal constraints.

Finally, the field of genetics is continuing to develop data about the impact of genes on health, including the genetic predispositions to certain diseases such as breast cancer (Turnbull & Rahman, 2008), the chances of becoming an alcoholic (McGue, 1999; Dick & Foroud, 2003), or the risk that a child may develop a mental illness (Insel, 2009; Insel & Wang, 2010). Miller et al. (2006) provide a comprehensive, biopsychosocial perspective on the impact of the field of genetics on individuals, couples, and families. As would be expected, this impact is evident in cases seen in therapy. For example, a white, cisgender mixed-sex couple seeks therapy for a presenting problem of being unable to decide whether to have a child. They avoid talking about the issues because the male partner is more ambivalent. They agree to a solution sequence where they will make a list of their pros and cons. When they next attend a session and show the list to the therapist, the male partner's list includes the fact that his mother is bipolar, and he does not want to pass that gene on to any child they might have. Knowing that the research supporting the diathesis-stress model (Hooley & Gotlib, 2000) emphasizes the interaction of both genetic and environmental factors in the development of mental illness, the therapist suggests that the couple obtain a genetic consultation regarding the matter. Making the referral keeps the therapist in a neutral, supportive position on an emotionally charged issue that might be clarified by expertise that is outside the scope of the therapist's practice. Following the genetic consultation, the couple decides not to conceive a child but to keep adoption as an option.

Spirituality

Spirituality is designated as a hypothesizing metaframework because it is the worldview through which many clients make meaning of their lives. Spirituality consists of "transcendent beliefs and practices within or outside formal religion" (Walsh, 2009, p. 3). In both cases, there is a sense of something beyond the material world of existence that is often described as a higher power or God. There is a sense of connectedness to something greater than oneself. Spirituality is a source of strength in the lives of many people. It can also be involved in ways that constrain the person or family. For example, a Jamaican American woman presented with depression. She reported that the depression worsens when she ruminates about losing her relationship with one of her adult children following a divorce years earlier. When asked if she wanted to find the child, she initially indicated that she did and agreed to googling the name of the child as a first step. In the next session, she reported that she did not do the search. When asked what kept her from doing the search, she replied that the spirits would bring the child back into her life if it were ordained that a reunion should occur. She had received no sign one way or another; therefore, she decided that she had to be patient and wait for a sign. The therapist then understood that to develop culturally appropriate solution sequences, the therapy would need to proceed within the client's spiritual frame of reference.

Managing Multiple Constraints

In the foregoing discussion of identifying constraints, the hypothesizing metaframeworks have been discussed one at a time which may suggest that there is just one constraint that prevents a successful implementation of the solution sequence. This scenario rarely occurs. Rather, the exploration of constraints more often reveals multiple constraints and sometimes a cascade of interlocking constraints that are progressively revealed as the therapist attempts to lift the original and subsequently revealed constraints. The therapist must, therefore, have a way to identify multiple constraints. This is facilitated by the therapist's growing knowledge about the hypothesizing metaframeworks, the skillful use of the constraint questions, and careful attention to client feedback including their reports, narratives, nonverbal communications, and interaction patterns. All the constraints can be mapped onto the *IST web of human experience*.

Each client will have a unique way of experiencing these constraints and will have narratives to explain them and how they are related to each other. Therapists must understand the narrative of each client and reconcile these narratives so that the clients can agree on a continuing effort to lift the constraints. For example, a family came to therapy with the presenting problem of conflict over expectations set by the mother. She expected everything to be in order, and the schedule had to unfold like clockwork. When it did not, she would become angry, and emotional outbursts among family members were common. The two teenagers and the father were exhausted trying to keep up with her demands and deal with her wrath. This constituted the problem sequence. When asked what kept her from modifying her expectations, she reported that she was born and raised in a European country, and that her family of origin was wealthy. Her father had been a perfectionist and constantly preached that to perform below the highest standards meant that a person was defective. She was a dedicated mother and wanted her children to succeed, so she believed she would be failing them were she to relax her standards. Regarding her husband, she believed he needed to adopt her values and standards so the parental messaging would be consistent. When she did get after him for falling short of perfection, she saw it as a "teaching moment" for him.

Thus, the mother's narrative of perfectionism was established. Over the course of several months, the therapist staged a series of sessions, meeting alone with the mother, with the couple, and with the whole family. These conversations were framed as discussions about the relative merits of personal perfection vs. family harmony. The couple came to realize how their marital closeness was compromised by sequences where the husband felt demeaned and consequently distanced himself from his wife. The children confessed that they often stayed away from the house or in their rooms rather than risk being caught in a moment of perfectionism. Gradually, the mother recognized that her parents' rigidity did come at a cost to family harmony, and that she had not had a happy childhood. Over time, the family agreed that there was a place for standards of performance, but it was more important to be happy as individuals and close as a group, than to be perfect. The mother committed to work in individual therapy on her perfectionism.

Conclusion

Therapists immersed in IST have made the ontological leap to conceptualize cases using the theory of constraints. For them, therapy is never repetitious because there is an infinite variety of ways that constraints can exist and interlock and keep a system from solving its problems. Therapists new to IST must make the conceptual leap to operate with the constraint pillar. Having done so, for some period, they will still need to practice asking themselves, "I wonder what is keeping them from...?" The information about what the constraint is and where within the biopsychosocial system it is located is embodied in the web of human experience (see Figure 1.4 in Chapter 1). Experience will often help the therapist identify the constraints, but a careful reading of client feedback is always the place to look for clues that help unlock the mystery of the system.

Exercises

1   Think about a solution sequence you are trying to enact in your personal life. Notice that it is not so easy to enact it. Ask yourself what keeps you from enacting it on a regular basis. Try to conceptualize your constraints with one or more of the hypothesizing metaframeworks.
2   Consider a case you are currently seeing. Craft a constraint question and ask it in session. Review the video recording of the session and imagine how you would feel if you were asked that question in the

tone it was asked. Consider whether you would modify your tone and delivery.

3 Consider a case you are currently seeing. Craft a constraint question and ask it in session. After the session, write down the client's response. What does that response tell you about the constraints? Do the clients' responses lead you to new hypotheses? If so, what are your thoughts? Considering the clients' responses, how do you feel the alliance was impacted by the question?

4 For a case you know well, construct a set of constraints that appear to keep or have kept the client(s) from solving their presenting problem. Consider at least four constraints in your formulation. Use the web of human experience to locate which constraints occur at what levels of the system.

References

Bateson, G. (1972). *Steps to an ecology of mind: Collected essays in anthropology, psychiatry, evolution, and epistemology.* Jason Aronson, Inc.

Bischoff, R. J., Springer, P. R., & Taylor, N. (2016). Global mental health in action: Reducing disparities one community at a time. *Journal of Marital and Family Therapy, 43*(2), 276–290. 10.1111/jmft.12202

Bowlby, J. (1979). The Bowlby-Ainsworth attachment theory. *The Behavioral and Brain Sciences, 2*(4), 637–638. 10.1017/S0140525X00064955

Breunlin, D. C. (1988). Oscillation theory and family development. *Family transitions, continuity and change over the life cycle*, 133–158. Guilford.

Breunlin, D. C. (1989). Clinical implications of oscillation theory: Family development and the process of change. In C. Ramsey (Ed.), *The science of family medicine* (pp. 135–149). Guilford.

Breunlin, D. C., Schwartz, R. C., & Mac Kune-Karrer, B. M. (1992). *Metaframeworks: Transcending the models of family therapy.* Jossey-Bass.

Breunlin, D. C., Schwartz, R. C., & Mac Kune-Karrer, B. M. (1997). *Metaframeworks: Transcending the models of family therapy.* Revised and Updated. Jossey-Bass.

Breunlin, D. C., Pinsof, W. M., Russell, W. P., & Lebow, J. L. (2011) Integrative problem centered metaframeworks (IPCM) therapy I: Core concepts and hypothesizing. *Family Process, 50*(3), 293–313. 10.1111/j.1545-5300.2011.01362.x

Brown, S. L., & Lin, I. F. (2012). The gray divorce revolution: Rising divorce among middle-aged and older adults. *Journals of Gerontology, 67*(6), 731–741.

Budge, S. L., Adelson, J. L., & Howard, K. A. S. (2013). Anxiety and depression in transgender individuals: The roles of transition status, loss, social support, and coping. *Journal of Consulting and Clinical Psychology, 81*(3), 545–557. 10.1037/a0031774

Burn, K., & Szoeke, C. (2016). Boomerang families and failure-to-launch: Commentary on adult children living at home. *Maturitas, 84*, 9–12. 10.1016/j.maturitas.2015.09.004

Carlson, D. L., Miller, A. J., Sassler, S., & Hanson, S. (2016). The gendered division of housework and couples' sexual relationships: A reexamination. *Journal of Marriage and Family, 78*(4), 975–995. 10.1111/jomf.12313

Centers for Disease Control and Prevention. (2020). *Coronavirus disease 2019 (COVID-19)-associated hospitalization surveillance network (COVID-NET).* U. S. Department of Health and Human Services. https://www.cdc.gov/coronavirus/2019-ncov/covid-data/covid-net/purpose-methods.html

Centers for Disease Control and Prevention. (2021). *Deaths involving coronavirus disease 2019 (COVID-19) by race and Hispanic origin group and age, by state.* U. S. Department of Health and Human Services. https://data.cdc.gov/NCHS/Deaths-involving-coronavirus-disease-2019-COVID-19/ks3g-spdg

Chun, K. M., & Akutsu, P. D. (2003). Acculturation among ethnic minority families. In K. M. Chun, P. Balls Organista, & G. Marin (Eds.), *Acculturation: Advances in theory, measurement, and applied research* (pp. 95–119). American Psychological Association. https://doi-org.turing.library.northwestern.edu/10.1037/10472-008

Cole, E. R. (2009). Intersectionality and research in psychology. *American psychologist, 64*(3), 170. 10.1037/a0014564

Crenshaw, K. (1989). Demarginalizing the intersection of race and sex: A black feminist critique of antidiscrimination doctrine, feminist theory and antiracist politics.

Daminger, A. (2020). De-gendered processes, gendered outcomes: How egalitarian couples make sense of non-egalitarian household practices. *American Sociological Review, 85*(5), 806–829. 10.1177/0003122420950208

Diamond, G. S., Diamond, G. M., & Levy, S. A. (2014). *Attachment-based family therapy for depressed adolescents* (1st ed.). American Psychological Association.

Dick, D. M., & Foroud, T. (2003). Candidate genes for alcohol dependence: A review of genetic evidence from human studies. *Alcoholism: Clinical and Experimental Research, 27*(5), 868–879. 10.1097/01.ALC.0000065436.24221.63

Doherty, W. J., McDaniel, S. H., & Hepworth, J. (1994). Medical family therapy: An emerging arena for family therapy. *Journal of Family Therapy, 16*(1), 31–46. 10.1111/j.1467-6427.1994.00775.x

Duvall, E. M. (1957). *Family development.* J. P. Lippincott.

Esmiol, E. E., Knudson-Martin, C., & Delgado, S. (2012). Developing a contextual consciousness: Learning to address gender, societal power, and culture in clinical practice. *Journal of Marital and Family Therapy, 38*(4), 573–588. 10.1111/j.1752-0606.2011.00232.x

Falicov, C. J. (2015). The multiculturalism and diversity of families. In T. L. Sexton, & J. Lebow (Eds.), *Handbook of family therapy* (pp. 102–129). Routledge.

Fishbane, M. D. (2007). Wired to connect: Neuroscience, relationships, and therapy. *Family Process, 46*, 395– 412.

Fishbane, M. D. (2013). *Loving with the brain in mind: Neurobiology and couple therapy.* Norton.

Fishman, H. C. (2013). *Intensive structural therapy: Treating families in their social context.* Basic Books. (Original work published 1993).

Goldner, V. (1988). Generation and gender: Normative and covert hierarchies. *Family Process, 27*, 17–31. 10.1111/j.1545-5300.1988.00017.x

Gottman, J. M. (1993). The roles of conflict engagement, escalation, and avoidance in marital interaction: a longitudinal view of five types of couples. *Journal of Consulting and Clinical Psychology, 61*(1), 6–15. 10.1037/0022-006X.61.1.6

Hadley, T. R., Jacob, T., Milliones, J., Caplan, J., & Spitz, D. (1974). The relationship between family developmental crisis and the appearance of symptoms in a family member. *Family Process, 13*(2), 207–214. 10.1111/j.1545-5300. 1974.00207.x

Haley, J. (1976). *Problem-solving therapy*. Jossey-Bass.

Haley, J. (1981). *Reflections on therapy and other essays*. Family Therapy Institute of Washington, D.C.

Hare-Mustin, R. T. (1978). A feminist approach to family therapy. *Family Process, 17*(2), 181–194.

Hernandez, P., Almeida, R., & Dolan-Del Vecchio, K. (2005). Critical consciousness, accountability, and empowerment: Key processes for helping families heal. *Family Process, 44*(1), 105–119. 10.1111/j.1545-5300.2005.00045.x

Hooley, J. M., & Gotlib, I. H. (2000). A diathesis-stress conceptualization of expressed emotion and clinical outcome. *Applied and Preventive Psychology, 9*, 135–152.

Insel T. R. (2009). Disruptive insights in psychiatry: Transforming a clinical discipline. *The Journal of Clinical Investigation, 119*(4), 700–705. 10.1172/JCI38832

Insel, T. R., & Wang, P. S. (2010). Rethinking mental illness. *Journal of the American Medical Association, 303*(19), 1970–1971. 10.1001/jama.2010.555

Kelly, S., Jérémie-Brink, G., Chambers, A. L., & Smith-Bynum, M. A. (2020). The Black Lives Matter movement: A call to action for couple and family therapists. *Family Process, 59*(4), 1353–1957. 10.1111/famp.12614

Kendler, K. S. (2013). What psychiatric genetics has taught us about the nature of psychiatric illness and what is left to learn. *Molecular psychiatry, 18*(10), 1058–1066.

Kernberg, O. F. (1976). *Object relations theory and clinical psychoanalysis*. Norton.

Kohlenberg, R. J., & Tsai, M. (2007). *Functional analytic psychotherapy: Creating intense and curative therapeutic relationships*. Springer.

Kohut, H. (1977). *The restoration of the self*. International Universities Press.

Kohut, H. (1984). *How does analysis cure?* The University of Chicago Press. 10.7208/chicago/9780226006147.001.0001

Krause, I. (ed.). (2012). *Culture and reflexivity in systemic psychotherapy: Mutual perspectives*. Routledge.

Lin, I. F., Brown, S. L., & Wright, M. R. (2018). Antecedents of gray divorce: A life course perspective. *Journals of Gerontology, 13*, 1022–1031.

Linehan, M. M. (2014). *DBT training manual*. The Guilford Press.

Madanes, C. (1981). *Strategic family therapy*. Jossey-Bass.

McDaniel, S. H., Doherty, W. J., & Hepworth, J. (2014). *Medical family therapy and integrated care* (2nd Ed.). American Psychological Association.

McDaniel, S. H., Hepworth, J., & Doherty, W. J. (1992). *Medical family therapy: A biopsychosocial approach to families with health problems*. Basic Books.

McDowell, T. (2005). Practicing with a critical multicultural lens. *Journal of Systemic Therapies*, *24*(1), 1–4. 10.1521/jsyt.2005.24.1.1

McGeorge, C. R., Coburn, K. O., & Walsdorf, A. A. (2021). Deconstructing cissexism: The journey of becoming an affirmative family therapist for transgender and nonbinary clients. *Journal of Marital and Family Therapy*, *47*, 785–802. 10.1111/jmft.12481.

McGoldrick, M., & Hardy, K. V. (2008). Introduction: Revisioning family therapy from a multicultural perspective. In M. McGoldrick, & K. V. Hardy (Eds.), *Re-visioning family therapy: Race, culture, and gender in clinical practice* (2nd ed., pp. 3–24). Guilford Press.

McGoldrick, M., Petro, N. G., & Carter, B. A. (2016). *The expanding family life cycle: Individual, family, and social perspectives* (5th ed.). Pearson.

McGue, M. (1999). The behavioral genetics of alcoholism. *Current Directions in Psychological Science*, *8*(4), 109–115. 10.1111/1467-8721.00026

McGuffin, P., & Murray, R. (2013). *The new genetics of mental illness*. Butterworth-Heinemann.

Miller, S., McDaniel, S. H., Rolland, J., & Feetham, S. (Eds.) (2006). *Individuals, families, and the new era of genetics: Biopsychosocial perspectives*. Norton.

Minuchin, S. (1974). *Families and family therapy*. Harvard University Press.

Minuchin, S., & Fishman, H. C. (1981). *Family therapy techniques*. Harvard University Press.

Otters, R. K., & Hollander, J. F. (2015). Leaving home and boomerang decisions: A family simulation protocol. *Marriage & Family Review*, *51*(1), 39–58, 10.1080/01494929.2014.963276

Patterson, J. E., Edwards, T. M., & Vakili, S. (2017). Global mental health: A call for increased awareness and action for family therapists. *Family Process*, *57*(1), 70–82. 10.1111/famp.12281

Pinsof, W., Breunlin, D., Russell, W., Lebow, J., Rampage, C., & Chambers, A. (2018). *Integrative systemic therapy: Metaframeworks for problem solving with individuals, couples, and families* (1st ed.). American Psychological Association. 10.1037/0000055-000

Prochaska, J. O., & DiClemente, C. C. (1984). *The transtheoretical approach: Crossing traditional boundaries of therapy*. Dow/Jones Irwin.

Rampage, C. (2002). Marriage in the 20th century: A feminist perspective. *Family Process*, *41*(2), 261–268. 10.1111/j.1545-5300.2002.41205.x

Rastogi, M. (2020). A systemic conceptualization of interventions with families in a global context. In K. S. Wampler, M. Rastogi, & R. Singh (Eds.), *The handbook of systemic family therapy*. Wiley. 10.1002/9781119438519.ch83

Rastogi, M., & Thomas, V. (Eds.). (2009). *Multicultural couple therapy*. Sage.

Rolland, J. S. (1994). *Families, illness and disability: A bio-psychosocial intervention model*. Perseus.

Rolland, J. (2019). The family, chronic illness, and disability: An integrated practice model. In B. H. Fiese, M. Celano, K. Deater-Deckard, E. N. Jouriles, & M. A. Wishman (Eds.), *APA handbook of contemporary family psychology: Applications and broad impact of family psychology* (pp. 85–102). American Psychological Association. 10.1037/0000100-006

Rolland, J. S., & Williams, K. W. (2005). Toward a biopsychosocial model for 21st century genetics. *Family Process*, *44*(1), 3–24. 10.1111/j.1545-5300.2005.00039.x

Schwartz, P. (1994). *Love between equals: How peer marriage really works*. The Free Press.

Schwartz, R. (2013). *Evolution of the internal family systems model*. Center for Self Leadership.

Seedall, R. B., Holtrop, K., & Parra-Cardona, J. R. (2014). Diversity, social justice and intersectionality trends in C/MFT: A content analysis of three family therapy journals, 2004-2011. *Journal of Marital and Family Therapy*, *40*(2), 139–151. 10.1111/jmft.12015

Simon-Rusinowitz, L., Wilson, L., Marks, L., Krach, C., & Welch, C. (1998). Reconfiguring retirement for baby boomers. *Journal of Mental Health Counseling*, *15*, 106–116.

Singh, A. A., & dickey, L. (2017). Affirmative counseling and psychological practice with transgender and gender nonconforming clients. In K. A. DeBord, A. R. Fischer, K. J. Bieshke, & R. M. Perez (Eds.), *Handbook of sexual orientation and gender diversity in counseling and psychotherapy* (pp. 157–182). American Psychological Association.

Stotzer, R. L. (2009). Violence against transgender people: A review of the United States. *Aggression and Violent Behavior*, *14*(3), 170–179. 10.1016/j.avb.2009.01.006

Toomey, R. B., Syvertsen, A. K., & Shramko, M. (2018). Transgender adolescent suicide behavior. *Pediatrics*, *142*(4). 10.1542/peds.2017-4218

Turnbull, C., & Rahman, N. (2008). Genetic predisposition to breast cancer: Past, present, and future. *Annual Review of Genomics and Human Genetics*, *9*, 321–345. 10.1146/annurev.genom.9.081307.164339

U.S. Bureau of Labor Statistics. (2019, April 20). Average hours per day parents spent caring for and helping household children as their main activity. Retrieved April 20, 2021, from https://www.bls.gov/charts/american-time-use/activity-by-parent.htm

Walsh, F. (2009). Religion, spirituality and the family: Multifaith perspectives. In F. Walsh (Eds.), *Spiritual resources in family therapy* (2nd ed., pp. 3–30). Guilford Press.

Watts-Jones, D. (2010). Location of self: Opening the door to dialogue on intersectionality in the therapy process. *Family Process*, *49*(3), 405–420. 10.1111/j.1545-5300.2010.01330.x

White, M. (1986). Negative explanation, restraint, and double description: A template for family therapy. *Family process*, *25*(2), 169–184. 10.1111/j.1545-5300.1986.00169.x

Wynne, L. C. (1984). The epigenesis of relational systems: A model for understanding family development. *Family Process*, *23*(3), 297–318. 10.1111/j.1545-5300.1984.00297.x

Chapter 8

Integrating Interventions to Address Constraints

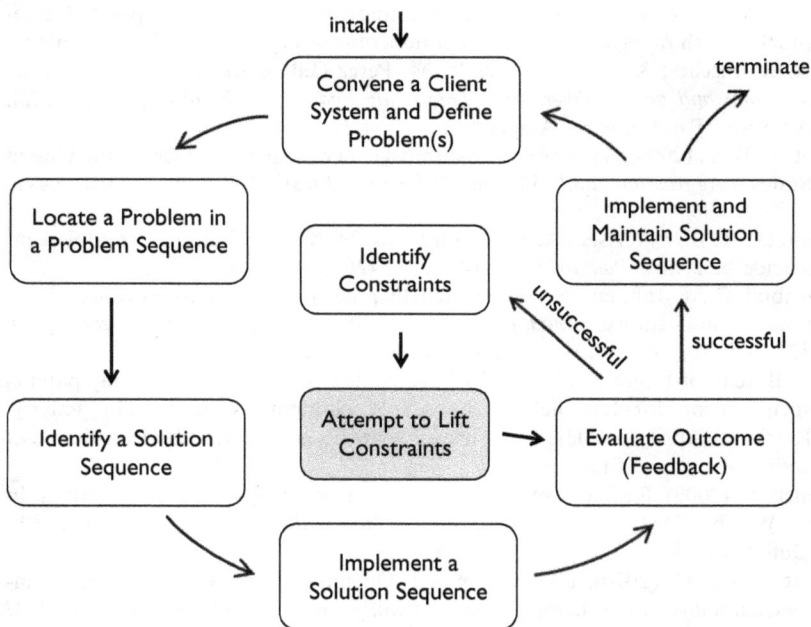

intake ↓

```
        Convene a Client                              terminate
        System and Define  ←                    ↗
           Problem(s)

Locate a Problem in                    Implement and
a Problem Sequence          Identify   Maintain Solution
                          Constraints     Sequence

                                      unsuccessful    successful ↑

Identify a Solution      Attempt to Lift  →  Evaluate Outcome
   Sequence               Constraints         (Feedback)

              Implement a
            Solution Sequence
```

IST Essence Diagram.

Objective

The objective of this chapter is to describe the essence step of selecting and applying strategies and interventions to address or remove constraints to solution sequences. The selection of strategies follows the IST guidelines for intervention represented on the IST matrix with an understanding that the prescribed progression may need to be modified in the face of a compelling hypothesis or a significant alliance issue. It is beyond the scope of this book (or any book) to describe all the strategies

DOI: 10.4324/9780429322273-8

and their related interventions in detail. This chapter outlines the process of selecting strategies, gives examples of interventions, and provides an extensive, but not exhaustive, list of IST strategies along with references for them.

Introduction

IST encourages therapists to focus the therapy on defining and modifying sequences of interaction that IST calls problem sequences. As solution sequences are agreed upon, the therapist works to help the family experiment with them and reads the feedback from the experiments to recognize their success or identify constraints to their implementation. Chapter 7 discussed in detail the process of identifying constraints. IST therapists begin by privileging hypotheses about constraints that are addressed by strategies that utilize more direct, less complex interventions. These interventions focus on here-and-now changes in clients' patterns of behavior and interaction. These initially preferred strategies may also involve modification of patterns of thinking and feeling. If various straightforward interventions fail to modify the constraints, the therapist begins to hypothesize about constraints related to biological factors or to the client's past experiences that constrain differentiation from the family of origin or are represented in the structure of a client's mind. Thus, IST provides guidelines for how to begin and progress with therapy. These guidelines are flexibly applied in that compelling hypotheses or strong client preferences may require a modification of the preferred order of intervention.

IST distinguishes strategies and interventions. Strategies state a general direction for solving a problem or removing a constraint. Interventions are specific ways of accomplishing the strategies. The strategies available to an IST therapist are limitless. They include any strategy currently in use by therapists and any strategy yet to be developed. The limitations on the selection of a strategy include whether it fits with the hypothesis about a constraint, is mindful of the IST guidelines, is considerate of the collaborative alliance, and is ethical. A strategy can be accomplished with multiple interventions. IST therapists choose interventions they have learned that fit the patterns of behavior and the needs of their clients. Further, if there are empirical findings for the efficacy or effectiveness of a certain intervention, that intervention is preferred to those without empirical support. Learning to practice IST includes learning both interventions and how interventions are applied within IST.

The IST Matrix (see Figure 1.5 in Chapter 1) depicts the way strategies are categorized, organized, and sequenced in therapy. The categories of strategies are called planning metaframeworks, and each of them contains strategies that share a common focus for problem resolution. For example, the action planning metaframework focuses on strategies that involve changing clients' patterns of action and interaction. Categorized by planning metaframework, a list of strategies, and associated intervention resources, are found in Appendix A. Though the list is not meant to be a complete list of all strategies used in IST, it does include a reasonably comprehensive set of strategies for each metaframework. Neither this chapter nor this book as a whole purport to explain all the strategies and interventions that can be accessed in IST. Rather, the intention is to clarify and illustrate the process by which interventions are integrated.

Once a strategy is identified, the therapist will need to choose an intervention that will fulfill the general strategy. General strategies for modifying constraints, however, can be accomplished by means of various interventions. For example, the meaning/emotion strategy of accessing contextually adaptive thoughts might lead to an intervention of circular questioning (Tomm, 1987), motivational interviewing (Miller & Rollnick, 2012), or externalizing the problem (White & Epston, 2004). The choice of intervention depends on the specific needs of the clients, their worldview, and therapist training. Interventions used to address constraints can vary from simple and readily applied interventions, such as reframing or referral for evaluation for psychotropic medication, to more complex modules of intervention, such as a formal exposure protocol or the application of an internal family systems therapy protocol. In IST, these interventions are imported into the work and utilized according to the collaborative process of the blueprint for therapy (see Figure 1.3). In other words, the IST therapist uses the intervention without having an ongoing commitment to seeing their work through the lens of the model from which the intervention came. So, an IST therapist, with proper training, can adopt an exposure protocol without becoming a cognitive-behavioral therapist or utilize an internal family systems (IFS) intervention without becoming an IFS therapist.

The therapist or supervisor (when the therapist is in training) must decide whether the therapist is adequately prepared to apply a particular intervention (Russell & Breunlin, 2019). Sometimes preparation can be as simple as reading about it and then discussing it in supervision or being taught a technique in supervision or class and role-playing it. Other times, more formalized training is required to perform the intervention. IST therapists embark on a career-long journey to attend workshops and training sessions and learn new interventions that can be integrated into their work. IST is not a therapy model or a treatment with a specific and limited set of interventions. It is an open system of ideas for organizing and systematically integrating the extant knowledge about individual, couple, and family therapy to fit the needs of each unique client system that presents for therapy.

Method

Modifying Who is in the Direct Client System

As a constraint is identified, the therapist begins to think about how to address it. The first consideration is who needs to attend therapy to address the constraint (direct client system). This may be the same direct client system as is currently attending therapy, or the approach to the constraint may require the attendance of other system members. For example, parents and three elementary-age children attend therapy that has been focused on emotion regulation and reducing conflict in the family. As the parents describe their attempts to establish new patterns in the household, the therapist learns that the kids spend time each week with their paternal grandmother who tends to react with high expressed emotion (hostile criticism) when the kids challenge her or have conflicts with each other. The therapist hypothesizes that the pattern of intense interaction with the grandmother is a likely constraint to the children learning new patterns of emotion regulation. The therapist will propose that the grandmother attends a few sessions so that they can all work together on the problem. The parents may readily agree, or they may need to discuss concerns or fears they have about this suggestion. If an agreement is reached to invite the grandmother, a plan is established. The therapist may explore questions with the clients such as who will propose it to the grandmother, what will they say, how will they respond if she is hesitant, and how will they help her feel comfortable attending the first session.

With the exceptions of physical or emotional safety or client refusal, it is recommended that the therapist convenes all those who are involved in the problem sequences and/or constraints. When this is not appropriate or possible, the therapist keeps the missing members of the family in mind and works with those who will attend the sessions. It is important not to communicate about the missing members in a judgmental manner. Clients are encouraged to manage their disappointment about other members without the added judgment of the therapists for the following reasons. First, the clients may have a deep loyalty to the missing members despite their disappointment, so in some cases, the alliance can be damaged by the therapist's judgment of the member not being present. Second, preliminary research suggests that how an important family member not attending the therapy feels about the therapy may be related to the rate and course of change (Schielke, 2013). It makes sense that when a client attending therapy (direct system client) says to the member not in therapy (indirect client system member) something like, "My therapist said that you are not helping the situation," the person on the receiving end of that comment will not likely be positively inclined toward the therapy. Thus, the therapist will need to exercise care in what is said about members in the indirect client system.

Importantly, ambivalent family members usually feel more comfortable committing to a few sessions than to an ongoing involvement in therapy. When a new member joins the therapy, it will be necessary for the therapist to back up a bit and briefly welcome the new member and contextualize the work.

Therapist: As you may know, we have been working on finding calmer ways of dealing with communication and conflict in the family. I understand that as a grandparent you are an important source of support and influence, so I thought it would be a good idea for you to join for a few sessions. Thank you for coming. Who would like to tell grandmother a little more about what we have been working on?

The therapist now has assembled the family members whose participation is needed to modify the patterns that constrain the development of the children's emotion regulation and the family's patterns of communication.

Addressing Constraints

Intervention in IST is dependent on a shared hypothesis between the therapist and client system that some factor constrains the clients from performing a solution sequence. Chapter 7 describes the process of identifying constraints in detail. Reaching an agreement that a constraint seems to exist begs the question of what will be done about it. In most cases, it is best to first ask the clients what they think about this. They may very well have some excellent ideas on how to proceed. For example, once the grandmother joined the effort to reduce conflict and improve emotion regulation, she introduced the traditional practice of counting to ten. This was something all members were able to understand and utilize. It was practiced in session and successfully adopted by the family as one of the techniques they would use.

If the client system does not have an idea for how they will address the constraint, they may directly or indirectly be looking to the therapist for guidance. Faced with a constraint and no obvious way to address it, clients' interest in the therapist's suggestions may well be increased. The therapist needs to respect that the identification of the constraint itself or a discussion of how to address it may be a source of embarrassment or concern for the client(s). For this reason, the therapist is careful to communicate on these matters with an attitude of respectful collaboration.

Some constraints are readily addressed as the identification and subsequent discussion of them brings sufficient awareness to allow clients to bypass the constraint and perform the solution sequence. Often, though, the therapist will need to access a more formal strategy. Although the therapy, according to IST guidelines, has already been action-focused as solution sequences have been tried, the therapist may still have an additional action strategy in mind. Just as likely, constraints of meaning and/or emotion may have been identified. Strategies that involve modifying action, meaning, or emotion are all found in the upper portion of the IST planning matrix (Chapter 1, Figure 1.5). These strategies, along with those located in the biobehavioral planning metaframework, all address constraints without regard to complex models of mind or the excavation of past experiences.

Before speculating that a client is not differentiated from their family of origin or that their past experiences have skewed their internal parts or mechanisms of mind, the IST therapist draws on the planning metaframeworks in the top half of the matrix. For example, if a client has agoraphobia, the IST therapist identifies the fear and seeks a way of managing it such that the client gradually works toward spending more time farther from home. In such a case, the therapist might draw on strategies that have to do with emotion regulation (meaning/emotion planning metaframework) and exposure (action planning metaframework). The therapist does not begin intervention by excavating family of origin experiences or working to address the internal representations of these experiences. Such interventions may be necessary at a later time if the more direct, here-and-now approaches are not effective.

In addressing constraints, two of the IST guidelines are particularly important to consider. First, the IST failure-driven guideline suggests that when interventions fail to modify the constraints sufficiently to allow implementation of the solution sequence, the therapy will need to shift to other interventions. As therapy progresses, this typically involves an additional or modified hypothesis about the constraints that calls for strategies drawn from planning metaframeworks that appear lower on the matrix. Second, the alliance priority guideline suggests that establishing and maintaining the therapy alliance takes priority over the preferred order for selecting strategies depicted in the matrix unless deferring to the alliance fundamentally compromises the efficacy or integrity of the therapy.

The Planning Metaframeworks

The planning metaframeworks are listed in the IST matrix in their generally preferred order (top to bottom) of application (see Figure 1.5 in Chapter 1). Examples of strategies that are contained in each of the planning metaframeworks are found in Appendix A. These strategies and the interventions associated with them each require a level of study and training for them to be implemented. This book does not discuss all strategies and interventions. Rather, it acknowledges that there are myriad strategies, provides an extensive list of them, and supports the process of selecting interventions to fit the strategies.

Action Planning Metaframework

Strategies housed in this metaframework are aimed at helping clients modify their patterns of action and interaction. The major working hypothesis associated with this metaframework is that clients have not been able to solve their concerns due to behavioral constraints such as inertia, habits of action and interaction, or just not knowing what else to do. Constraints of meaning or emotion at this stage of intervention are not hypothesized to be strong enough to prevent a change in action. Establishing an action plan, however, does require mutual understanding between therapist and clients which occurs in the realm of meaning and emotion, but the central focus of these strategies is to initiate change through action.

The action metaframework draws strategies and interventions from social learning (Bandura, 1991), behavioral and cognitive-behavioral approaches (Barlow et al., 1989; Baucom et al., 1990; Craske, 1999; Jacobson & Margolin, 1979; Patterson et al., 1992), dialectical behavior therapy (Linehan, 2015; Linehan & Wilks, 2015), structural family therapy (Minuchin & Fishman, 1981), strategic therapy (Haley, 1987; Watzlawick et al., 1974) and solution-focused therapy (Berg, 1994). Additionally, research findings and established practices that transcend models are rich sources for strategies and interventions.

Meaning/Emotion Planning Metaframework

These strategies and their related interventions are primarily focused on modifying meaning (thoughts, beliefs, narratives) and emotion. Although meaning and emotion are present in every moment of therapy, they become the basis for a strategy when one or the other seems to constrain a client or clients from performing a solution sequence. Resting on this hypothesis, IST therapists seek to develop adaptive cognitions or narratives, heighten adaptive emotions, or regulate constraining emotions. The meaning/emotion planning metaframework includes cognitive-behavioral (Beck, 2011), integrative-behavioral (Baucom et al., 2002; Christensen et al., 1995), emotion-focused (Greenberg, 2011; Johnson, 2015), narrative (White & Epston, 1990), dialectical behavioral (Linehan, 2015; Linehan & Wilks, 2015), acceptance and commitment (Hayes et al., 1999), psychoeducational (Gottman, 2001), vulnerability cycle (Scheinkman & Fishbane, 2004), and experiential (Safran et al., 1988) strategies and interventions. The meaning/emotion strategies are organized into two categories: Those that target specific sequences of mind and those that involve a more complex system of intervention.

Biobehavioral Planning Metaframework

The strategies contained in this metaframework are designed to address the hypotheses that clients have been unable to solve their presenting problems due to biological constraints such as illness, biological components of mental illness, anxiety states, and physiological reactions that occur during conflictual sequences. Strategies for addressing these constraints include both biological and behavioral means of impacting the biological component of the biopsychosocial system. Biobehavioral strategies include exercise (Otto & Smits, 2011), mindfulness/meditation (Tang, 2017), coordinating interpersonal neurobiology (Fishbane, 2007, 2013), and biofeedback, as well as medical strategies such as psychopharmacological intervention (Holtzheimer et al., 2010) or acupuncture.

Family of Origin Planning Metaframework

Family of origin strategies are used when the therapist hypothesizes that solutions are constrained by a lack of differentiation of an adult client from their family of origin. These strategies aim to facilitate differentiation of self and mature interdependence. The focus is often on the development of insight into how the family of origin issues impact current relationships or individual functioning. This metaframework can also focus on working directly with a client and the family of origin to modify relational patterns that constrain the client. The family of origin metaframework draws strategies from the work of family therapy pioneers Murray Bowen (Bowen, 1974), Ivan Boszormenyi-Nagy (Boszormenyi-Nagy & Spark, 1973), and James Framo (Framo, 1992), as well as current-day theorists Mona Fishbane (2015, 2016) and Monica McGoldrick (McGoldrick et al., 2008).

Internal Representation Planning Metaframework

Internal Representation strategies address internalized mental representations of early relational experiences and family figures. They seek to modify internal (mental) objects or parts, the relationships among them, and/or the relationship between objects/parts and other people. The internal representation metaframework uses strategies derived from internal family systems (IFS) therapy (Schwartz, 2013), object relations theory (Guntrip & Rudnytsky, 2013; Scharff, 1995), and other psychodynamic therapies. Strategies in this metaframework address hypotheses based on an M2 model of the mind that describes how the components of mind are organized.

Self Planning Metaframework

IST's self planning metaframework provides strategies that are designed to address the M3 level of mind by means of intensive work focused primarily on the interactions between the therapist and client. These strategies and interventions, derived traditionally from self-psychology (Kohut, 1977, 984; Hagman, 2019) and more recently from functional analytic psychotherapy (Kohlenberg & Tsai, 2007), are aimed at the development of adaptive coping and relating that Kohut described as a stronger, more flexible, less vulnerable self. The therapeutic relationship is the primary source of change. Without positing a self, functional analytic therapy (a contextual, behavioral approach) addresses the interpersonal behaviors associated with M3 constraints by working on how the client behaves with the therapist. When the therapist has worked extensively with other planning metaframeworks, but constraints of mind continue to prevent solution sequences, individual therapy that addresses the strengthening of what Kohut referred to as the self is recommended. Although the strategies associated with this metaframework were designed for individual therapy, some of them (e.g., modeling rupture and repair skills within the therapeutic relationship) can be integrated into couple or family work.

Integrating Interventions to Address Constraints

Addressing Constraints of Mind

Mind, of course, has been the focus of traditional psychotherapy since its inception; hence, many theories of mind and their associated strategies of intervention exist in the literature. IST does not posit or endorse one approach to mind; rather, it organizes a set of strategies associated with a variety of theories of psychotherapy and makes them available for the therapist to draw upon to meet the needs of a specific client. As stated in Chapter 7, IST considers three levels of analysis of mind: M1 (thoughts, feelings, sequences of thoughts and feelings, narratives), M2 (model of the mind that addresses the organization of its components), and M3 (model of the mind that addresses the development of self).

The M1 level of analysis is addressed by the meaning/emotion planning metaframework, which provides many strategies (see Appendix A), each of which contains multiple interventions. Graduate-level training introduces students to a variety of interventions, but interventions are continually learned and adopted over the course of a career. Having more options for intervening with M1 patterns allows therapists to be more flexible in the way they intervene, which provides more freedom to find what fits best for the clients instead of rigidly adhering to the therapist's preferences (Lebow, 2014).

Intervening with M1s begins with identifying and labeling the thoughts or feelings that may be constraining a solution sequence. This typically comes about in one of four ways. First, the therapist asks clients if they think anything will get in the way of implementing the solution sequence. Second, once they have had difficulty implementing a solution sequence, the therapist asks the clients what kept them from doing it. Third, a client is talking in session about an event that occurred or a plan to do something (action talk) and the therapist decides to learn more about how the client is feeling or what they are thinking about it. And fourth, the client expresses a part of a sequence of mind and the therapist decides to explore in greater detail how the full sequence of thinking and feeling works and how it influences the client's actions or interactions. For example, if a client whose presenting problem is depression provides a problem-saturated narration of events and outlook, the therapist will likely wonder how the pattern of mind impacts mood and problem-solving. The therapist will attend carefully to what the client says and use client feedback to see if they can move toward a shared hypothesis that a pattern of mind functions as a constraint. "I appreciate you sharing that. How does that feeling affect what you do about (the problem)?" Or "Do you think those thoughts will get in the way of trying this experiment?" Or "I think what you are describing is important because it may get in the way of things you might do to feel better."

The therapist can also interrupt or supportively challenge thoughts, feelings, or narratives. For example, when a couple in conflict begins to get angry, the therapist may interrupt the conflict and ask both parties to take a deep breath and focus on what they are experiencing in the moment. Having the clients describe such experiences as "disregarded" or "disrespected" can be a starting point for modifying an interaction. Another example would involve interrupting the expression of hostile criticism (expressed emotion; Butzlaff & Hooley, 1998) in session and asking the person to consider the effects of such criticism. A therapist might say something like, "I know you care deeply about your daughter and that her success in school is very important to you, but have you considered how she is affected by what you have been saying in the last few minutes?"

IST therapists seek new views to support new patterns of action and interaction. This involves helping clients to notice, experience, and express thoughts and narratives that are contextually adaptive in that they facilitate a solution sequence. This can be accomplished through reframing or suggesting a new view of the problem. For example, "I think when your partner complains, they are reaching out to you." Or the therapist can ask, "Have you ever thought there might be a different way to view this?" Other interventions within this strategy are more complex. They include systems for asking questions that aim for reappraisal or deeper understanding, including Socratic questions (Overholser, 2018), circular questioning (Tomm, 1987), externalizing the problem (White & Epston, 2004), and motivational interviewing (Miller & Rollnick, 2012).

An M1 pattern can also be addressed in the realm of emotion. The strategies include heightening adaptive emotion (Greenberg, 2017; Johnson, 2020), facilitating direct emotional expression (Greenberg, 2017; Johnson, 2020), providing psychoeducation on emotion (Goldman & Greenberg, 2019; Gottman, 2001), and regulating constraining emotions (Gross & Thompson, 2007; Linehan, 2015). An example of an emotion that constrains a solution sequence is found in the case of a single parent who gets overwhelmed with feelings of guilt about neglecting the children several years earlier when she was using drugs. The guilt keeps her from holding the limits with the children. As the therapist supports her in recognizing and attending to the feelings of guilt, she begins to uphold rules and create greater harmony in the family.

Conflict in couple and family systems is often sustained by the respective secondary (defensive) emotions and fixed ideas of participants. These emotions and ideas are often generated to protect the parties from feeling hurt, diminished, or abandoned. Accessing and communicating primary (vulnerable) emotions in the structured, safe context of therapy can help couples and families develop alternative adaptive sequences of interaction (solutions). This work is most fully articulated in the emotion-focused (Greenberg, 2017) and emotionally focused (Johnson, 2020) models of therapy, both of which provide useful modules or components of work that can be integrated into IST.

Complex patterns of meanings and emotions that cluster around or comprise clinical presentations may require more complex meaning/ emotion strategies. Examples of these strategies include integrating traumatic experiences, facilitating forgiveness, or facilitating grief and adaptation to loss (Pinsof et al., 2018; Appendix A of this book). These strategies involve multiple steps or an ongoing process of work with meaning and emotion over time. Associated interventions sometimes address an M2 level of mind, but not necessarily. There is powerful work to be done at the M1 level with what clients see and feel about their world, their relationships, and their problems.

When patterns of mind are constraining and interventions aimed at M1 patterns have not been successful, the IST therapist begins to hypothesize at the level of M2, which uses a model of mind that describes how its components fit together. To address M2 hypotheses, the therapist utilizes strategies from the internal representation metaframework (See Appendix A). These strategies aim to address internalized representations of past experiences, including representation of self, parts of self and internalized early attachment figures. These strategies and their corresponding interventions address the various parts of mind, often linking them to childhood or other formative experiences. The strategies of this planning metaframework derive primarily from the Internal Family Systems (IFS) approach (Schwartz, 2013) and the object relations approach (Luborsky & Barrett, 2006; Scharff & Scharff, 2005; Scharff & de Varela, 2005). Some IST practitioners become adept at both approaches, but most select one or the other with which to understand the structure of the mind. The description of these approaches and their related strategies is beyond the scope of this book, but a case example may illustrate their utility with respect to a solution sequence.

Val and Jo are a white, cisgender, lesbian couple in their late 30s. Jo recently took a job that required travel for work. Val was getting highly anxious and drinking too much when Jo traveled. The therapist asked a series of questions about Val's drinking and found that she did not otherwise exhibit any problems with alcohol (past or present). The drinking caused significant concern for them as Jo noted Val's significant impairment in their phone conversations. The therapy, involving both partners, initially focused on what to do about the drinking. A solution sequence that involved substituting other activities for alcohol had limited, short-term success, but proved not to be sustainable. The therapist probed further and learned more about Val's M1 sequence involving separation, anxiety, and catastrophic worries that constrained the solution sequence. The therapist utilized cognitive-behavioral interventions for Val to reduce her anxiety and worries and worked on the patterns of communication between the partners. As this work was not sufficiently effective in addressing the anxiety, the therapist began to introduce the language of parts (Schwartz, 2013) into the therapy. The conversation identified a part of Val that was highly anxious about being left alone and upon separation felt out of control with fear. She felt very ashamed of that part. The drinking was attributed to a *firefighter* part that stepped in to help her deal with the fear. The therapist helped Val access these parts and supported her in establishing a relationship with her *exiled* fearful part via dialog in session in which she alternately took the part of her *self* and the *exiled* part. With intensive coaching over several sessions, Val was able to support and soothe the fearful part and assure the *firefighter* that she was appreciated but not needed when Jo traveled. After this work, Val began tolerating Jo's travel without the use of alcohol.

When M2 strategies and interventions have not been successful in removing a constraint of mind, the therapist may utilize an M3 analysis of mind to describe the constraint. At this level of analysis, the therapist wonders if a client's self is too fragile to work directly and effectively on their internal representations. When the client is self-harming, highly impulsive, strongly reactive to perceived criticism or rejection, or satisfies the diagnostic description of borderline personality, the preferred treatment is referral to a dialectical behavior therapy program (Linehan, 2015). In other cases, when M3 constraints seem operative, therapy can utilize the strategies of the self planning metaframework (See Appendix A) which create change primarily through work that occurs within the therapeutic relationship. One approach to this is functional analytic psychotherapy (Kohlenberg & Tsai, 2007) which derives from the radical behavioral tradition, but is classified in IST's self planning metaframework because functional analytic therapy works in vivo with the client's problem sequences as they occur with the therapist. Change is produced by identifying problematic behaviors that occur in individual therapy sessions and developing and reinforcing new ways of relating to the therapist that transfer to the client's other relationships. Learning the strategies and interventions of this approach requires specialized training.

A more traditional approach to the self planning metaframework is self-psychology (Kohut, 1977), which seeks to strengthen the client's self through deepening the therapeutic bond, managing the vicissitudes of the therapist-client relationship, tolerating dependency and emotional intensity with the client, and awakening the self to embrace disowned parts. Some of the strategies of the self-planning metaframework can be integrated directly into IST therapy, for example, the strategy of empathically linking the client's struggle with a solution sequence to the vulnerability of the self, or the strategy of recognizing and repairing tears in the therapeutic alliance (Pinsof et al., 2018). However, most of this work is done in individual therapy with someone trained in self-psychology. This is a long-term therapy that IST does not recommend until a wide variety of other strategies and interventions have been tried.

Addressing Organizational Constraints

Hypotheses about how a system's components fit together are described with concepts contained in the organization hypothesizing metaframework. The way the components fit together, including the dimensions of boundaries and leadership, can constrain families from adopting and maintaining solution sequences. Such constraints are most often addressed by strategies drawn from the action and meaning/emotion planning metaframeworks.

Chapter 7 mentioned a family consisting of a grandmother, a single mother, and her children. The presenting problem was that two of the children were not applying themselves sufficiently to their schoolwork. A solution sequence was formulated that involved the children beginning their homework right after school, which was before the mother arrived at home. The mother would ask the grandmother, who was not attending sessions, to structure these homework sessions. At the next session, when it was reported that the kids did not often follow the new structure, the therapist asked what kept that from happening and the kids reported that their grandmother said it was okay to play outside after school. The therapist hypothesized that the leadership in the family was constrained in that the mother and grandmother were not on the same page. The therapist asked the mother to invite the grandmother to the next session and, if possible from a childcare perspective, have a session with just the adults. This was an attempt to work with those responsible for the leadership patterns of the family. It is worth noting that some families lack the social support or the financial means to secure childcare, which may require that the children be in the session.

The therapist's job in the next session was to join with the grandmother and help her feel comfortable in the session. The starting point was to welcome her to the session, tell the story of the therapy thus far, and state how important her participation would be in finding a solution to the school achievement issue. Then the therapist opened the discussion on the expectations for the completion of homework. The mom wanted it done right after school. The grandmother believed it was best for the children to get outside and "blow off some steam" before doing their homework. The therapist asked what they do in situations like this when they have different views. What emerged was a description of two regimes under one roof that seemed to alternate depending on which of them was home and actively engaged with the children. The therapist asked what they thought this was like for the kids. "Confusing" and "they get away with murder" were among their responses. This led the therapist to say, "Let's talk about how you see your roles and how you work together for the advancement of the kids' education." A conversation ensued about how they would lead the children to greater success in school, but this conversation was also about how they would be leaders together and what roles they would each take. At some point, the therapist can make this more explicit. "We have a plan for the homework now and it seems to be working. I wonder if we also need to talk more about how the two of you will work together on other parenting issues?"

Sometimes, addressing leadership constraints is straightforward, and other times it may be more complex with challenges such as the early traumatic experiences of a caregiver or the long-standing conflict between caregivers. Such constraints may require a significant detour in the therapy or a referral to another therapist to address them. In such cases, the therapist considers the question, "Can I work with this complex constraint while maintaining my alliance with all of the family members?" In IST, the answer is most often "yes." If the answer is "no," then an additional therapist will be needed to handle a portion of the case.

In the case of the mother and grandmother, discussion with the therapist may lead to specific plans for managing homework but also a change in the way they work together—an organizational change. Note that IST discusses leadership functions but does not prescribe a particular pattern for how those functions are accomplished. Rather, the therapist collaborates with families to develop patterns of leadership that, upon experimentation, the clients feel work better. The IST therapist will be mindful and respectful of family traditions and cultural factors and share, as applicable, ideas from organizational theory such as the importance of clarifying who the leaders are and how they work together to manage the functions of leadership that were discussed in Chapter 7. In IST, the therapist does not set out to assess and reform the family with respect to all these factors. Rather, the focus is on which, if any, of these factors are constraining a solution sequence or are identified as a matter of concern by the family.

The organization metaframework also addresses boundaries (level of communication and involvement) among members and subsystems. Based on client reports and direct observations by the therapist (feedback) the therapist may hypothesize that the level of involvement is high in a way that constrains the development or autonomy of a member, or that the level of involvement between or among members is too low to allow sufficient connectedness and support. For example, a diffuse boundary between father and son may allow the father to communicate significant detail about the parents' marital problems to the son. This communication may interfere with the son's relationship with his mother and/or his own development. A hypothesis that a solution sequence is constrained by a boundary issue leads the therapist to initiate the conversation about the possible link between the boundary issue and the presenting concern. Questions for the son might include: "I wonder what it is like for you to hear what your dad has to say about your mom?" Or "How is this information affecting your relationship with your mom?" Or "What do you do when you feel uncomfortable with what you are hearing?" And the therapist might ask the father: "What is it like to hear your son say this makes him feel uncomfortable?" Or "I understand that the marital concerns are important to you. What would it be like for you if you were not talking to your son about them?" The therapist can take positions as well. For example, the therapist can say to the father, "Now that I hear how this works, I think it is important that you discontinue talking with your son about the marriage. Can you see how this would be to his benefit?" and "I am concerned about you, too. Do you have another outlet for your feelings?"

The conversation based on the therapist's questions and suggestions can lead to a new view that supports modification of the boundary. The father and son may come to see that it is better not to talk about the marital relationship. Changes in patterns of action that comprise a modification of boundaries or leadership patterns require a justification or purpose. Why else would clients want to make the changes that the therapist suggests? A new meaning (idea, view, value) sets the stage for the new boundary which requires new patterns of interaction. The meaning is reinforced by further discussion of it and by a plan to enact it. To the father: "Now that you have decided not to talk with your son about the marital issues, I think it will be a good idea to talk with him about this decision." As the conversation progresses, the therapist may have other questions. To the son: "How will it feel to not hear about this?" and "Do you think your dad can handle his feelings about his relationship with your mom without your support?" Then the new boundary is enacted between sessions and the therapist checks in on it in subsequent sessions by asking such questions as: "How is that boundary working?" "Are you finding other things to talk about?" "How are each of you coping with the change?" Following up on the outcome of their efforts is important because the establishment and maintenance of the new boundary can have far-reaching implications for how the family functions.

Addressing Developmental Constraints

As discussed in Chapter 7, human systems proceed through developmental transitions and stages. The development metaframework includes the vast and evolving territory of knowledge that pertains to the development at the individual, relational, familial, community, and societal levels of the system. Therapists cannot master all this knowledge. Rather, they incorporate new knowledge continually through training and practice and build the skills of accessing new knowledge with respect to specific cases they see. This is an ongoing process of lifelong learning.

The stage of development of a family and its members, along with the fit among members with respect to their development, has an important impact on therapy. First, it informs the therapist about which solution sequences and interventions are appropriate. For example, the cognitive development of children will influence what we ask them to do in and between sessions. Another example would be the need for a couple to establish trust in their relationship as a precondition of emotional intimacy. These examples demonstrate how developmental issues provide limits to what is feasible in therapy. Second, the therapist will need to address developmental factors that constrain a solution sequence from being successful. For example, a plan to spend family time may be constrained by the competing social interests and demands of adolescence.

The key to working with constraints of development is making a link between a developmental issue and what is being worked on in therapy. This typically involves such meaning/emotion strategies as providing psychoeducation about the developmental issue, giving an interpretation of how a developmental issue seems to be impacting the problem, or reframing a dilemma in developmental terms. For example, in a case where parents were overly critical of an adolescent son's behavior, "Your son is highly intelligent, but he is just 15. His brain is not yet fully developed, and it won't be until he is about 25, so it is expected for him to be less thoughtful about the way he responds or to make judgment calls that don't always make sense to you." In this way, the therapist brings in the research on adolescent brain development (Casey et al., 2008) and can tailor the explanation of it to the family's level of interest in science.

Knowledge about family development can be used to normalize dilemmas. A couple with three children between two and six presented with concerns about the reduction of the couple's emotional and sexual intimacy over the course of their partnership. The therapist explores the concerns and meanings they have about their intimacy and since they do not seem to be polarized on the intimacy issue, the therapist asks whether they see their life stage as a constraint on intimacy. They do, of course, and the therapist responds with empathy and by sharing research findings on the subject. For example, the therapist might begin this by saying, "Though painful, it is understandable and normal that couples experience some loss of intimacy as they face the demands of parenthood." There is a lot that can be said about this, and it can set the stage not just for moderated expectations, but for realistic ways to maintain and enhance intimacy in their relationship. Exploration of the rhythm and routine of the household can be a springboard for finding opportunities to manage some of the stage-related constraints and find more opportunity for intimacy.

The developmental needs of a family member can bring challenges as well. For example, a family with an autistic child may see launching postponed, and retirement of the parents may also be postponed due to the need to provide support for their adult child. For parents experiencing an ambiguous loss (Bravo-Benítez et al., 2019) related to this developmental challenge, the therapist may draw on IST's complex meaning/emotion strategies of acceptance or adaptation to loss (See Table A in the Appendix). Family members who have spent years avoiding painful feelings can be helped to experience and share these feelings. Dilemmas such as these will need to be grieved and accepted. Additionally, the therapist may initiate work to facilitate the development of an adaptive narrative that acknowledges what is and provides meaning and direction for the clients.

Development can be constrained by factors described in other meta-frameworks. For example, a family with a highly anxious parent and diffuse boundaries may find it difficult to extend certain freedoms to an adolescent. A similar constraint may occur in a family who has immigrated to a country that has a different conception of adolescence than is generally held in the host country. These constraints need to be addressed to work with the developmental constraints. As is often the case, the therapist's work will need to consider multiple, interlocking constraints.

Addressing Constraints Related to Culture

The culture metaframework recognizes that people draw their identity, in part, from membership in certain groups and exclusion from others. These memberships, or sociocultural contexts, are described by such categories as race, ethnicity, religion, economic status, education, geographic region, gender identity, sexual orientation, and age. Membership in a context, the intersectionality of contexts, or the fit of a person's contexts with other levels of the system can facilitate development and problem solving but can sometimes be constraining. For example, a couple who moves from a big city to a small town where one of them grew up may find that the other partner has difficulty developing a sense of belonging in the town due to educational background, interests, political opinions, or socioeconomic status.

Culture is a relevant consideration for every problem-solving task of the essence diagram. We have seen, for example in Chapter 5, its importance in the selection of a solution sequence. Factors described in the culture metaframework are also useful in identifying certain constraints, which then are typically addressed by strategies primarily drawn from the meaning/emotion planning metaframework. In some cases, the constraints may require work derived from the family of origin or internal representation planning metaframeworks. Importantly, culture influences the nature of family boundaries and leadership (organization), the approach to spirituality, beliefs about disease (biology), and the views of what is expected with respect to developmental stages, gender identity, and gender roles. This means that work on constraints related to culture will typically be accompanied by attention to other hypothesizing metaframeworks.

Clients will sometimes comment on their culture and link it to the presenting concern. For example, a 27-year-old Irish American, cisgender, straight man cites culture as a partial explanation for the challenge of abstaining from alcohol. This cultural issue may become part of the dialog such that the issue is changed from how a person stays sober to how an Irish American man stays sober (change in meaning). It might be even further defined as how a twenty-something Irish American man stays sober. In this way, the challenges related to identity and social network are better addressed. For example, the client may be tasked to find other sober folks who are Irish Americans and talk with them (new action) about how sobriety is reached and maintained. This approach accepts the client's view of himself and incorporates it into the process of developing a workable way forward.

Clients will not always mention a cultural issue, but the therapist can initiate a discussion about a cultural context or intersectionality. One way to explore and modify meanings related to culture is circular questioning

(Selvini-Palazzoli et al., 1980) which provides clients the opportunity to broaden their understanding of the multiple levels of their context and better understand the views of others within it. The therapist asks a series of questions about relationships and differences among members with respect to the presenting problem and factors that may be related to it. In the case of a cisgender adolescent girl whose parents immigrated to the United States, the therapist asked the following question, "What is it like to be both a member of a family that is fairly new to the U.S. and a teenager in the neighborhood?" The question begins to get at the current level of fit between the family and the community and between the daughter and the parents. These are differences the family can discuss, and such discussions may create a new understanding of dilemmas that constrain the teenager and the family. This may lead to changes in patterns of action, such as a modification in rules or expectations for the adolescent and her siblings.

Many constraints derive from a lack of influence or access to resources. Since therapists with privilege do not experience these types of constraints, it is essential for them to be sensitive to the limitations that have been imposed on their clients due to economic disadvantage, race, ethnicity, sexual orientation, or gender identity. For example, clients whose incomes fall in the lowest income bracket may reside in a food desert with limited access to nutritious food, so it can be shame-inducing for them if the therapist makes assumptions about the availability or affordability of nutritious food. Such assumptions can constrain or damage the therapeutic alliance. IST requires a systemic view that includes a focus on community and societal factors that constrain equity and inclusion and marginalize people and communities. The therapist must seek to understand how societal constraints impact their clients, assume the role of ally with respect to the constraints the clients face, and bear witness to the strengths clients bring to managing their challenges.

Lastly, issues of difference and fit are important in the relationship between therapist and clients. A meta-analytic review focused on therapist and client racial-ethnic matching found no significant differences between ethnically matched and non-ethnically matched therapist-client dyads (Shin et al., 2005). Yet, therapist attention to a cultural goodness of fit remains a salient indicator of therapeutic success and calls for therapists to remain mindful of their cultural differences with their clients and encourages efforts to modify goals and strategies to fit the needs of clients from non-dominant populations (Sue et al., 2019).

Differences may be particularly salient for clients who are working with therapists who are from a more dominant race, ethnicity, or gender identity, or when there are distinct differences in abilities or age (Sue et al., 2019). Thus, the therapist needs to acknowledge factors and differences related to race, ethnicity, sexual orientation, sexual identity and ability/disability, and assure that such factors are part of what clients can discuss in therapy. Rather than conceptualizing this as just another therapeutic task, it is asserted here that being a therapist requires an ongoing commitment to the cultivation of cultural competence (Awosan et al., 2018; Kelly et al., 2014). This journey involves developing awareness of one's own cultural contexts and privilege that can prevent awareness of what clients experience as well as developing openness to the cultural identities most important to clients (Hook et al., 2013). Cultural humility, respect, and curiosity combine with the use of the IST blueprint to assure that client feedback is solicited, heard, and integrated into the plan for therapy.

Case Example of Addressing a Culture-related Constraint

Jejomar and Norjannah initiated therapy at the request of their fourteen-year-old daughter, Narges, who was a first-year student in high school. They were a Pilipino (Filipino) American family, practicing Catholics, with the parents having lived in the U.S. for 17 years. The family also included Narges' two adult brothers, Arman and Cristano, who were born in the Philippines. The parents and Narges attended the first session. Narges explained that despite good grades, she struggled with low self-esteem and often thought of herself as "incapable" or "stupid." She had initially requested individual therapy, but she and her parents agreed with the therapist's suggestion of a plan for family as well as individual sessions.

The therapist met with Narges for an individual session, and Narges shared openly about the pressures she felt within the family to excel in school. She revealed that she felt extreme pressure to take AP courses and excel in all aspects of her schoolwork. Her older brothers had made some poor choices and did not do that well in high school. She felt that she was held to a much higher standard by her parents. They often reminded her of the demanding work they had done to migrate to the U.S. and provide a better life for her and her brothers. She appreciated their sacrifices and wanted to do well but found herself obsessing over her academic performance to a point where she had difficulty sleeping at night.

In a subsequent session with Narges and the parents, Jejomar stated that if Narges would work hard, the work would bear fruit and she would feel better. Norjannah shared that she was concerned about how her daughter was feeling, but felt it was important for her to achieve at the highest level and limit her socializing to school events and immediate neighborhood friends. When Narges brought up her brothers, Arman and Cristano, Norjannah said, "Don't worry about your brothers and what they do. It is your responsibility to do better." Jejomar said, "You waste too much time. How will you get into a good university?"

The therapist hypothesized that the parents' rigid patterns of thought (work harder) were constraining Narges adaptation and wondered why the daughter's stress level did not lead to the parents easing up a bit. The therapist drew strategies from the action planning metaframework to attempt to modify the sequences of interaction between the parents and Narges. New meanings, such as the idea that Narges was already highly motivated, were introduced to support changes in interaction patterns, but the redundant pattern of the parents emphasizing hard work continued. The therapist hypothesized that there was power in the narrative of the parents' immigration story that kept the family from modifying their patterns and asked, "Jejomar and Norjannah, have you ever told Narges the story of your migration to the US?" The parents were uncertain about what they had shared and not shared throughout the years. The therapist then turned to Narges and asked, "What have your parents told you about life in the Philippines and their decision to come to the U.S.?" The therapist established that the story was referred to but never fully explained to the children and this led to a proposal to meet in a full family session to discuss this important aspect of the family's background. The therapist planned to utilize the meaning-focused strategy of facilitating the development of an adaptive narrative (White & Epston, 1990).

In the next session, in the presence of their three children, Jejomar and Norjannah took their time to tell the story of how they decided to leave the Philippines and how they struggled to gain a foothold in their adopted country where they had found fellow Pilipinos, but also faced discrimination. They shared that they felt they had failed their sons (adults now) by not knowing how to guide them in the U.S., but they agreed that it was essential that they make sure that their daughter (who they worried was vulnerable as a young woman) would be successful. The therapist brought Narges, Arman, and Cristano into the conversation and encouraged them to ask questions. Their questions helped the parents fully formulate where their preoccupation with Narges' success had come from. The conversation continued for an additional session with more back and forth and Narges shared what it was like to grow up in the family and to feel the pressure she felt. Norjannah suddenly and emotionally shared that her sister had been raped when she was a young teenager and as Norjannah shared her deep pain about this family secret, she began to see the connection of it to her efforts to protect her daughter. A shared understanding of how a history of poverty, trauma, and immigration continued to affect the family in the present was emerging.

After these two sessions, the parents were able to begin to talk differently with Narges about what they expected, and they relaxed some of their rules. Narges acknowledged that she had come to see that her parents' rigidity stemmed from their fears and their need to protect her from danger and poverty. She reported feeling more supported by them.

As therapy continued, she began to speak differently to them and found an effective way of reassuring them that she would succeed. And with that, her confidence began to improve and her stress level decreased.

Addressing Constraints Related to Gender

There is a range of issues related to gender that can constrain clients from solving their presenting concerns. Sources of constraints include rigid gender roles, gender-based power, and invalidation of transgender or gender non-conforming persons. Oppression and invalidation can occur for individuals whose gender identity is not supported by family, community, and society. An affirmative therapist for transgender and nonbinary clients (McGeorge et al., 2021; Singh & Dickey, 2017) can begin to address these constraints with meaning or emotion strategies, focusing on the client's experience, narrative, and self-statements. The therapist may explore current patterns of interaction within the family of origin as well as other contexts (work, school, friends) and utilize action strategies to help the client make modifications in sequences of interaction. Strategies of differentiation drawn from the family of origin planning metaframework may appeal to some clients when their families continue to demonstrate ambivalence about their gender identity. Differentiation involves progressively being oneself with behaviors, opinions, or values that differ from others in the family while maintaining an emotional connection to them. Work on this may involve convening sessions conducted with the client and family of origin members or coaching an individual client on how to modify their position and interactions in the family.

In the case of constraints related to rigid gender roles or gender-based power, the therapist draws the clients out in relation to their beliefs about organizational factors such as roles, decision-making, and access to resources. Questions can be used to invite the couple or family to consider such things as how they each learned about roles and leadership, where they agree and disagree on these matters, and whether they have seen an evolution in their thinking in recent years. The therapist asks questions that are targeted toward the specific constraint hypothesized. Considering this in the context of couple therapy, the therapist might say something like, "I see that there is some strain around housework. I would like to learn more about how that works. How do you handle the distribution of responsibilities, and who does what?" Then, when each party has responded, "How do you each feel about how things are done?" And then, "What are the effects of the current arrangement on your relationship?" And "Have you ever considered changing this?" This may lead to a realization that there is inequality with respect to effort and responsibility, and that the couple can benefit by a commitment to a change in the realm of action that amounts to some redistribution of responsibilities.

If the therapist hypothesizes that a couple is constrained by a gendered power imbalance, questions that address decision-making and access to resources are indicated. "I find it helpful to understand how couples make decisions. Would you mind if I asked you some questions about that?" Then, with their permission, "How do you decide things like where to live, who will work, where the kids will go to school, what grades to expect of them?" And "How do you make decisions about spending?" Or "What is the means by which you each access money?" This process leads to a shared understanding of how power and influence works for the couple. It leads to a discussion of how they think and feel about the arrangement, as well as the effects it has on them as a couple and as individuals. These effects form a reason for change as the therapist uncovers and acknowledges the impact of the constraint of inequality. Discussion of gendered power in relationships can also trigger emotion and defensive coping mechanisms (mind hypothesizing metaframework) along with associated conflictual sequences which will require modification. Once these sequences are clearly described, the therapist will need to choose a strategy or strategies to address them. One strategy would be to help the partners access and communicate the primary emotions (Greenberg, 2011) that underlie the defensive coping mechanisms and the conflict. Ultimately, the couple may choose to modify their patterns of leadership, which will involve a return to the action planning metaframework to implement changes in behavior.

Issues of development can influence how gender is handled in a family. For example, some cisgender, heterosexual couples, as they begin to have children, skew their roles toward the man being the primary income earner and the woman being the primary homemaker. They may have considered this adaptation to be a necessary arrangement at a certain time in their relationship, but it may have had a lasting impact on roles, and on equity, which constrains satisfaction in the relationship and impacts the connection between the partners. Intervention, therefore, may benefit from a historical view of how their roles developed and whether they still fit for the couple and family.

Culture often has an impact on the view of gender roles and gender-based power, and can sometimes be a factor in the invalidation of gender and sexual minorities. The understanding of family beliefs and culture of origin traditions with respect to gender is a necessary step in helping a family, couple, or individual place their concern or dilemma in its full context. Working in the realm of meaning, the therapist can ask many questions about traditions and beliefs and contrast them with evolving current-day and current-place conceptions. Such questions are interventions in and of themselves. The therapist can formulate the contrast between the *there-and-then* and the *here-and-now* and challenge couples and families to accommodate the needs of all their members. Importantly, families can be encouraged to honor some traditions and evolve with respect to others.

Addressing Biological Constraints

A biological factor or condition is sometimes the presenting problem. In such cases, it is clearly a focus of therapy. For example, a person is diagnosed with multiple sclerosis and seeks therapy to cope with this challenging fact of their life. In other cases, a biological factor becomes part of the therapy as the client(s) or therapist hypothesizes that it limits the range of solution sequences that can be established or constrains a solution that is being tried. For example, a man's physiological arousal during disagreements with his partner constrains him from listening to his partner and sometimes leads him to storm out of the room or explode in anger. Or, a child's type 1 diabetes may constrain the level of autonomy parents are comfortable extending to them. Biological constraints include factors such as illness and disability, aging, sleep difficulties, depressed mood, irritability, anxiety, and individual and relational neurobiological challenges. None of these factors are 100% biological, as they exist in a multi-level biopsychosocial context, but they all have a biological component. Addressing the constraint includes one or more of the following three strategies: (1) doing something to modify what is happening on a biological level; (2) helping clients understand and accept the impact of the biological constraint; and (3) helping clients take action to manage the constraint. Thus, the IST therapist draws primarily from the biobehavioral and meaning/emotion planning metaframeworks to address biological constraints.

There is a range of strategies in the biobehavioral planning metaframework to draw upon. Biobehavioral psychoeducation is often the starting point, as the therapist can help clients see the role of the constraint in their problem sequences and share knowledge they have on the constraint. This is straightforward when it comes to sharing general findings such as the well-established effects of exercise on mood (Stathopoulou et al., 2006; Blumenthal et al., 2007), but more indirect when it comes to physical illness in which case the therapist will encourage the client to seek appropriate education and information from their doctor and/or the medical setting in which they are being treated.

Some strategies target mood, anxiety, or physiological arousal. They include exercise and fitness, relaxation exercises, and mindfulness. These are important resources that can improve problem-solving and enhance overall health. The therapist's job here is to orchestrate a conversation that leads to the idea that mood, anxiety, or physiological arousal constrains them from doing the solution sequence. The logic is: *You want this outcome. We decided that this solution could bring it. You seem to be having trouble with the solution due to this factor (biology). Therefore, let's consider what to do about this biological factor.*

For example, in the case of a man who gets so physiologically aroused in a conflict that he is unable to listen, the therapist might say, "I notice when you are talking together you seem tense, Ted. Do you feel tense right now?" Then, "Ok, can you tell me what it feels like?" And "Once you feel that way, what is the conversation like for you? Are you able to listen carefully?" The therapist looks to create an opening to talk about the arousal in the context of the relationship(s) and begin to address it with calming strategies that can be taught and then utilized in session when arousal begins to escalate.

Other strategies seek further information about the constraints by making referrals for evaluations. A medical evaluation should always be utilized when there are somatic complaints. A neuropsychological evaluation is often important for children suspected of having a cognitive or learning issue, for aging adults who seem to be exhibiting a cognitive deficit, and for adults who are struggling with executive function or attention. An addiction evaluation is useful when a client or family member shares concerning information about their substance use. An evaluation for psychopharmacological intervention is typically indicated for major mental illness or for possible biological constraints that underlie anxiety or mood issues that do not respond to action, meaning/emotion, or other biobehavioral strategies. When a psychotropic medication is prescribed, the therapist is in an advantageous position to see how it impacts the constraint and should work collaboratively with the psychiatrist to assure this feedback is considered.

Not surprisingly, biology interacts with factors described in other hypothesizing metaframeworks. An illness or condition can have a significant impact on psychological functioning, family organization, and individual or family development. Facing biological constraints can be challenging, and clients may need to grieve the loss of their sense of invulnerability or a particular role that is important to them. A woman who developed macular degeneration had to come to terms with the progressive loss of her vision. Her grieving began as she lost her ability to drive. She shared what driving had meant to her—independence, strength, and ability. The therapist helped facilitate the grieving process and met with the woman and her husband to discuss the process of adaptation to the loss of sight. The therapist also referred her to an organization that provides programs and services for the visually impaired.

Factors described in various other metaframeworks impact biological constraints as well. Patterns of mind will impact how someone copes with illness, injury, or disability. Culture and spirituality can have a strong influence on how illness is viewed and experienced. Given this influence, it is important for the therapist to ask clients about their beliefs and traditions regarding illness: "I believe that every family has a tradition for how to see illness. Would you be okay sharing how illness is viewed in your family tradition?" For couples, even when partners are from the same racial, ethnic and regional backgrounds, it is common to find that they have two quite different views on how much attention should be given to a family member who is sick. Such differences can bring disappointment and hurt to couples. The therapist can normalize each tradition and invite the couple to see the difference in a more benign way and to make changes to accommodate each other.

Some family traditions include a hesitancy to disagree with authority figures such as doctors, but this does not mean that family members necessarily intend to follow the treatment plan. Some families carry a tradition of feeling shame over the weakness associated with illness. Other traditions may view illness as God's plan or even a kind of punishment for past mistakes. It is important for the therapist to explore the clients' beliefs and learn how important they are in the overall scheme of their cultural background and religious or spiritual life. If views are strong enough, the therapist will need to work within the bounds of the established beliefs. Importantly, both culture and spirituality are the source of great strengths that can be brought to bear on the challenges of illness and disability.

Addressing Constraints Related to Spirituality

Spiritual beliefs and practices are a significant resource for many clients who face adversity (Walsh, 2009). The sustaining power of faith or the healing power of a transcendent focus provides great strength for many people. For example, a woman with five children discovers that her husband, who travels extensively for work, has been having an affair. When she confronts him, he commits to ending the affair. She is in crisis, but she says, "I feel God is with me and gives me strength to accept where I am today. I know I have difficult decisions ahead of me, but I do not need to make any major decisions right now." Although certain beliefs or practices in particular families may be constraining, much of the research on religious and spiritual practices suggests that they play a role in preventing physical and mental illness, improving how people cope with illness, and facilitating recovery (Ellison & Levin, 1998; Miller & Thoresen, 2003; Koenig, 2015). Thus, the therapist is wise to acknowledge the clients' spirituality as a strength to draw upon.

Spiritual traditions and practices overlap with the province of therapy because they address such issues as loss, forgiveness, acceptance, hope, and letting go. This commonality, along with the high proportion of people who hold religious or spiritual views, suggests that the therapist learn how important the clients' religious or spiritual involvement is to them (Walsh, 2009). Important questions include, "Is your spirituality a source of strength when you face adversity?" and "Do your beliefs affect how you see or what you do about the things that bring you to therapy?" The answers to such questions help the therapist consider clients' beliefs when proposing a solution sequence. For example, a client presents with concerns about anxiety. As the client discloses the importance of her spiritual life, the therapist hypothesizes that a self-calming strategy might best be constructed as prayerful meditation as opposed to a secular approach to mindfulness or progressive muscle relaxation.

In addition to being a strength, spirituality can also function as a constraint. In some cases, this is due to the particular way someone uses a spiritual precept. For example, a cisgender man who participated in the Alcoholics Anonymous program seemed to interpret the important spiritual practice of acceptance in an overly broad manner such that he would turn things over to a higher power that he could, and perhaps should, manage. This practice served the function of avoiding the stress associated with trying to change or manage something; however, it often caused stress for family members who felt uncomfortable with his lack of engagement in problem-solving. As his sobriety was well-established, the therapist probed for a deeper examination of the client's use of the serenity prayer (Sherman, 2017) to consider more carefully what was in his control and what was not. This work employed strategies that addressed his meaning system and the way he managed his emotions, but it had significant implications for the reassessment of the actions for which the client would ultimately decide to take responsibility.

Differences in beliefs within a family, religious-based patriarchy, and rigid beliefs about gender or sexuality constrain some client systems. The work with these constraints is done primarily with meaning-based interventions such as reframing (Watzlawick et al., 1974), circular questioning (Tomm, 1987), or motivational interviewing (Miller & Rollnick, 2012). Externalizing (White & Epston, 2004) the difference and exploring its impact on the family can bring new meaning to the dilemma. In these ways, the therapist explores whether the clients can come to see and experience their beliefs and their dilemma in a new way. These are delicate matters, so the therapist must have good intentions and seek to be respectful without flinching in asking difficult questions. Finding commonality among members' values or beliefs despite differences and finding compassion for each other are possible ways forward. In more extreme cases of alienation due to differences in beliefs or oppressive effects of beliefs, the family of origin strategy of differentiation may be necessary when family members do not agree to disagree.

In working with spirituality, several principles are important to keep in mind. First, clients may hesitate to discuss spiritual beliefs, as they may have learned that religion is not to be discussed in public. Therapists will need to open space for clients to discuss what they believe and how it may impact the problem-solving process. Second, therapists must not presume to understand what a client means by the term "God" (Griffith & Griffith, 2003); rather, they need to learn what the client means by this term. Third, therapists must avoid subtle or overt ways of imposing their own spirituality on the clients. For example, saying "God bless you" to clients without knowing how this fits for them constitutes an abuse of power by the therapist in that it communicates the expectation that the clients should believe what the therapist believes to participate in the relationship. Fourth, the therapist may ask clients to think through the likely future consequences of a constraining belief. In such a case, the therapist does not oppose the belief, but highlights the dilemma the clients have with it. Fifth, the therapist can consult with the clients' priest, rabbi, minister, mullah, or monk to better understand the nature of the spiritual constraint. This is particularly helpful when the therapist hypothesizes that the clients may have adopted a more fundamentalist position than the cleric. An example of this is a father who stopped communicating with his daughter because she had moved in with her boyfriend despite the familial and religious expectation that cohabitation does not precede marriage. In consultation, the Catholic priest supported the father's wish to uphold a principle but did not sanction the cut-off. This led to a deeper discussion of the father's feelings about his daughter not fulfilling his expectations.

Due to the personal nature of spiritual practices and religious beliefs, clients are understandably sensitive to such conversations. With respect for this sensitivity and for clients' beliefs, Doherty (2009) discusses degrees of intensity for intervention in spiritual matters. The lower levels of intensity, including exploring and acknowledging clients' spirituality, are the most frequently utilized strategies. When a client's spiritual belief constrains the goals of therapy, the therapist can summarize the dilemma that the belief poses, including the impact of it on members of the system. In the above example, the father had a dilemma in that he wanted a relationship with his daughter, and he did not want to cause her distress, but he believed it was his duty to refuse to communicate with her since she was cohabitating with her partner. The strategy at the highest level of intensity is reserved for situations in which a belief is damaging to relationships or wounding to an individual and when other interventions have not resolved the situation. At that point, the therapist can respectfully articulate the dilemma, speak to the damage being done, and share their personal beliefs about the situation (Doherty, 2009).

Spirituality can have an impact on factors described in other hypothesizing metaframeworks. Certainly, it can impact the process of mind in that spiritual thoughts will be part of various sequences of mind and may function importantly in how people cope mentally. Spirituality can influence organization and development in families as well. The stronger clients feel about their spirituality, the more likely spirituality interacts with other metaframeworks, and the more necessary it is for therapists to explore this realm of their clients' lives.

Acknowledging and exploring clients' religious and spiritual beliefs and practices may strengthen the therapeutic alliance. The more important spirituality is to them, the more the therapist needs to know about it. Throughout the process of accessing spiritual strengths and identifying and addressing spiritual constraints, the therapist monitors the alliance. This is a matter of reading feedback from the clients and hypothesizing about alliance considerations. To this end, therapists can ask themselves questions such as: "Am I being respectful of their beliefs?" "Is the client with me on this suggestion or might it go against their spirituality?" "I wonder what it means that the client did not attend this week after I had suggested she invite her highly religious parents to an upcoming session?" It is particularly important to be sensitive to how an intervention might be experienced by clients from the standpoint of their familial, cultural, and spiritual traditions. The interventions available to an IST therapist are diverse and virtually limitless, but they all have in common the requirement of maintaining a therapeutic alliance.

Conclusion

The therapist addresses hypotheses about constraints by gathering the system members needed, selecting a strategy that fits the constraint, and proposing an intervention that serves the strategy. The strategies of IST, abstracted from therapy models and best practices, are organized into planning metaframeworks based on foci and mechanisms of change. Strategies are accomplished by a variety of interventions. The selection of an intervention is influenced by therapist training and preference as well as the needs and views of the clients. Proposing an intervention requires the therapist to provide a rationale for what the clients are being asked to do. As with the proposal of a solution sequence, the therapist must be careful that the intervention chosen fits for the clients. Cultural factors and the intersectionality of identities will influence the range of interventions that are appropriate for them.

The planning matrix depicts a generally preferred order of intervention based on the IST guidelines that encourage the therapist to begin working in an interpersonal context when possible and appropriate with an initial focus on here-and-now action-oriented strategies. This work often requires that the therapist also address current sequences of meaning and emotion. More complex strategies, such as those that address the internalized effects of past experience, are reserved for cases that do not respond to basic problem-solving approaches. The order of progression suggested by the matrix is flexible in that a therapist's compelling hypothesis or a client's strong preference will override it.

When therapists and clients collaborate in addressing constraints, there will be an outcome that provides feedback for the direction of therapy.

Chapter 9 will discuss how to utilize this feedback, evaluate treatment progress, and modify treatment planning as needed.

Exercises

1   Think of one of your cases or, if you are not practicing yet, a case you have heard or read about. Be prepared to write or type your thoughts about it. Identify a solution sequence and then a factor that seems to constrain it. Write down both the solution sequence and the constraint. Consider a strategy to address the constraint. Then choose an intervention to fulfill the strategy. Write down both the strategy and the intervention. Now, think about how you might talk to the client(s) about the strategy, developing a rationale for it. Record the rationale on the page as well. You are hypothesizing and planning.

2   Take the first exercise a step further (if you are seeing clients): Discuss the constraint and your plan to address it with the client(s). Ask them to share their reactions to your idea. Pay careful attention to their response. Then you will be conversing and reading the feedback. Perhaps the feedback will lead you to change your hypothesis and plan. Or, maybe you will get a green light and proceed ahead with the intervention.

3   For each of the action, meaning/emotion, biobehavioral, and family of origin planning metaframeworks, review the list of strategies in Appendix A. Write down the strategies for which you know an intervention and record the intervention you know how to do under that strategy. Notice the strategies for which you still need an intervention. Have you heard of an intervention that fits that strategy? List the interventions you feel you should learn in a separate column alongside those you had recorded. Pick one and discuss with your supervisor or co-worker how you can acquire competence in that intervention. For advanced practitioners: Though you already have interventions for each strategy, consider additional interventions that may be useful in your practice.

4   Review the strategies listed in the internal representation planning metaframework. Consider how you think about these intrapsychic processes. Is there a psychodynamic model that interests you (e.g., internal family systems, object relations)? Discuss this interest with a supervisor or co-worker.

References

Awosan, C. I., Curiel, Y. S., & Rastogi, M. (2018). Cultural competency in couple and family therapy. In J. L. Lebow, A. L. Chambers, & D. C. Breunlin (Eds.), *Encyclopedia of couple and family therapy*. Springer. 10.1007/978-3-319-49425-8_472

Bandura, A. (1991). Social cognitive theory of self-regulation. *Organizational Behavior and Human Decision Processes, 50*(2), 248–287.

Barlow, D. H., Craske, M. G., Cerny, J. A., & Klosko, J. S. (1989). Behavioral treatment of panic disorder. *Behavior Therapy, 20*(2), 261–282

Baucom, D. H., Epstein, N. B., & Norman, B. (1990). *Cognitive-behavioral marital therapy*. Brunner/Mazel.

Baucom, D. H., Epstein, N. B., LaTaillade, J. J. & Kirby, J. S. (2002). Cognitive-behavioral couple therapy. In A. S. Gurman & N. S. Jacobson (Eds.), *Clinical handbook of couple therapy* (3rd ed., pp. 31–72). Guilford Press.

Beck, J. S. (2011). *Cognitive behavior therapy: Basics and beyond* (2nd ed.). Guilford Press.

Berg, I. K. (1994). *Family-based services: A solution-focused approach*. W. W. Norton.

Blumenthal, J. A., Babyak, M. A., Doraiswamy, P. M., Watkins, L., Hoffman, B. M., Barbour, K. A., Herman, S., Craighead, W. E., Brosse, A. L., Waugh, R., Hinderliter, A., & Sherwood, A. (2007). Exercise and pharmacotherapy in the treatment of major depressive disorder. *Psychosomatic Medicine, 69*(7), 587–596. 10.1097/PSY.0b013e318148c19a

Boszormenyi-Nagy, I., & Spark, G. M. (1973). *Invisible loyalties: Reciprocity in intergenerational family therapy*. Harper & Row.

Bowen, M. (1974). Toward the differentiation of self in one's family of origin. *Georgetown Family Symposium, 1*, 222–242.

Bravo-Benítez, J., Pérez-Marfil, M. N., Román-Alegre, B., & Cruz-Quintana, F. (2019). Grief experiences in family caregivers of children with autism spectrum disorder (ASD). *International Journal of Environmental Research and Public Health, 16*(23), 4821. 10.3390/ijerph16234821

Butzlaff, R. L., & Hooley, J. M. (1998). Expressed emotion and psychiatric relapse: A meta-analysis. *Archives of General Psychiatry, 55*(6), 547–552. 10.1001/archpsyc.55.6.547

Casey, B. J., Getz, S., & Galvan, A. (2008). The adolescent brain. *Developmental Review, 28*, 62–77.

Christensen, A., Jacobson, N. S., & Babcock, J. C. (1995). *Integrative behavioral couple therapy*. Guilford.

Craske, M. G. (1999). *Anxiety disorders: Psychological approaches to theory and treatment*. Basic Books.

Doherty, W. J. (2009). Morality and spirituality in therapy. *Spiritual resources in family therapy* (2nd ed., pp. 215–228). Guilford Press.

Ellison, C. G., & Levin, J. S. (1998). The religion-health connection: Evidence, theory, and future directions. *Health Education & Behavior, 25*(6), 700–720. 10.1177/109019819802500603

Fishbane, M. D. (2007). Wired to connect: Neuroscience, relationships, and therapy. *Family Process, 46*, 395–412.

Fishbane, M. D. (2013). *Loving with the brain in mind: Neurobiology and couple therapy*. Norton.

Fishbane, M. D. (2015). Couple therapy and interpersonal neurobiology. In A. S. Gurman, J. Lebow, & D. Snyder (Eds.), *Clinical handbook of couple therapy* (5th ed.). Guilford.

Fishbane, M. D. (2016). The neurobiology of relationships. In J. Lebow & T. Sexton (Eds.), *Handbook of family therapy* (4th ed.). Routledge.

Framo, J. L. (1992). *Family-of-origin therapy: An intergenerational approach.* Psychology Press.

Gottman, J. M. (2001). Meta-emotion, children's emotional intelligence, and buffering children from marital conflict. In C. D. Ryff & B. H. Singer (Eds.), *Emotion, social relationships, and health series in affective science* (pp. 23–40). Oxford University Press.

Goldman, R. N., & Greenberg, L. S. (2019). Enduring themes and future developments in emotion-focused therapy. In L. S. Greenberg & R. N. Goldman (Eds.), *Clinical handbook of emotion-focused therapy* (pp. 513–520). American Psychological Association. 10.1037/0000112-023

Greenberg, L. S. (2011). *Emotion-focused therapy: Theory and practice.* American Psychological Association.

Greenberg, L. S. (2017). *Emotion-focused therapy* (Rev. ed.). American Psychological Association.

Griffith, J. L., & Griffith, M. E. (2003). *Encountering the sacred in psychotherapy: How to talk with people about their spiritual lives.* The Guilford Press.

Gross, J. J., & Thompson, R. A. (2007). Emotion regulation: Conceptual foundations. In J. J. Gross (Ed.) *Handbook of Emotion Regulation* (pp. 3–24). Guilford Press.

Guntrip, A. S., & Rudnytsky, P. L. (2013). *The psychoanalytic vocation: Rank, Winnicott, and the legacy of Freud.* Routledge.

Hagman, G., Paul, H., & Zimmermann, P. B. (2019). *Intersubjective self psychology: A primer.* Routledge.

Haley, J. (1987). *Problem-solving therapy* (2nd ed.). Jossey-Bass.

Hayes, S. C., Strosahl, K., & Wilson, K. G. (1999). *Acceptance and commitment therapy: An experiential approach to behavior change.* Guilford Press.

Holtzheimer, P. E. III, Snowden, M., & Roy-Byrne, P. P. (2010). Psychopharmacological treatments for patients with neuropsychiatric disorders. In S. C. Yudofsky & R. E. Hales (Eds.), *Essentials of neuropsychiatry and behavioral neurosciences* (2nd ed., pp. 495–530). American Psychiatric Publishing.

Hook, J. N., Davis, D. E., Owen, J., Worthington Jr., E. L., & Utsey, S. O. (2013). Cultural humility: Measuring openness to culturally diverse clients. *Journal of Counseling Psychology, 60*(30), 353–366. 10.1037/a0032595

Jacobson, N. S., & Margolin, G. (1979). *Marital therapy: Strategies based on social learning and behavior exchange principles.* Brunner/Mazel.

Johnson, S. M. (2015). Emotionally focused couple therapy. In A. Gurman, J. Lebow, & D. K. Snyder (Eds.), *Clinical handbook of couple therapy* (5th ed., pp. 97–128). Guilford.

Johnson, S. M. (2020). *The practice of emotionally focused couple therapy: Creating connection* (3rd ed.). Routledge.

Kelly, S., Bhagwat, R., Maynigo, P., & Moses, E. (2014). Couple and marital therapy: The complement and expansion provided by multicultural approaches. In F. T. L. Leong, L. Comas-Diaz, G. C. Nagayama Hall, V. C. McLoyd, & J. E. Trimble (Eds.), *APA handbook of multicultural psychology, Vol. 2: Applications and training* (pp. 479–497). American Psychological Association. 10.1037/14187-027

Kohlenberg, R. J., & Tsai, M. (2007). *Functional analytic psychotherapy: Creating intense and curative therapeutic relationships*. Springer.

Kohut, H. (1977). *The restoration of the self*. International Universities Press.

Kohut, H. (1984). *How does analysis cure?* The University of Chicago Press. 10. 7208/chicago/9780226006147.001.0001

Koenig H. G. (2015). Religion, spirituality, and health: A review and update. *Advances in Mind- Body Medicine, 29*(3), 19–26.

Lebow, J. L. (2014). *Couple and family therapy: An integrative map of the territory*. American Psychological Association.

Linehan, M. M. (2015). *DBT skills training manual* (2nd ed.). Guilford Press.

Linehan, M. M., & Wilks, C. R. (2015). The course and evolution of dialectical behavior therapy. *American Journal of Psychotherapy, 69*(2), 97–110. 10.1176/ appi.psychotherapy.2015.69.2.97.

Luborsky, L., & Barrett, M. S. (2006). History and empirical status of key psychoanalytic concepts. *Annual Review of Clinical Psychology, 2*, 1–19. 10.1146/ annurev.clinpsy.2.022305.095328

McGeorge, C., Coburn, K., & Walsdorf, A. (2021). Deconstructing cissexism: The journey of becoming an affirmative family therapist for transgender and nonbinary clients. *Journal of Marital and Family Therapy, 47*, 785–802. 10.1111/jmft.12481

McGoldrick, M., Gerson, R., & Petry, S. S. (2008). *Genograms: Assessment and intervention*. W. W. Norton.

Miller, W. R., & Thoresen, C. E. (2003). Spirituality, religion and health: An emerging research field. *American Psychologist, 58*(1), 24–35.

Miller, W. R. & Rollnick, S. (2012). *Motivational interviewing: Helping people change*, (3rd ed.). Guilford.

Minuchin, S. & Fishman, H. C. (1981). *Family therapy techniques*. Harvard University Press.

Otto, M., & Smits, J. A. J. (2011). *Exercise for mood and anxiety: Proven strategies for overcoming depression and enhancing well-being*. Oxford University Press.

Overholser, J. (2018). *The Socratic Method of Psychotherapy*. Columbia University Press.

Patterson, G. R., Reid, J. B., & Dishion, T. J. (1992). *Antisocial boys: A social interactional approach*. Castalia.

Pinsof, W., Breunlin, D., Russell, W., Lebow, J., Rampage, C., & Chambers, A. (2018). *Integrative systemic therapy: Metaframeworks for problem solving with individuals, couples, and families*(1st ed.). American Psychological Association. 10.1037/0000055-000

Russell, B., & Breunlin, D. (2019). Transcending therapy models and managing complexity: Suggestions from integrative systemic therapy. *Family Process, 58*(3), 641–655. 10.1111/famp.12482

Safran, J. D., Greenberg, L. S., & Rice, L. N. (1988). Integrating psychotherapy research and practice: Modeling the change process. *Psychotherapy Theory Research & Practice, 25*(1), 1–17. 10.1037/h0085305

Scharff, M. E. D. (Ed.). (1995). *Object relations theory and practice: An introduction*. Jason Aronson.

Scharff, D. E., & Scharff, J. S. (2005). Psychodynamic couple therapy. In G. O. Gobbard, J. S. Beck, & J. Holmes (Eds.), *Oxford textbook of psychotherapy* (pp. 67–75). Oxford University Press.

Scharff, D. E., & de Varela, Y. (2005). Object Relations Couple Therapy. In M. Harway (Ed.), *Handbook of couples' therapy* (pp. 141–156). John Wiley & Sons.

Scheinkman, M., & Fishbane, M. (2004). The vulnerability cycle: Working with impasses in couple therapy. *Family Process, 43*(3), 279–299. 10.1111/j.1545-5300.2004.00023.x

Schielke, H. (2013). *Systemic Alliance and Progress in Individual Therapy: The Influence of Indirect Client System Alliance on Process and Progress in Individual Therapy*. [Doctoral dissertation, Miami University). Ohio Link Electronic Theses and Dissertation Center.

Schwartz, R. (2013). *Evolution of the internal family systems model*. Center for Self Leadership.

Selvini-Palazzoli, M., Cecchin, G., Prata, G., & Boscolo, L. (1980). Hypothesizing, circularity, and neutrality: Three guidelines for the conductor of the session. *Family Process, 19*, 3–12. 10.1111/j.1545-5300.1980.00003.x

Sherman, J. E. (2017). The serenity prayer and 16 variations. *Psychology Today*. https://www.psychologytoday.com/us/blog/ambigamy/201703/the-serenity-prayer-and-16-variations

Shin, S., Chow, C., Camacho-Gonsalves, T., Levy, R., Allen, I., & Leff, H. (2005). A meta-analytic review of racial-ethnic matching for African American and Caucasian American clients and clinicians. *Journal of Counseling Psychology, 52*(1), 45–56. 10.1037/0022-0167.52.1.45

Singh, A., & Dickey, L. (2017). *Affirmative counseling and psychological practice with transgender and gender nonconforming clients*. American Psychological Association.

Stathopoulou, G., Powers, M. B., Berry, A. C., Smits, J. A. J., & Otto, M. W. (2006). Exercise interventions for mental health: A quantitative and qualitative review. *Clinical Psychology: Science and Practice, 13*(2), 179–193. 10.1111/j.1468-2850.2006.00021.x

Sue, D., Sue, D., Neville, H., & Smith, L. (2019). *Counseling the culturally diverse: Theory and practice* (8th ed.). John Wiley & Sons, Inc.

Tang, Y. (2017). *The neuroscience of mindfulness meditation: How the body and mind work together to change our behaviour* (1st ed.). Springer International Publishing. 10.1007/978-3-319-46322-3

Tomm, K. (1987). Interventive interviewing: Part II. Intending to ask lineal, circular, strategic, or reflexive questions? *Family Process, 27*, 1–15.

Walsh, F. (2009). Religion, spirituality and the family: Multifaith perspectives. In F. Walsh (Eds.), *Spiritual resources in family therapy* (2nd ed., pp. 3–30). Guilford Press.

Watzlawick, P., Weakland, J. H., & Fisch, R. (1974). *Change: Principles of problem formation and problem resolution*. Norton.

White, M., & Epston, D. (1990). *Narrative means to therapeutic ends*. Norton.

White, M., & Epston, D. (2004). Externalizing the problem. *Relating Experience: Stories from Health and Social Care, 1*(88), 88–94.

Evaluating Treatment Progress and Modifying Plans

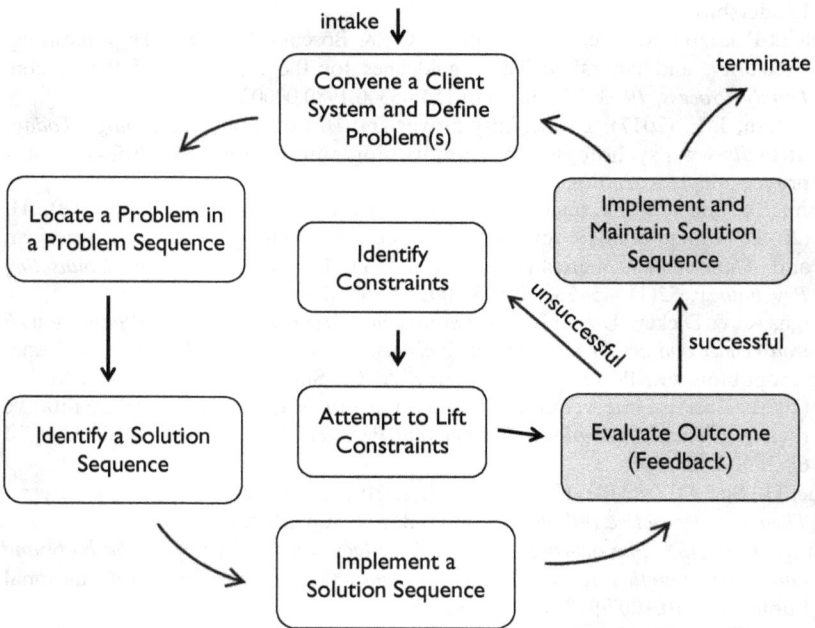

IST Essence Diagram.

Objective

This chapter will present the IST perspective on how to evaluate therapy progress and modify treatment planning. This includes evaluating the appropriateness of and client fidelity to the solution sequences, the success of interventions to remove constraints, and the path for determining if other constraints are still present. The intricacies of the evaluation process are discussed in relation to particular interventions as well as the overall progress of therapy. Special emphasis is given to the discussion of

DOI: 10.4324/9780429322273-9

client feedback and how it can lead to the modification of a plan, which is a hallmark of the IST approach.

Introduction

Like any therapy, IST is not a simple linear process that proceeds precisely according to the descriptions in books and articles. Even manualized treatments must be adjusted based on the emerging circumstances of a case, but IST is considerably more fluid than manualized treatments. While there is an overarching structure for IST that is grounded in the essence diagram, the solution sequences designed to solve the presenting problem and the methods chosen to remove constraints are all constructed to fit the case and are not derivative of any one model. IST is client system-centered and not model-driven. Hence, while the essence diagram always serves as the standard road map for IST, therapists will need to hypothesize and improvise to accomplish the essence steps given the unique nature of each case.

The essence diagram (see Figure 1.2 in Chapter 1) has a step that calls for the therapist to evaluate the outcome of a solution sequence as a step toward solving the problem, but then when the solution sequence is not deployed or fails, to move to the step of determining what the constraints are that kept it from being successful. Once one or more constraints have been identified, the next step is to develop interventions that are designed to lift the constraints. Chapter 8 presented a host of strategies and interventions designed for this purpose.

IST is an integrative therapy built on the failure-driven premise: what do you do when what you are doing isn't working? The process of evaluating progress is crucial to the decision to stay the course or modify the direction of therapy. The therapist is always asking: Is what I am doing producing progress in the therapy? IST is committed to helping clients solve the presenting problems that propel them to seek therapy. When the approach being taken isn't showing progress, the IST therapist has a plethora of alternatives to which to turn. The way the therapist changes course, however, is driven by a set of principles.

IST does not view the evaluation of outcome in a pass/fail framework. Rather, evaluation is couched in a framework of progress. Effort and partial success both count as progress. And, lack of progress is framed as an opportunity to learn more about what needs to be addressed in therapy. Progress places the therapy in a positive light. Of course, if progress is too slow, clients may lose motivation and conclude that the change is too small or too late in coming. In such a case, the task (the intervention) and the goal (solve the problem) components of the alliance suffer which may result in the clients withdrawing from therapy. Thus, it is essential to solicit feedback, track progress, and collaborate with clients on whether to affirm or modify the direction of therapy.

The Time it Takes to See Progress

As seen in Appendix A, IST's six planning metaframeworks are each associated with a set of strategies. A variety of interventions for implementing a given strategy can be selected from the many models of therapy and informed by the research on pantheoretical variables generally referred to as common factors (Davis et al., 2012; Sprenkle & Blow, 2004; Sprenkle et al., 2009). When a constraint is identified that is keeping the solution sequence from working, the therapist selects a planning metaframework, a strategy from that planning metaframework, and an intervention to implement the strategy. Sometimes the intervention can be implemented and evaluated during the session, but more often the implementation occurs between sessions. In these situations, the intervention can be evaluated in the next session. For example, one of the partners in a same-sex relationship complained that most of the housekeeping was done by her even though both women worked. The therapist initially addressed this presenting problem by suggesting the clients make a list of domestic tasks and divide them equally. They did this in the session and planned to implement it at home that week. During the next session, the therapist learned that nothing had changed. When the partner who did less housekeeping was asked what kept her from attending to the items on her list, she said that she had been raised in a home in another country where there were servants who did all things domestic. She did not remember her parents ever doing domestic chores and she and her siblings were not asked to help. She confessed that on some level she still had the feeling that it was beneath" her to do the work of a servant. Since it was out of the question financially for the women to solve the problem with domestic help, they had to find another way to lift this cultural constraint. In this situation, the therapist intervened, evaluated the intervention, and found a constraint in one week's time.

At other times, the intervention takes time to unfold over the course of several weeks or even months; hence, evaluation of the intervention cannot occur until it has had sufficient time to work. For example, the parents of two children (six and eight) sought therapy because the children often ignored the parents' requests (to take a bath, put on pajamas, come to dinner, etc.). The problem sequence was as follows: Parents make a request of the children, the children ignore the request, the parents push, the children ignore and then one of the parents steps in and gets involved in completing the requested behavior. For a solution sequence, in a family therapy session, the therapist asked the parents to pick three behaviors for which they wanted to see better compliance and explain this to the children. The children were on board, and the parents agreed to post the behaviors on the refrigerator. In the next session, the parents reported that the solution sequence had not been successful. When asked what kept it from working, the father noted that his wife did not believe in punishment so there were no consequences to the noncompliance. Based on further discussion, the therapist hypothesized that the mother's beliefs about parenting prevented the use of consequences. Respecting this, the therapist decided on a strategy of introducing consequences but in the form of positive reinforcement rather than punishment. The use of a contingency contract was chosen as the intervention to accomplish the strategy. The therapist used psychoeducation to explain contingency contracting to the parents, and they agreed to implement a star chart for each child. The children were involved in selecting the reward they would receive once they had achieved the requisite number of stars. Knowing that it takes, on average, about 66 days to establish a new pattern (Lally et al., 2009), the therapist monitored the parents' commitment to it weekly and asked about progress. The progress was initially somewhat sporadic both at the parents' end (failing to put the stars on the chart) and the children's end (still some noncompliance). During the session in the sixth week of the intervention, the therapist requested that the parents bring the coming week's star chart to the next session. The children were asked to bring any rewards they had received to show the therapist. In the next session, a simple count revealed an 80% compliance rate for the target behaviors, and the children had both chosen special time with a parent as their reward. The mother noted that an adage used by the therapist, "catch them being good," resonated with her. Overall, the therapist's evaluation was that the constraints had been lifted, but given the research on habit formation, it was wise to monitor the success of the intervention for a couple more weeks.

Method

Tracking Progress

Regardless of the type of therapy or how its outcomes are defined, research suggests that better outcomes are achieved when the therapist monitors the therapy's progress (Harmon et al., 2005; Lambert et al., 2001; Lambert et al., 2004; Lambert et al., 2018; Pinsof et al., 2012; Tasca et al., 2019). There are three general ways to track progress. The first is for the therapist to simply ask the clients about progress. This can be done on a session-by-session basis: "So let's talk about how the session went today," or periodically, "So we have had five sessions so far. Let's talk for a minute about how you think we are doing." The second way is to use informal measures of progress such as scaling. Scaling can informally measure the frequency, intensity, or duration of a variable such as the level of conflict in a fight. If any of those variables scale in the right direction, some progress is being made.

The third way to monitor progress is to use a validated progress instrument that can be administered for each session or episodically. These instruments reflect client (rather than therapist) perspectives on progress. The client's view is important because it enables the therapist's collaboration and, interestingly, some research suggests that therapists themselves are not particularly good judges of progress, especially when a case is not going well (Lambert, 2013). The most well-known progress instruments have been developed primarily for individual therapy. They include the Outcome Questionnaire-45 (OQ-45) (Lambert et al., 2001), the Outcome Rating Scale for adults (ORS) (Miller et al., 2003), and the Child Outcome Rating Scale for children (CORS) (Duncan et al., 2006), as well as an instrument for couples therapy, the Partners for Change Outcome Management System (PCOMS) (Miller et al., 2005).

Progress instruments provide the therapist with feedback that is used to track progress, but also to affirm or modify the direction of therapy. For example, a 35-year-old Chinese American cisgender heterosexual woman presented for individual therapy for depression. At the therapist's request, she agreed to complete a weekly instrument that tracks progress at the individual, couple, and family level of the system and also tracks the alliances in therapy (Systemic Therapy Inventory of Change; Pinsof et al., 2009). The client lived with her mother in a conflicted relationship. The two had come to the United States many years ago. The daughter considered herself to be Chinese American, while she reported that her mother thought of herself as Chinese and seemed to want the daughter to think of herself in that way. The two had many conflicts, resulting in the daughter largely subjugating her identity to fit the needs of her mother.

A scale on the progress instrument measures negative affect. As the daughter used therapy to validate her Chinese American identity, her progress feedback on the negative affect scale moved farther into the clinical range (meaning more negative affect). When the therapist asked the daughter why she thought the scale was going in that direction, she said that she was finally becoming her own person and felt guilty knowing that the mother would not approve of the choices she was making to embrace the American part of her identity. When the therapist and woman discussed the concept of differentiation, the woman understood her ambivalence better. The therapist helped her use parts language to articulate that a part of her knew she needed to differentiate for the sake of her identity, while another part of her felt guilty that she was abandoning what she believed her mother wanted her to be.

It is interesting that one of the alliance scales that measures what a client thinks family members who do not participate in the therapy feel about the therapy continued to deteriorate over this same period. This suggested that the mother did not support the goals of the therapy. The daughter confirmed that this was the case. The mother saw the therapy as taking her daughter further toward the identity of an Asian American woman and further away from that of a Chinese-born woman. The therapist decided that it was essential to hold sessions with the daughter and the mother in the hope that the mother would come to a different understanding of her daughter's dilemma and be more accepting of the direction of the therapy. Thus, progress was tracked and the plan for the therapy was modified, in part, based on feedback from the client's completion of a validated progress instrument.

Evaluation Using Informal Measures of Progress

IST evaluation focuses on the ongoing progress of the case. In addition to formal progress measures discussed earlier in the chapter, there are several additional ways to measure progress. Which one is adopted depends on both the nature of the constraint being lifted and the type of intervention being used. The first type of measure is *scaling*. It is appropriate for a variable associated with a constraint that varies in magnitude much as the temperature does. Usually, the variable can be measured in terms of its frequency (how often are there hot or cold days in a given location), intensity (how hot or cold does it get) and duration (how long does it stay very hot or cold). Frequency and duration can be measured simply by tracking how often something occurs and how long it lasts. Intensity can be measured on a 10-point scale. For example, a couple sought therapy to address frequent arguing that usually culminated in intense shouting (intensity). They reported that they had such arguments about five times a week (frequency). When asked to put the intensity on a ten-point scale, they said that a typical fight would get to a seven, but they had been known to go as high as a nine or ten. They maintained that physical violence never occurred. They also said that when the argument ended, they usually did not speak to one another for the rest of the day, or longer if the argument was at an elevated level of intensity.

The therapist noted that the arguments were symptomatic of some underlying distress in their relationship and added that therapy could not address that distress until they were able to communicate without such intense arguing. They agreed. In IST language, de-escalating conflict was the strategy and the therapist chose "time out" as the intervention, noting that once one of them reached a five on the intensity scale, they would agree to stop the conversation for 15 minutes and then resume it if the intensity for both of them had abated.

In the next session, they reported that they had failed, but when the therapist tracked the variables of frequency, intensity, and duration, it was clear that they had been successful. The couple only had two arguments, as opposed to their average five, the intensity never got above a five and while they still could not resume the conversation, the duration of the arguments was shortened. The couple also reported that they were getting along a few hours after the arguments rather than stonewalling each other. Framed this way, the couple could see they were making progress.

Adoption of frequency, intensity, and duration as measures of progress is often indicated when the client is seeking symptomatic relief. In many of these cases, a more realistic outcome is to moderate the problem rather than completely eliminate it. The problem can be anxiety, depression, pain, or excessive involvement in a behavior such as working, eating, or substance use. As progress is measured over time, the client(s) and therapist decide whether the progress is sufficient.

The second type of measurable change involves the addition or subtraction of a behavior that is part of an intervention. The measure of progress is the extent to which the clients add or eliminate the behaviors. Again, trying something new and partially succeeding rather than demonstrating proficiency in the new behavior is sufficient to provide a positive assessment that progress is being made. For example, a couple was consistently critical of each other while still professing that they wanted to work on their relationship. Using the strategy of increasing positivity in the relationship, the therapist introduced the 5:1 ratio derived from Gottman's research on couples (Gottman, 1993) that showed that stable relationships evidence five positive statements to each negative. The couple readily acknowledged that their ratio was nowhere near 5:1. The couple and therapist agreed that the couple would work on improving their ratio. They returned for the next session and admitted that they said a few positive things but did not come close to the 5:1 ratio. Still, they had internalized the strategy to increase their positivity. The therapist praised them for a good start and encouraged them to renew their efforts. Over the course of several sessions, they continued to improve their ratio.

The third measurement of progress focuses on an organizational constraint described with a concept from the organization metaframework. When the organizational constraint is lifted, the organizational parameters that regulate the system function better which facilitates the resolution of the problem. The organizational issue often involves boundaries and/or leadership in the client system. Progress is deemed to have occurred when the organizational variable begins to approximate what would be considered functional. Of course, what is deemed functional is determined as much by the cultural norms of the client system as by the hypothesis about how the parts of the system fit together (organization).

For example, a couple in their 60s recently retired and sought therapy to address a concern that they were growing apart despite retirement affording them more time together. They agreed with their therapist on a solution sequence to do something together at least twice a week. When they returned for the next session, they had not done anything together. When asked what kept them from spending time together, they reported that their adult children dominated their lives, which precluded the time they needed to be a couple. The therapist asked them to explain how the constraint worked. They explained that they had four adult children. Two of the children were cited as the most problematic. The first was a daughter in her early 30s who continued to live at home and was not working. She often sought out her mother for companionship, and the mother would rarely turn her down. She would use the kitchen and leave it for the mother to clean up. She monopolized the public spaces, thus keeping the couple from having privacy. The second daughter in her mid-30s had two children. She would bring them to the couple's house most days. Entering unannounced, she would leave the children in their care for the entire day.

The therapist read all of this feedback to hypothesize that one of the constraints was a constraint of organization involving loose boundaries that kept the couple from having sufficient time together. The opportunity created by retirement to enrich their relationship had been hijacked by the time demanded from their adult children. As the constraint was clarified, the couple agreed that they wished to address it. Lifting this constraint required many sessions. The therapy goal was to establish clear boundaries that placed limits on the time the parents would devote to their adult children. Over the course of several months, sessions were held with the couple, the whole family, the couple and each daughter, and each daughter separately.

Ultimately, the daughter living at home agreed to get a job, clean up after herself, and establish a plan for independent living. The daughter who brought her children over to babysit agreed to limit the amount of time to twice a week for three hours each time. The couple was delighted to have their lives back and reported feeling much closer to each other. These outcomes served as the measure that considerable progress had been made toward the goal of defining clearer boundaries. Furthermore, progress in lifting the organizational constraint of diffuse boundaries had facilitated the solution to the couple's presenting problem.

It is worth noting here that lifting the boundary constraint required a change in the behavior of both daughters. This required identifying constraints they presented, lifting them, and evaluating the progress. The following illustrates how the constraint lifting process in IST requires the continued application of the blueprint.

First, when the therapist discussed with the couple what kept the daughter living with them from establishing more of her own adult life, they reported that she had always performed poorly at school. She dropped out of college in her first year and held several jobs for short periods of time. What was keeping her from being more successful? After meeting with her and the parents, the therapist hypothesized that she had attention deficit hyperactivity disorder (ADHD). A referral to a psychiatrist confirmed this diagnosis, and she was placed on a stimulant medication to which she had a positive response. With the ADHD managed, a plan was made for her to enter the workforce part-time, complete her schooling and eventually get a job that would allow her to live independently. The therapist monitored and evaluated her progress at each step. She did see the psychiatrist and took the prescribed medicine. She did get a part-time job and took courses at a local community college. When she did have free time, she volunteered to go to her sister's house to provide childcare. It was clear that she was taking steps to reclaim her life. She was making progress with each component of her plan. As she spent more and more time away from the parents' house, the parents were able to spend time together.

Constraints also existed for the daughter who dropped off her children every day. She had been in a serious accident that caused damage to her spine and left her in chronic pain. She dealt with this by reducing the demands of her life, which included leaning on her parents to provide childcare for her children. The daughter's husband had a constraining view of his role in childcare. Based on his experience in his family of origin, he did not believe men needed to participate substantially in the daily caretaking of the children. He also did not seem to understand the extent of his wife's disability. The therapist met with the daughter and her husband and helped the husband understand that his wife needed more assistance. He changed the schedule of his work so he could provide more childcare. The result was that the daughter relied less heavily on her parents.

When asked about the extent of her injury, it was clear that the daughter did not fully grasp the nature of it. Employing a biobehavioral strategy, the therapist facilitated her referral to a spine specialist who provided several options, including surgery for reducing her pain. After much discussion, she elected the surgery. The recovery was long and arduous, but the family pulled together to help her. As she recovered, she progressively relied less on her parents to the point where she used them for childcare only when they were willing and able.

This case required the therapist to track progress on each of the constraints as well as on the originally identified problem of the parent's lack of connection. The therapist used the blueprint to collect information (feedback) and hypothesize about the constraints at various subsystems of the family system. Strategies and interventions (plans) were selected for each constraint and the therapist used client feedback to evaluate progress. As the constraints were lifted the parents were able to enact new patterns (solution sequences) that led to their feeling more connected.

A Decision Tree for Progress Evaluation

There are several crucial junctures in the course of practicing IST that call for sound judgment by the therapist. This judgment is guided by the therapist's reading of the feedback both in sessions and between sessions. These junctures include evaluating the relative success of the solution sequence and deciding whether to modify it, evaluating the success of an attempt to lift a constraint, managing two or more constraints, and working with intractable constraints.

Evaluating the Solution Sequence

For a solution sequence to impact the presenting problem, the clients must have a good grasp of what they are to do, be fully committed to doing it, and have the time to do it. It is the responsibility of the therapist to assure that the clients are on board in these ways and to be thorough with the who, what, when, where, and why of the solution sequence. When the therapist and clients meet next following the scheduled employment of the solution sequence, it is useful to invite the clients to talk about their experience of performing it. The therapist should be prepared for some version of the classic "life happens" scenario. For example, "I came down with a bad cold early in the week, so we never got to try it" or "His work made him travel this week, so we never found a good time to try it." Both explanations seem reasonable, and the therapist's judgment might be to take them at face value. If, however, variants of excuses are offered several times, the therapist will begin to question whether something is keeping the couple from trying the solution sequence. This judgment would lead to a constraint question: "It seems like it has been difficult for you to find time to try this experiment. Do you think something might be keeping you from trying it?"

If the clients tried the solution sequence but had partial success or failure, it is important to first review its parameters to be sure there are no flaws in it that preclude it from working. If flaws are discovered, it is worth making adjustments and then asking if the clients are willing to try again. For example, if a parent has agreed to assist with homework in a less hovering way but has not done it because the student has not brought the assignment home, the parent might add a step of calling the teacher to develop a plan that assures that the assignment makes it into the student's backpack or is available in digital form.

If the clients still have been unable to perform the solution sequence after several adjustments, the therapist hypothesizes that a constraint exists that keeps the clients from doing the solution sequence. The therapist next asks a variant of the constraint question, for example, "Can you think of anything that might be keeping you from being able to do the experiment on which we agreed?" The clients will provide feedback. Sometimes the response is easy to interpret in the language of constraints. For example, a woman in a committed relationship with her partner owned a piece of property that she had purchased many years ago with the dream of someday building a home on it. The partners came to therapy with the problem that their future was clouded by the woman's insistence that they could mingle their assets except for this property. The woman wanted the property to remain titled in her name alone. This was greatly upsetting to her partner who could not see how this property should be an exception. The strong emotions generated whenever this discussion came up resulted in a pattern of avoidance of the subject. The result was that their relationship always seemed at risk. An initial solution sequence was to eliminate the avoidance pattern and to have a conversation where the goal was simply to state their opinions about the issue pertaining to the property. The couple had two chances to enact this solution sequence, but did not do so on either occasion, due to what seemed like avoidance on the part of the woman.

The therapist hypothesized that the woman attached some special meaning to the property that she could not or would not articulate. The original solution sequence had been drawn from the action planning metaframework with the strategy to reduce avoidance by enabling direct communication. It was not working. The therapist shifted to an M1 (mind metaframework) hypothesis that the property represented an important meaning for the woman that was woven into her self narrative. In the next session, drawing on the meaning/emotion planning metaframework, the therapist said to the woman, "I wonder if there might be some special meaning that you attach to the property that makes you want it to be exclusively yours and prevents you from being able to discuss it with your partner?" The woman sat silently for several minutes and then told the story that the property had been willed to her by her father whose own great grandfather had owned the property and held enslaved people during the time of slavery. The woman felt extremely guilty about this legacy but had a dream that one day she would return to the property and do something with it that would foster social justice in that community. She had never told her partner anything about this part of her history and feared that discussing the property would open Pandora's Box and lead to her partner abandoning her.

So, just how should the constraint be described? The constraint involves the family legacy of involvement in slavery, the meaning she attaches to the property that is a part of that legacy, and the fear she has that revealing anything about it will irrevocably damage her relationship with her partner.

Evaluating the Success of an Attempt to Lift a Constraint

In the example above, when the constraint no longer keeps the solution sequence from solving the presenting problem, it is considered lifted. Once a constraint has been identified, the first step for the therapist is to evaluate whether simply describing it has a positive effect. In the example, staying in the meaning/emotion planning metaframework, the therapist wondered if naming the constraint had impacted its power to silence the woman on the topic of the property. Of course, fear reduction, in this case, is relational. It depends, in part, on the response of the partner to hearing about it. The therapist decided to inquire about the partner's response first. Fortunately, as this brief segment of dialogue illustrates, the partner was supportive:

Partner: "I can see this property holds a lot of meaning for you and what you just shared makes me understand just how complicated the issue is for you."

Woman: "I was so afraid that you would just outright reject me if you knew about my family's past. So is it true that my past won't be a deal breaker for our relationship?"

Partner: "I assure you that is not possible. I love you, which is why I want us to be on the same page going forward about our assets."

At this point, the therapist has to read the feedback and hypothesize about the constraint. The partner seemed open and was not asking to grill the woman about her past. The therapist concluded that going back to the solution sequence and asking them to resume their talks about assets was appropriate. This is an example of why the matrix diagram has a small arrow pointing back toward the top of the diagram. Often, once a constraint is lifted, the originally planned work can be resumed.

As the couple worked through the issues about the property, the woman expressed a preference to keep the property in her name so she could be free to do with it as she pleased. The couple found a way to balance the assets, and both felt comfortable with the solution they had achieved.

Managing Two or More Constraints

It is common to identify two or more constraints that interfere with a successful implementation of the solution sequence. Sometimes multiple constraints are uncovered as a cluster at one time, while at other times they emerge sequentially. Simultaneously emerging constraints require the therapist to prioritize which of the constraints receives attention.

Sequentially emerging constraints also require the therapist to decide whether to put a pause on the constraint being addressed at the moment and to prioritize the newly revealed constraint. Prioritization is based on two principles. First is the impact of the constraint on the health and safety of a family member. Second is the therapist's hypothesis about the relative strength of the constraint in preventing solutions. For example, parent functioning—both individual and relational—profoundly affects a child's development. Consequently, the therapist may prioritize certain parental constraints when working with child problems.

A family entered therapy to address their seven-year-old son's adjustment to school. He did not get along well with the other children and was frequently resistant to lessons and assignments. An evaluation had revealed a learning disability, which clearly was a constraint. The son had also been born prematurely. As a result, his parents had been very protective of him since birth. He was somewhat immature for his age and had spent little time socializing with other children prior to entering school. His level of social and emotional development served as a second constraint. The therapist worked with the school to take these factors into account and, as part of his Individual Education Plan (IEP), he was assigned time to work with a classroom assistant.

He seemed to be doing better but during this time, the mother was pregnant. She gave birth and developed postpartum depression. The therapist hypothesized that two additional constraints had emerged. One was developmental and involved the jealousy the boy felt for feeling displaced by a new baby in the house. The other involved the loss of presence of the mother created by the postpartum depression. The boy began to act out at school, and the teachers felt even greater concern.

Of the four constraints in play (learning disability, social/emotional immaturity, postpartum depression, and the family life-cycle transition of a new baby), the therapist decided to focus first on the depression by consulting with the mother's obstetrician-gynecologist and providing a referral to a psychiatrist to address the postpartum depression. This was an obvious choice, but one that demonstrates that constraints can be prioritized according to 1) their impact on health and safety and 2) the relative strength of the constraint in preventing solutions. Postpartum depression satisfied both conditions. With proper medication and guidance, the mother was able to manage the depression. To address the son's reaction to having a new sibling, family therapy sessions were held that included all four family members. The son, in a developmentally appropriate way, was able to express his feelings of abandonment and jealousy. He was also validated as the big brother and taught to take pride in his ability to be helpful in the care of his new sibling. This work had the added benefit of advancing his maturity.

Intractable Constraints

The IST essence diagram calls for therapists to work with clients to lift constraints. There are times, however, when the constraints are intractable. A constraint is intractable when the client system in which it is embedded does not have the influence or the resources to lift it. In these situations, while the constraint cannot be lifted, the client system can learn to manage it in a way that is less problematic so that solution sequences can be identified and implemented. When working with intractable constraints, the therapist must first ascertain that the constraint is, in fact, intractable for that client system, then identify the problem sequence adopted by the client system to deal with it, and lastly find a more adaptive solution sequence that improves the way it is managed. Progress in therapy is assessed in relation to these three tasks and thankfully not by the therapy's impact on the intractable. Of the various types of intractable constraints common in therapy, three examples will be addressed: unresolvable relationship issues, trauma, and biological constraints.

Unresolvable Relationship Issues

Gottman's (1993) research has established that 69% of issues around which couples have conflict never go away, yet couples often find themselves embroiled in arguments about these issues that can inflict serious damage to their relationships. It is as if a couple embarks on an argument saying to themselves, "This is the time when I am going to convince my partner to do something differently," only to, once again, find out that it is not going to happen. Their problem sequences seem to treat an unsolvable problem or difference as if it is solvable. Referred to by Gottman as perpetual problems, unresolvable relational issues are typically based on differences in personal characteristics. Examples include differences in patterns of punctuality, money management, privacy, and differences on the spectrum of introversion-extroversion.

To deal more effectively with an unresolvable issue, a couple must first accept it as such. In support of acceptance, the therapist can provide psychoeducation based on Gottman's research that suggests that all couples have unresolvable differences. It is often helpful to establish that certain things are in a person's nature—for example, one party may crave social situations and the other may much prefer to stay at home. There can be disappointments, frustrations, or conflict related to such a difference, but a characteristic is not essentially a sign of disregard or disrespect. Once a perpetual difference is accepted, it will continue to exist, but it can be less of a source of conflict and disappointment as the couple accepts that discussions about it need not escalate because the issue is not going to change. At this point, the therapist can guide the couple to search for more adaptive ways to manage the difference and encourage them to view the difference in light of the overall value of the relationship and the positive characteristics of each partner.

Trauma

Estimates are that 70% of individuals will experience at least one traumatic event during their lifetime (Benjet et al., 2016). A significant percentage of those individuals will experience complex trauma involving repetition of the behavior causing the trauma (Courtois & Ford, 2016), for example, sexual abuse repeated over a period of years. Today, trauma is considered so relevant to a person's mental health that some models of therapy are centered on the treatment of trauma. Trauma as a historical fact is intractable. Its sequelae may or may not be. When trauma is revealed as a constraint, it must be thoroughly addressed.

A distinction should be made here between the trauma, itself, and the impact it has on an individual. Regarding the former, the event of the past cannot be undone; hence, traumatized clients must forever reckon with the terrible things that have happened. Moreover, complex trauma can alter physiological aspects of a person's functioning (Osterman & Chemtob, 1999; van der Kolk, 2015; Courtois & Ford, 2016). For some individuals, trauma has ravaged their lives. For others, they possess a resiliency that enables them to be relatively or virtually unmarred by the trauma, with some reporting a sense of growth subsequent to it.

From an IST perspective, there are several considerations in determining whether trauma will become a focus in therapy. First, is the client presenting with an interest in working directly on a trauma or in mitigating the way it influences their lives? In other words, is it the presenting problem? Second, if the trauma is not the presenting problem, how constraining is it to what the client system is working on? Is it necessary to address the trauma in order to resolve the constraint? Third, if the work can proceed without directly addressing the trauma, then it is still possible that the initial discussion of it leads the client to want to address it in therapy. In this way, trauma can become an additional presenting problem within the therapy or a reason to provide a referral for work on it.

An IST therapist working with trauma will slow down the process of problem-solving and pay much closer attention to emotional safety within the therapeutic environment. This is consistent with several trauma models that have specified a first stage of therapy such as creating a context for change and providing a refuge (Barrett & Fish, 2014), establishing safety (Herman, 2015), and safety and stabilization (Courtois & Ford, 2016) as well as approaches that emphasize establishing emotional and relational safety (Armstrong, 2019; Goelitz, 2021). Further intervention follows the establishment of a sense of safety with the therapist. Clients are helped to manage symptomatology and are given a clear sense that they can control the pace of therapy in the context of a collaborative alliance. The current-day manifestation of the post-traumatic experience is understood in terms of internal sequences of intrusive and avoidant responses, physiological manifestations, the narrative of the traumatic events and their aftermath, and the interactional sequences in the client's relationships with family members, friends, co-workers, and the therapist.

When trauma has a lasting negative impact on a person, competent therapy that attends to it is required. The IST planning metaframeworks have strategies that can be utilized to address trauma, and their corresponding specific interventions (listed in Appendix A), typically from empirically-supported treatments, can be integrated into the work. Addressing these strategies and interventions is beyond the scope of this book, but it is worth emphasizing that substantive training is required in order to utilize them. If, after substantive and intensive treatment, the sequelae of traumatic events prove to be intractable, the individual and the family system will need to accept the family member's condition, increase social support, learn means of managing the symptoms together, and develop the flexibility to manage the waxing and waning of post-traumatic symptomatology.

Biology

There are myriad aspects of our biology that constitute constraints, and many of them are intractable. Progressive and permanent illnesses keep family members from achieving many goals in life. The aging of a family member often involves home care that can upend the balance of a family. The impending loss is excruciating, time demands are extensive, and coordinating family resources can divide families. Injuries with permanent sequelae can destroy the dreams of the injured client as well as those of loved ones. For example, a 21-year-old had a motorcycle accident that left him a quadriplegic. The family entered therapy with the tasks of mourning the loss of potential while simultaneously planning for his care. In other cases, the injuries occur years prior to the therapy and the family has obviously made some adaptation to it, but when the information about the injury surfaces, the therapist must read the feedback and wonder whether the injury plays a role in constraining the family from solving the problem that brought them to therapy.

Death is the ultimate biological constraint. Though death is obviously intractable, grief is not, though it can be extraordinarily challenging. The grief spawned by the loss of a loved one can ripple through relationships in silent but impactful ways. Constraints associated with loss can have far-reaching effects on relationships. For example, Lisa, a 30-year-old white, cisgender woman sought therapy to address the lack of purpose in her life. She had attended college but was indifferent to her major, and she had been dissatisfied with the jobs she had taken since graduation. She reported having no hobbies or special interests. The primary question in therapy became, "What keeps you from finding something in life about which you can be passionate?" At some point, Lisa shared that her parents had lost an infant boy early in their marriage, and that she believed that she served as a replacement for the lost son. Further, she felt that her father had a gender bias in favor of males, and she believed he was deeply disappointed not to have a son to be the successor to his business. Hence, as she saw it, nothing she pursued could serve as a replacement for her deceased brother.

The therapist hypothesized that Lisa had not sufficiently differentiated from her family of origin; hence, she never learned how to independently search for her own passions. The therapist thought that a plan to address the constraint of lack of differentiation would have several components. First, Lisa needed to examine and revise her narrative that she was nothing more than a second-best replacement child. Drawing from the meaning/emotion planning metaframework, the therapist would utilize interventions from narrative therapy. Once her narrative embraced the idea that she was a person in her own right and not a replacement for her brother, she may be able to work more directly on finding her interests and passion. As the work progressed, the therapist referred her to a psychologist who administered an occupational interest inventory and aptitude testing. Next, the therapist helped her plan a meeting with her parents to discuss the lost brother and its impact on her. This proved to be an effective step in the process of differentiating from her family of origin. After the constraints related to the family process and narrative were addressed, Lisa was able to work productively on finding direction for her life.

Conducting Therapy Over Time

As the previous example suggests, therapy is a planful activity that uses the blueprint to read feedback, hypothesize and plan how to accomplish the tasks of the IST essence. Careful attention is paid to the therapeutic conversation and the maintenance of the alliance. The goals of therapy are defined and pursued. Constraints that emerge along the way are identified and lifted.

Like other therapies, IST can be said to have a middle stage. At this stage, the work has been laid out and agreed upon by the clients and the therapist and the task is to keep working through it. Each model of therapy specifies what there is to work through. In IST, the working-through process is likely to continue to involve new discoveries. This is the case due to IST's constraint pillar which encourages progressive identification of new constraints and to IST's guideline that assessment continues throughout therapy. New discoveries lead to a further understanding of client strengths as well as constraints that must be lifted or, if they are intractable, managed in a healthier way. Since this work is in the service of the clients' goals for therapy, there is a continual return to the themes and solution sequences associated with those goals.

Always, IST is geared to treat a client system; hence, the therapist and clients decide who will participate in the direct client system and why. The decisions about who attends sessions and when are continually driven by the discovery of who is needed to participate in a solution sequence or to lift a constraint. Thus, the direct client system is not a static entity as the decisions about who attends therapy may continue throughout the early, middle, and later stages of the work.

Evaluation of the progress of therapy during this middle phase centers on an assessment of the progress being made toward the lifting of key constraints. As discussed in the Methods section above, there are a variety of ways to measure progress. In addition to the measurement(s) utilized, the therapist should periodically inquire about the progress clients feel they are making. Again, the primary indicator of success is progress more so than specific outcomes. If the therapist and clients ascertain that sufficient progress is being made toward the goals, therapy can continue in the direction it is going until there is sufficient progress to consider termination. If the client is not feeling that enough progress is being made, the therapist will explore the direction of therapy including the current hypotheses and the plan or plans that have been made to address them. Sometimes over the course of therapy clients will ask to work on a different problem. In general, IST therapists would agree with this shift with the caveat that the current goals are being shelved rather than abandoned.

Addressing the state of the alliances is vital to maintaining the prospect of a positive outcome. Recall that when doing relational therapy there are several alliances. The alliance one partner believes the therapist has with the other partner can be as important as the alliance that partner has with the therapist. For example, if Jan wants to address her partner Amanda's level of alcohol consumption, but Amanda is not ready to discuss it (precontemplation stage of change), then pushing this issue to the forefront of therapy will potentially damage the therapist's alliance with Amanda. It also may impact Jan's alliance with the therapist, even though Jan had been the one to initiate the focus on alcohol. In other words, Jan may be concerned that the therapist is not maintaining a good alliance with Amanda.

Conclusion

All therapy should include an evaluative component. Because IST operates with a failure-driven premise (what do you do when what you are doing is not working?), it is essential that the therapist continually solicits client feedback and assesses progress. When progress is not being made, the integrative nature of IST provides the clinical pathway to do something different. The steps of the essence diagram depict where evaluation is required: Is the solution sequence working? Are constraints being lifted? Is the therapy identifying additional problems? Is the overall progress of therapy adequate? The answer to any of these questions may require that the therapist modify a hypothesis or the plan to address it. Such shifts are expected in IST, and they are a source of the flexibility required to fit a therapy to the client system's patterns and needs. This process of evaluation and the shifting of therapeutic direction has been the subject of this chapter. The next chapter will discuss the termination of therapy.

Exercises

Consider these questions. Discuss with a colleague or record your answers by one means or another.

1   How do you determine whether your clients are making progress?
2   Pick one of your cases and evaluate your most recent intervention with it. Did you get enough feedback from the client to evaluate the outcome of the intervention? Do you think the intervention contributed to progress with the case?
3   Pick one of your cases and evaluate the overall progress with the case? What is improving? What is not? Are you satisfied with the progress?
4   Do you regularly ask your clients whether they feel progress is being made in their therapy? If you don't, given the research that indicates feedback improves progress, what might be keeping you from doing so? Supervision is a good place to work on this issue, as person-of-the-therapist issues are often the constraining factor in not asking clients how the therapy is working for them.

A Project

If you do not use a standardized instrument to measure progress, do you think it might be valuable to locate one and try it with some of your cases? If so, select one and learn how to use it. Use it with a few of your cases and compare your experience with those cases to that of a comparable group of cases with which you don't use a progress instrument. Evaluate whether it makes a difference in your work.

References

Armstrong, C. (2019). *Rethinking trauma treatment: Attachment, memory reconsolidation, and resilience.* Norton & Company.

Barrett, M. J., & Fish, L. S. (2014). *Treating complex trauma: A relational blueprint for collaboration and change.* Routledge.

Benjet, C., Bromet, E., Karam, E. G., Kessler, R. C., McLaughlin, K. A., Ruscio, A. M., Shahly, V., Stein, D. J., Petukhova, M., Hill, E., Alonso, J., Atwoli, L., Bunting, B., Bruffaerts, R., Caldas-de-Almeida, J. M., de Girolamo, G., Florescu, S., Gureje, O., Huang, Y., ... Koenen, K. C. (2016). The epidemiology of traumatic event exposure worldwide: Results from the World Mental Health Survey Consortium. *Psychological Medicine, 46*(2), 327–343. 10.1017/S0033291715001981

Courtois, C. A., & Ford, J. D. (2016). *The treatment of complex trauma.* Guilford Press.

Davis, S. D., Lebow, J. L., & Sprenkle, D. H. (2012). Common factors of change in couple therapy. *Behavior Therapy, 43*(1), 36–48. 10.1016/j.beth.2011.01.009

Duncan, B. L., Sparks, J., Miller, S. D., Bohanske, R. T., & Claud, D. A. (2006). Giving youth a voice: A preliminary study of the reliability and validity of a brief outcome measure. https://www.scottdmiller.com/wp-content/uploads/CORS%20JBT%20(2).pdf

Goelitz, A. (2021). *From trauma to healing: A social worker's guide to working with survivors* (2nd ed.). Routledge.

Gottman, J. M. (1993). The roles of conflict engagement, escalation, and avoidance in marital interaction: a longitudinal view of five types of couples. *Journal of Consulting and Clinical Psychology, 61*(1), 6–15. 10.1037/0022-006X.61.1.6

Harmon, C., Hawkins, E. J., Lambert, M. J., Slade, K., & Whipple, J. S. (2005). Improving outcomes for poorly responding clients: The use of clinical support tools and feedback to clients. *Journal of Clinical Psychology, 61*(2), 175–185. 10.1002/jclp.20109.

Herman, J. L. (2015). *Trauma and recovery: The aftermath of violence – from domestic abuse to political terror.* Basic Books.

Lally, P., Van Jaarsveld, C. H., Potts, H. W., & Wardle, J. (2009). How are habits formed: Modelling habit formation in the real world. *European Journal of Social Psychology, 40*(6), 998–1009.

Lambert, M. J., Hansen, N. B., & Finch, A. E. (2001). Patient-focused research: Using patient outcome data to enhance treatment effects. *Journal of Consulting and Clinical Psychology, 69*(2), 159–172. 10.1037/0022-006X.69.2.159

Lambert, M. J., Harmon, C., Slade, K., Whipple, J. L., & Hawkins, E. J. (2004). Providing feedback to psychotherapists on their patients' progress: Clinical results and practice suggestions. *Journal of Clinical Psychology, 61*(2), 165–174. 10.1002/jclp.20113

Lambert, M. J. (2013). Outcome in psychotherapy: The past and important advances. *Psychotherapy, 50*(1), 42–51. 10.1037/a0030682

Lambert, M. J., Whipple, J. L., & Kleinstäuber, M. (2018). Collecting and delivering progress feedback: A meta-analysis of routine outcome monitoring. *Psychotherapy 55*(4), 520 –537.

Miller, S. D., Duncan, B. L., Brown, J., Sparks, J. A., & Claud, D. A. (2003). The outcome rating scale: A preliminary study of the reliability, validity, and feasibility of a brief visual analog measure. *Journal of Brief Therapy*, *2*(2), 91–100.

Miller, S. D., Duncan, B. L., Sorrell, R., & Brown, G. S. (2005). The partners for change outcome management system. *Journal of Clinical Psychology*, *61*(2), 199–208. 10.1002/jclp.20111

Osterman, J. E., & Chemtob, C. M. (1999). Emergency intervention for acute traumatic stress. *Psychiatric services (Washington, D.C.)*, *50*(6), 739–740. 10.1176/ps.50.6.739

Pinsof, W. M., Zinbarg, R. E., Lebow, J. L., Knobloch-Fedders, L. M., Durbin, E., Chambers, A., Latta, T., Karam, E., Goldsmith, J., & Friedman, G. (2009). Laying the foundation for progress research in family, couple, and individual therapy: The development and psychometric features of the initial systemic therapy inventory of change. *Psychotherapy Research*, *19*(2), 143–156. 10.1080/10503300802669973

Pinsof, W. M., Goldsmith, J. Z., & Latta, T. A. (2012). Information technology and feedback research can bridge the scientist–practitioner gap: A couple therapy example. *Couple and Family Psychology: Research and Practice*, *1*(4), 253–273. 10.1037/a0031023

Sprenkle, D. H., Davis, S. D., & Lebow, J. L. (2009). *Common factors in couple and family therapy: The overlooked foundation for effective practice*. Guilford Press.

Sprenkle, D. H., & Blow, A. J. (2004). Common factors and our sacred models. *Journal of Marital and Family Therapy*, *30*(2), 113–129.

Tasca, G. A., Angus, L., Bonli, R., Drapeau, M., Fitzparick, M., Hunsley, J., & Knoll, M. (2019). Outcome and progress monitoring in psychotherapy: Report of a Canadian psychological association task force. *Canadian Psychology/Psychologie Canadienne*, *60*(3), 165–177.

Van der Kolk, B. A. (2015). *The body keeps the score: Brain, mind and body in the healing of trauma*. Penguin Books.

Chapter 10

The Decision to End Therapy

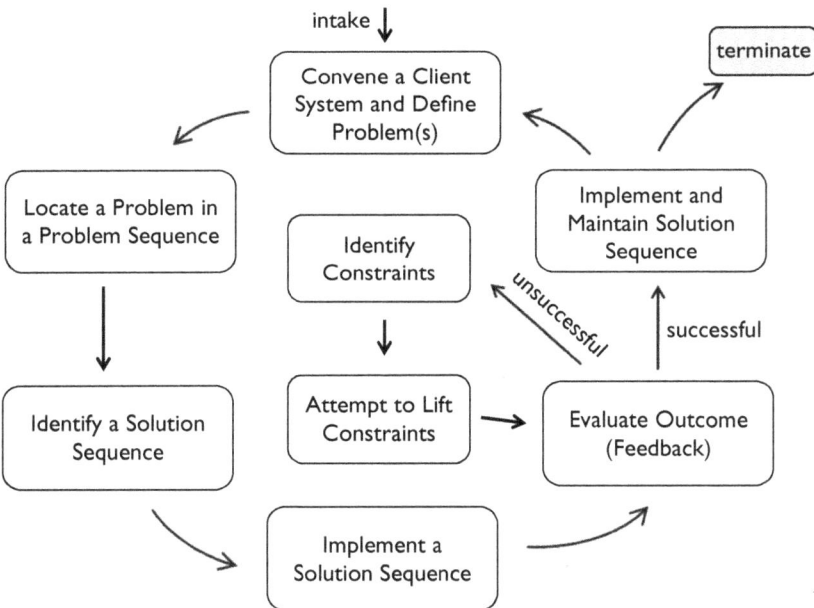

intake ↓

Convene a Client System and Define Problem(s)

terminate

Locate a Problem in a Problem Sequence

Identify Constraints

Implement and Maintain Solution Sequence

unsuccessful successful

Identify a Solution Sequence

Attempt to Lift Constraints

Evaluate Outcome (Feedback)

Implement a Solution Sequence

IST Essence Diagram.

Objective

This chapter will discuss and illustrate the IST process of ending therapy. The dimensions of termination addressed include evaluating with the clients whether they have achieved their goals, planning for their management of issues going forward, reflecting on the work and the therapeutic relationship, discussing the conditions under which another episode of therapy might be relevant, and saying goodbye. Prior to this phase in the therapeutic process, the therapist and the clients have routinely evaluated progress in relation to specific goals and periodically

DOI: 10.4324/9780429322273-10

discussed overall progress; however, the termination process is distinct in that it involves a more comprehensive evaluation of therapeutic progress and examines the implications of ending the therapy.

Introduction

In the PBS television series, *Downton Abbey*, the privileged and cantankerous Dowager Countess makes the following statement: "All life is a series of problems which we must try and solve, first one and then the next, until at last we die" (Fellowes et al., 2010). This description leaves out the love, joy, and pleasure of life, of course, and it could be more optimistically restated as one solution or one opportunity after another, but it does speak to the problem-solving dimension of life. When clients present for therapy, they are involving the therapist in their problem-solving process. The work has that "first one and then the next" nature to it as each problem and its constraints are addressed until the episode of therapy is completed. Clients will leave the episode of therapy with tools they can apply to solve additional problems that will inevitably arise. Since these new concerns sometimes require another episode of therapy, the process of termination includes an invitation to the clients to seek therapy again if they feel stuck. Where possible, the clients will often return to the same therapist.

The creators of IST practiced in the same community for decades and saw parts or all of the client systems for multiple episodes of therapy. For example, a couple sought therapy to work on their relationship. Some years later they returned for family therapy when one of their adult children struggled to get a foothold in life. They sought therapy a third time when one of their mothers was diagnosed with Alzheimer's disease. Unless constrained by circumstances, the therapist may have the extraordinarily gratifying experience of providing therapy to families at various stages of their lives. Of course, this is not possible for some therapists, since they may change jobs, move to new communities, or focus their work in specialized ways that preclude working with returning clients. And some clients are constrained by one factor or another from returning to the same therapist years later.

Although termination in IST is often "goodbye for now" rather than "goodbye," an IST therapist pays careful attention to the termination process. One definition of termination is "the ethically and clinically appropriate process by which a professional relationship is ended" (Younggren & Gottlieb, 2008, p. 500). Termination has also been described as "an intentional process that occurs over time when a client has achieved most of the goals of treatment, and/or when psychotherapy must end for other reasons" (Vasquez et al., 2008, p. 653). Research has found that there are a number of distinct hallmarks of the termination phase of treatment that are commonly accepted regardless of the therapist's model (Norcross et al., 2017), including collaborating on the decision to terminate the therapeutic relationship, identifying and discussing areas of the client system's growth, fostering favorable perspectives on the therapeutic process, empowering the client system's ability to own their gains, looking ahead and planning accordingly, and remaining mindful of ethical guidelines of the therapeutic relationship. IST endorses the incorporation of each of these hallmarks into the process of termination.

Specific to IST, the most relevant termination question is: Are the clients satisfied that the problem for which they sought treatment has been adequately addressed? Related to the answer to this question are considerations about the sustainability of the solution sequence and the durability of constraint modification. For example, a beleaguered family enveloped in childcare demands to develop a solution sequence where the primary wage earner, who had been working about 70 hours per week, agreed to moderate their work hours and demands. The therapist wondered whether the primary wage earner would sustain that change over time or slowly drift back to the 70-hour week, thus undoing the solution sequence. The therapist addressed the issue of drift and led a discussion on how to prevent it.

The amount of time and attention given to termination is correlated with the length of therapy because the bond component of the alliance tends to deepen over time. Clients who attend a handful of sessions do not require as formal a process. In longer-term work, ending therapy means ending a relationship that may be especially important to the client(s). This constitutes a loss that must be addressed. In such instances, termination is conducted over several sessions and, perhaps, over an extended period of time, if sessions are held less frequently in the termination phase. The therapist will directly advise on guidelines for termination, but clients are asked to collaborate in establishing a plan and schedule for the termination sessions.

Method

Maintaining a Solution Sequence(s) and Soliciting Feedback on Overall Progress

As shown in Chapter 9, maintaining a successful solution sequence is an important part of the process of addressing each problem defined in therapy. The decision to terminate involves a collaborative evaluation of whether the presenting problem and any other identified problems have been sufficiently addressed. The therapist relies to a significant extent on the clients' sense of their overall progress but brings to these conversations knowledge and expertise on problem-solving and human functioning. The IST therapist will facilitate discussion of overall progress by creating the space for the client system to reflect on their growth and change with respect to the goals of therapy. Below is an example of a dialogue between a client and therapist in which progress is discussed. The client has expressed ambivalence about some aspects of the therapy and has indirectly implied that therapy should be terminated. Having read this feedback, the therapist initiates a discussion on the overall progress of therapy.

Therapist: We have been working together to address your fears and anxieties about commitment in relationships. How do you feel about the progress you have made?

Client: I think therapy has been helpful overall, but I can't exactly say how. I still have the same fears about commitment.

Therapist: If you reflect on our work together on the issue of commitment, what would you say has worked so far and what has not?

Client: Umm… I'm not really sure. I think when we began to talk about my parents' relationship and me finding out when I was 12 that they were both seeing other people, I realized that it messed with me and made me think that's why I don't trust when someone says they're committed. I can't really believe them. I get where this comes from, but that's just never going to change for me. I don't think it was helpful when you suggested that I call my mom and talk to her about what I learned when I was 12.

Therapist: I remember your disappointment with that. I am sorry you had a negative experience with your mom. I could have given more thought to the possible negative outcomes that could result from that conversation. Would you say talking to your mom about your experience of finding out about their affairs revealed a problem in your relationship with your mom?

Client: Yes! I mean I can see how it would be related to my own commitment issues and all, but now not only do I not know how to fix my own commitment issues, but now my mom and I are mad at each other, and I'm just left feeling angry with my parents without knowing how to even deal with it. I am just staying away from her at this point because the smallest thing just sets me off.

The therapist identifies the sequence of avoidance behavior with her mother which seems similar to the client's problem sequence of avoidance within intimate partner relationships.

Therapist: Where would you say you are stuck in talking to your mom?

Client: My anger. I just lose my temper and hang up the phone. I just can't hold a conversation with her because she immediately becomes the victim and starts accusing me of things because she feels like I am accusing her. I just don't have any patience for it. She always has to be a victim. If my father were alive, he would probably be easier to talk to about this. I don't know anymore. I'm just tired. I just feel like my problems are multiplying.

Therapist: I can imagine how difficult it must be to try to hold those conversations with your mom, given how you were affected by the affairs. I never intended for you to have a falling out with your mom. Would you like to improve your relationship with her? What do you think of us doing that work together?

Client: That really scares me, but my mom used to be a source of support and I wish I could get that back. Tell me what you have in mind.

Therapist: Well, first of all, I would be much more cautious this time before we agree to any plan. When you are ready and we have prepared, I think I could help you talk with her if she joined us for a session. I will be there to moderate anytime things become too tense for you. What do you think? Would you be willing to try?

Client: I'm nervous about this, but it may be worth thinking about. I guess I can do one session with her and see what happens from there.

Therapist: We will plan all the steps together, even how you extend the invitation to her. I am also worried about your pessimism about your fears about commitment. There is a lot more that we can do about that problem so I would like to give it another try. How about we commit to another six sessions and then re-evaluate the progress of therapy again?

Client: OK, that makes sense.

In this example of client-therapist dialogue, the client reflected on the course of therapy. The therapist collaborated with the client to pinpoint where the therapy was stuck and stated how a new problem sequence had developed based on attempting a solution sequence suggested by the therapist. Following the path of the new problem sequence, the therapist was able to identify that the mother should be brought into the direct system. The therapy evolved to include the mother and daughter in an exploration of the underlying issue of trust and mistrust in relationships.

This effort also moved the client from feeling stuck and considering termination to a new effort to address the presenting problem from a different therapeutic angle.

Solution sequences can include behavior change, cognitive shifts, and/ or new ways of processing emotions. Maintaining the solution sequence is an important aspect of the work leading up to termination. Utilizing one or more of the means of measuring progress discussed in Chapter 9, the therapist can see if a solution is holding up over time. This may involve some further work to address factors that continue to constrain the solution. In the discussion of overall progress, the therapist ascertains whether other issues or problems have emerged that the client would like to address in therapy.

The therapist is also interested in the extent to which the clients are able to manage challenges to the solution sequence. In IST, one common way of testing this is to begin to space the sessions out. Meeting twice per month, monthly, or every other month at an advanced stage of therapy can help the therapist determine whether the clients are ready to terminate. The essential question is: Can the clients maintain successful adaptation without the weekly involvement of the therapist? In the case of a woman who presented with depression and isolation, in preparation for termination, the appointments were scheduled less frequently, and the therapist tracked her mood, her involvement with others, and specific solution sequences related to her daily routine and engagement in activities.

The Ways That Therapy Ends

A course of therapy can end in several ways. Clients may decide precipitously to end it, the therapist may initiate it for reasons of lack of progress or other concerns, or the therapist and clients may agree that the therapy has accomplished what it needs to accomplish. Termination is distinguished from psychotherapy dropout where the client ends treatment prematurely. The latter involves clients ending therapy prior to resolving the problem that led to their seeking treatment (Swift & Greenberg, 2015). Premature termination can result from several different factors including, but not limited to, a tear in the therapeutic alliance, lack of client motivation, and external factors such as changes in the client's circumstances that reduce the need for therapy or make it more difficult to attend.

In instances where the client discontinues therapy prematurely without any contact or closure, the IST therapist typically will contact the client by phone or other secure communication means. The goal is to have a conversation about the progress of therapy and the therapeutic relationship in order to see if there has been a rupture in the alliance that might be repairable. Sometimes a client will attend therapy or call to request a phone conversation with the agenda of terminating with the therapist. In such cases, the therapist listens carefully to the reason for termination and is open to hearing whether the client is dissatisfied with the progress or has hurt feelings about what the therapist has done or said. Person-of-the-therapist issues may well arise in these conversations, especially when clients are indeed dissatisfied. When a client is dissatisfied, the therapist will need to manage any defensiveness and ensure that the client has the space and platform to express any feelings of hurt they may have. Understanding and validating the client's experience may lead to an opportunity to repair the alliance. If the therapy can be shifted in some way in recognition of client needs or concerns, that may provide a way forward in the work. If not, the therapist assesses the need for a referral.

For client-initiated terminations that occur prior to the accomplishment of therapy goals, the therapist asks the clients about their experience with therapy. Was the work focused on what they wanted to accomplish? Were gains made? What things were left undone? Did they feel judged or pressured by the therapist? The therapist should respond empathically to the client's experience. Whatever the client's response, the therapist can summarize any progress observed and, of course, mention the strengths manifested by the client. The therapist can also share recommendations or cautions with the client based on the problem sequences and constraints that have been identified.

If the termination is a result of financial or larger systemic constraints such as insurance-related issues or changes in accessibility based on transportation issues, it is the duty of the therapist to ensure the client is not abandoned from therapy when still in need of it. The therapist will need to provide an appropriate termination process and give the client a referral that is reasonable in terms of cost and accessibility.

Some clients seeking an unanticipated termination are satisfied with the therapy and feel it has been worthwhile. Enough of the work is done and they have competing demands for their time and money, or they think of themselves as independent people who only use as much help as they need. The therapist can invite them to a more formal conversation about the progress made and explore any challenges they are likely to face. The client(s) can also be invited to check in with the therapist in a few months to see if their gains are holding and if other issues have arisen.

Many clients do resolve the presenting problems that brought them into therapy and do not leave therapy precipitously. This makes a planned termination possible. As mentioned, the plan may well allow for decreasing the frequency of sessions over time until the decision is made to end the therapy. During the process of termination, there will be additional opportunities for the client and therapist to work on maintaining solution sequences and addressing additional constraints that are identified. One example of an additional constraint occurs when family members do not all agree about their readiness to terminate therapy. In such instances, the therapist ensures that all members can express the reasoning for their position and helps them discuss possible avenues for the therapy. In the following example, given different levels of readiness to terminate therapy, the therapist reflects what each family member has been saying and helps them find their way forward.

Therapist: I have been listening to your conversation and taking in what each of you are saying. As I understand it, both Dad and Isabelle (12-year-old daughter) feel ready and confident to move forward without therapy. I hear they are feeling good about their skills in reducing and managing conflict. I sense that Seoma (11-year-old son) is showing me with his body language, that he may not be too excited about Isabelle and Dad's idea to terminate at this point. Are my observations correct?

The therapist waits to receive feedback about the hypothesis and continues to probe for more dialogue about the observed differences while encouraging the members of the family to be curious about one another's thoughts about termination. The family's original goals were to reduce conflict and spend more time together. Since all members agree conflict has been reduced, the therapist wonders if the amount of time spent together might still be an issue for Seoma who appears more resistant or apprehensive about the prospect of terminating.

Therapist: Seoma, can you tell me what you have most enjoyed about coming to family therapy with your dad and sister?"

This question helped Seoma admit that therapy provided the opportunity to spend time together. They rode in the car together, had their session, and sometimes stopped for dinner on the way home. He liked the uninterrupted time together. His father and sister reassured him they would find the time to be together. The therapist, concerned that good intentions don't always translate into sustained action, entered the process and guided them to construct a plan for how they would regularly find time together. Once the plan was in place, Seoma felt more comfortable with termination.

Reflecting on the Therapy

During the termination process, the therapist leads a discussion of the course and outcome of therapy. This includes asking the clients what the experience was like for them, what they feel they accomplished, and what they need to continue to work on. It is often helpful for the therapist to frame the conversation with a brief statement about the clients' entry into therapy and what they had said they wanted to work on.

Therapist: Once upon a time you walked into our waiting room for the first time. That was 18 months ago. I remember our first session. You said that you wanted some help with decision-making as a couple. Would you be willing to tell your story of the therapy?

Examples of other questions that can be asked include the following.

Therapist: I am interested in hearing what this therapy has been like for you.

Therapist: Can you talk a bit about what you feel you accomplished in therapy?

Therapist: Can you talk about something that you feel was a key to your success?

Therapist: I am interested in what you have learned about yourself and your partner (family) in this process?

Therapist: Are some things left undone?

Therapist: As you look ahead, what challenges do you see on the horizon?

Therapist: How will each of you use your takeaways to work together on things that will challenge you in the future?

IST follows the family therapy tradition of empowering clients to own the gains they make in therapy. The therapist appreciates the clients' gratitude, but ultimately credits the clients' strengths and hard work for the gains made in therapy. Following is an example of an IST therapist's statement to a couple that acknowledges strengths and gains.

Therapist: In the last 18 months of working together, I have seen your courage and commitment to hear and understand each other even when what was being said was challenging to hear. I know it wasn't easy to have some of the discussions, particularly those about boundaries with your families of origin, and the conversations about raising your children in an interfaith marriage. But you always came back to one crucial point and that was your commitment to one another and to the life you have built together. Along the way, I believe you made some important changes.

Discussion of What Would Signal a Need to Return to Therapy

Development assures that client systems will continue to evolve and change over time. For example, children become adolescents, graduates go to college, marriages sometimes end in divorce, and older adults face health crises. Any of these nodal events can create a problem for the client system and point it toward another episode of therapy (Greenberg, 2002). Successful solution sequences do not always hold in the face of loss, illness, life cycle changes, significant changes in routine, or periodic emergence of intrapsychic and interpersonal reactions that begin to degrade the solutions. Interaction patterns may regress to the mean. Constraints can reemerge. New constraints present themselves. The therapist should make a point of normalizing challenges and regression. They are expected and may comprise a reason to return to therapy.

The therapist can ask the clients to share how they will know when it is time for further therapy. If this is difficult for them to imagine, the therapist can remind them to think of how they knew it was time to start the therapy they are now terminating. The therapist can also share that when they encounter distress again, they may be able to successfully reinstate solutions they learned in therapy or create new solutions using the skills they have developed. In such cases, they would not need to return to therapy. However, if they are unable to reinstate a solution or instate a new one and they are experiencing distress, it would be time to reenter therapy at least for a consultation.

Diversity, Inclusion, and Social Justice

Like any step in the therapeutic process, the termination process is influenced by intersectionality, equity, and inclusion. In considering the post-termination challenges the client system will face, it is important to consider the constraints clients feel they may face in relation to their ethnicity, race, economic status, immigration status, religion, sexual orientation, or gender identity. The therapist will need to ask whether the clients think that factors related to their intersectionality will make it challenging to maintain solution sequences over time. For example, how will a client's mood be affected by continued exposure to racially-motivated violence and other aspects of systemic racism, including inequality of power, opportunity, and economic resources?

Focus on clients' specific sequences of interaction as well as the meanings and emotions related to them is certainly important, but societal and community factors that impair social justice have far-reaching implications. For example, in the discussion of how to know when to return to therapy, the therapist needs to be aware of the financial and geographic barriers that the client may face. A client with resources may have a reasonable chance of returning to the same therapist, but when a client is seen in an agency setting where staff turnover is high, sadly there may be no way back to that therapist. Similarly, if a client changes jobs or loses a job, the new insurance coverage may preclude seeing the former therapist. In the process of terminating, therapists must be aware of the impact of inequities and constraints to inclusion and be allies in the search for the resources clients need.

Conclusion

Clients terminate for a variety of reasons. In all cases, the therapist seeks a conversation about the termination that considers the progress of therapy and the state of the alliance. In client-initiated termination, the therapist seeks to determine if there has been a rupture in the alliance or if clients are terminating for other reasons that can be addressed. IST therapists seek to collaborate on the decision to terminate and how to terminate. Oftentimes, the frequency of sessions will be reduced as part of the plan to maintain the solution sequences in the face of life circumstances that play out over time. Termination in IST empowers clients to own the changes they have made and invites them to a conversation that forecasts the constraints and challenges they encounter going forward, including a discussion of what would be a sign that they need to return to therapy. The therapist says goodbye, and in a context that will allow for it, it may be "goodbye for now" as the client is welcome to reach out to the therapist in the future.

Exercises

Review the case scenarios provided below. With the information provided in those scenarios, reflect on the following questions for each case.

1   Formulate and write down some questions you might ask the client(s) as a means of evaluating the course of therapy.
2   Consider the questions you would ask and statements you might make to address the challenges the clients may face post-termination.
3   What do you see as your person-of-the-therapist feelings or issues that may get in the way of discussing termination with your clients when their problems have been resolved?

Family: Saeed is a 48-year-old single father of two children, 12-year-old Amir, and 9-year-old Suri. They have been coming to therapy for the past year to work through the grief and loss of losing the children's mother and Saeed's true love, Setareh, due to cancer one year prior to the start of family therapy. The family has done an incredible amount of work toward healing this immense loss. They have also worked on their communication with one another and report feeling closer than ever to each other and able to move forward in making new memories as a family while reminiscing and keeping the memories of Setareh close by. The family has been showing consistency in maintaining the solution sequences that they had worked on together for some time, yet they have said nothing about wanting to end therapy. You as the therapist have found yourself attached to the family's story and their degree of resilience, and really look forward to seeing them every week, but you do not hear that the family has any remaining goals for therapy at this time. Please address the questions listed above in the case examples.

Individual: 32-year-old Natalia has been working with you for several years on adaptation to the loss of her mother and the traumatic events she experienced in her previous relationship. She has been maintaining key solution sequences and effectively managing new constraints that she encounters. For example, she has had the courage to start dating again and be vulnerable within her current relationship without the emergence of previous anxieties and related problem sequences of self-sabotage. You have been working closely with her since she moved to the United States and have watched her throughout the years build a new life for herself in her new home. The dilemma you face, however, is that when you have begun to talk about termination or reducing the frequency of the sessions, she develops increased anxiety about her life and future. You hypothesize that the anxiety arises in relation to the prospect of termination. She is one of your favorite clients and you find yourself feeling that if you had never been her therapist, you could be good friends. How will you address the sequence of termination/frequency talk being followed by increased anxiety? What things are there to say or ask that move the conversation along? Also, make sure to address the questions listed above these two case examples.

References

Fellowes, J., Naeme, G., & Eaton, R. (Executive Producers). (2010–2011). *Downton Abbey* [TV series]. Carnival Films & Television; Masterpiece Theater.

Greenberg, L. S. (2002). Termination of experiential therapy. *Journal of Psychotherapy Integration, 12*(3), 358–363. 10.1037/1053-0479.12.3.358

Norcross, J. C., Zimmerman, B. E., Greenberg, R. P., & Swift, J. K. (2017). Do all therapists do that when saying goodbye? A study of commonalities in termination behaviors. *Psychotherapy, 54*(1), 66–75. 10.1037/pst0000097

Swift, J. K., & Greenberg, R. P. (2015). *Premature termination in psychotherapy: Strategies for engaging clients and improving outcomes.* American Psychological Association. 10.1037/14469-000

Vasquez, M. J. T., Bingham, R. P., & Barnett, J. E. (2008). Psychotherapy termination: clinical and ethical responsibilities. *Journal of Clinical Psychology*, *64*(5), 653–665. 10.1002/jclp.20478

Younggren, J. N., & Gottlieb, M. C. (2008). Termination and abandonment: History, risk, and risk management. *Professional Psychology: Research and Practice*, *39*(5), 498–504. 10.1037/0735-7028.39.5.498

Chapter 11

Pathways within Integrative Systemic Therapy

Objective

The objective of this chapter is to consider the various pathways IST can take depending on variables related to client situations, the therapist's work context, and personal characteristics of the therapist. Client-related variables of risk issues and mandated therapy are explored with an emphasis on importing standards of best practice into IST. The impact of the work context on the actual practice of IST is discussed, including some commentary on its application to case management and inpatient or residential programs. Lastly, the chapter proposes that the practice of IST allows for a unique developmental path that is a function of a therapist's own style and preferences within IST, as well as their own journey in the development of the person-of-the-therapist.

Introduction

IST provides therapists with a set of general problem-solving steps (essence), a collaborative process for planning and intervening (blueprint), storehouses of concepts and interventions housed in the blueprint components, and guidelines for therapy. IST does not specify how to intervene with certain types of problems, situations, or populations. Rather, it provides a set of concepts and procedures that support the therapist in taking a systemic and integrative approach to tailoring therapy to the clients who present for therapy. Practitioners trained in IST have many commonalities in their work, but their practice will also be a function of who they are and will invariably reflect a set of preferences (Pinsof et al., 2018). Their work is also influenced by the context within which they practice. The style and preferences of the therapist, the influence of the workplace, and the unique nature of each client system suggest that IST can take different pathways. This chapter will focus on pathways within IST that may result from the following factors: Clinical situations that require modification of essence steps; the context in which the therapy

DOI: 10.4324/9780429322273-11

takes place; and the therapist's development, including continuing training and the development of the self-of-the-therapist (person-of-the-therapist).

Client Situations Requiring Modification of Essence Steps

Risk Issues

The alliance is a central concern in therapy and, as has been discussed and demonstrated in prior chapters, developing and preserving it is given a high priority. Alliance considerations override the therapist's hypothesis and the preferred order of intervention specified by the planning matrix. Not surprisingly, issues of risk and danger are of such importance that they supersede even the alliance. Simply put, safety first, safety last. In this regard, the IST therapist shares a common purpose and responsibility with all therapists in giving the highest priority to safety (including the monitoring of the risks of self-harm, suicidality, danger to others, domestic violence, human trafficking, sexual assault, and elder abuse/neglect) and to the protection of children from abuse and neglect.

In IST, the presenting problem is defined largely by the clients as the therapist asks a set of questions and makes clarifying comments or suggestions. Concern about risk may be directly presented by clients, too, but this is not necessarily so. Parents who abuse their children do not generally present abuse as a problem to work on in therapy. Even in court-referred cases, the abusing parent often enters therapy denying or minimizing the abuse. In the case of clients who may be dangerous to themselves or others, they do not always seek help for the risk issue, and often in cases involving psychosis, they do not even recognize that they are in a psychotic state. Thus, when risk may be involved, the therapist unilaterally elevates it to the status of the primary presenting problem by virtue of the therapist's judgment and responsibility. The therapist can explain this focus by saying they are concerned about safety and are required to assess and intervene as needed. The therapist may seek to minimize damage to the alliance, but the alliance is in all cases secondary to safety concerns.

In the case of risk, the solution sequence is constructed to address the risk. When necessary, the therapist enacts a solution of contacting outside community agents such as the state department of child protection, the police department, or a mental health facility to address a safety concern. Other times the solution sequence is a set of actions a client commits to as part of a safety plan. IST does not provide a specific approach to assessing and managing danger and risk. Rather, the IST therapist integrates standards of practice consistent with the laws of their country and state, their professional ethics, and the policies and procedures of their agency or practice.

Within legal and ethical requirements and standards of practice, the therapist can utilize the IST blueprint (hypothesizing, planning, conversing, and reading feedback) to inform the moment-to-moment conversation about issues of risk or child abuse/neglect. For example, Sara was seeing a blended family in family therapy. One week, the mother and stepfather attended the session without the children. They reported the stepfather had responded to the 12-year-old son's defiance by hitting the boy with his fist. Sara discussed this event in detail with them. They reported that the boy was not talking with the stepfather, but was doing well physically, though he had some bruising on his cheek. The parents stated that this was the first time something like this had happened. The stepfather expressed regret, but also frustration that the boy did not give him respect. Sara understood that she was required to report this event to the state Department of Children and Family Services (DCFS). She thought that making the report would be damaging to the alliance but hoped that openness and respect might mitigate some of the damage (hypothesis). She considered whether telling the parents about her requirement to report would create a danger for anyone and concluded that there was nothing that she knew about the stepfather or other family members that would suggest that (hypothesis). She decided to tell the parents that a report to DCFS was necessary and to propose that she make the report in their presence (plan).

Sara stated that their openness was appreciated and that it showed good faith in the process of therapy (conversing). The stepfather reiterated that he was sorry this had happened and that it would not happen again (feedback). The couple agreed that the event had created significant stress between them, but they were beginning to heal from it. Sara then told them that she was glad to hear these things but that she had a legal obligation to report the event to DCFS. The mother and stepfather looked at each other and Sara could feel the stress in that moment. The stepfather then said, "How does this work? Can I make the call?" (feedback). Sara said, "Sure, we can do it now. I will also have to make a report during the call and will do so right after you do." Based on the stepfather's proposal and Sara's understanding of her responsibilities, there was a consensus on how the call would be made (plan).

Sara was aware that the balance of confidentiality and mandate to report would suggest that the report be limited to what is relevant to the decision to report and to factors directly relevant to what is reported. It is worth noting here, however, that since the specific requirements for reporting may vary from country to country or from state to state, therapists need to be clear on the requirements for reporting as well as their professional values and standards with respect to confidentiality.

When Sara learned about the act of violence, it became the immediate presenting problem. She was free to handle the conversation and establish a plan in several ways that would have fulfilled her obligation to report it. Her direct, open, and collaborative approach via the blueprint led to a report to DCFS that, in this case, minimized the damage to the therapeutic alliance. Still, there was alliance repair to do, which began at the end of that session with an initial discussion about how each parent felt about the call and what they feared may come of it. Then, with an agreement to continue therapy together, the repair within the family would begin.

Mandated Therapy

This section pertains to mandated referrals for therapy and not to mandated evaluations or assessments for which IST has not been adapted. When therapy is mandated, there is an essential change in the interpersonal dynamic of the therapy. It is typically not a matter of clients feeling, "I want (or need) this therapy," but more a matter of "I have to do this therapy." Sometimes, a mandated client system enters therapy with the idea that they want something from it. And if not, sometimes they can move to "I want this" over the course of therapy. Their starting point, though, is clearly different from that of clients who have come to terms with the need to seek help and initiate it on that basis. Self-initiating clients may be ambivalent about entering therapy or unsure of what can come from it, but they are not being forced to attend. All may agree that people don't like to be forced to do things. This is especially the case when the thing they are forced to do may seem to involve discomfort, emotional vulnerability, or legal risk.

Mandated clients are referred by societal systems such as child protective services, juvenile court, and divorce court. The goals of the referrals include such things as improved mental health of a juvenile or adult, treatment of addiction, family reunification, resolution of parental alienation, and reduction of parental conflict. A school may suggest therapy in a way that the parent or parents feel is tantamount to it being mandated. For example, it may be suggested that the child's educational placement may need to be modified if the child's behavior in school does not improve and, further, that therapy is a way of improving the child's behavior. Similarly, an employer may expect an employee to enter therapy as they are given the opportunity to correct certain workplace behaviors.

The literature on mandated clients addresses ethics and values pertaining to mandated clients (Barsky, 2010), strategies of intervention (Rooney, 2009), the importance of cultural sensitivity (Baker, 1999), alliance challenges in high-conflict custody or visitation disputes (Lebow &

Rekart, 2007), and motivational interviewing with addiction (Lincourt et al., 2002). Learning to work with mandated clients requires training or supervision, as well as careful attention to the policies of the agency within which the therapy is conducted. Although IST does not provide a specific model for how to work with mandated clients, the IST therapist integrates existing practices and guidelines into the IST frameworks and thinks systemically about the mandate.

In mandated therapy, the therapist agrees to accommodate a triangular system of the client, mandating agent, and therapist. In this context, the mandating agent, at one level of specificity or another, defines the presenting problem. The client, in turn, reacts and responds to the mandate with refusal (which will carry some consequence for them) or some level of compliance. Since IST typically begins with a discussion of what the client wants to accomplish in therapy and begins to build the therapeutic alliance on that, the work with mandated cases begins differently. The therapist needs to establish a clear understanding with both the client and the mandating agent of the purpose and requirements of therapy, including whether the therapist would be committing to provide a report or reports on client participation or progress. The therapist next initiates a discussion with the clients about how they feel and what they think about the mandate. The therapist can acknowledge their feelings or concerns and attend carefully to what it must be like to be forced into therapy. This conversation leads to the question of whether there is something that the client wants to accomplish in therapy. The goal is to bridge from the mandate to something within the mandate that the clients agree they would like to work on. For example, a couple who had been referred by the court to work on managing their conflict had some feelings of resentment about the referral, but in conversation with the therapist, agreed that it would be a good idea for the sake of their kids for them to fight less. This was a starting place.

Motivational Interviewing (Miller & Rollnick, 2012; Miller & Rose, 2009) provides some helpful procedures for dealing with the dilemmas of motivation and readiness. Once the mandated requirements and reporting expectations are clarified, and once the clients have identified something to work on in therapy, the therapist can proceed with IST's problem-solving tasks as outlined in the essence diagram. If clients do not specify a goal to work on, then the therapist can propose something that is within the mandate. "Well, the court specified that you work on issues related to substance use, so if you are open to it, we can begin discussing that. Are you open to that?" Without the client agreeing to work on something, it is reasonable for the therapist to decline further work and/ or report to the mandating agent if that is the agreement of all parties and the release forms have been signed.

Contexts of Therapy That Impact IST Practice

Workplace Requirements and Constraints

Working in an agency or practice involves participating in a culture. The culture includes mission, values and traditions, as well as patterns of interaction among the staff. There are also the requirements of funding sources or third-party payers such as health insurance companies. Further, agencies and practices have standards of care that also inform policy and procedures. Some of these conventions may not be the most natural fit for an IST therapist. Among these are the notions of identified patient and diagnosis, as well as requirements in some agencies for extensive social histories and assessments.

As a systemic therapy, IST does not naturally lend itself to the idea that one person in a family is the client. It is more natural to think of a family system as a client, with those who attend the therapy being in the direct client system, and those who do not attend being in the indirect client system. In individual therapy, the person attending is clearly the client, but even then, the therapist maintains the awareness that the client is part of a system and the therapy of an individual both impacts and is impacted by the system. In couple or family therapy, the IST therapist would not naturally think to name one member as the patient. However, therapists generally practice in contexts where the designation of a person as the patient or client is required. This is a long-standing dilemma that family therapists have faced over the years for which the solution has historically been to accept the requirement of naming a client. The therapist can communicate to clients that there needs to be an identified client, but that the therapy is for all of them and that all of their interests will be equal in the context of the therapy. There are exceptions to this approach in certain agencies or circumstances. For example, the U.S. Veterans Administration (V.A.) prioritizes the needs of veterans over their family members who participate in therapy. The veterans are the patients. In this case, the mission of the V.A. will need to be communicated to the family members at the very beginning, and it should be made clear that the service is being provided primarily for the veteran's benefit. Hopefully, all members will benefit, and outcomes that benefit the family system can certainly benefit the veteran.

Another convention that systemic therapists have become accustomed to is the requirement to diagnose the client. The therapist needs to understand and speak the language of a categorical diagnostic system such as DSM-5 or ICD-10 and use it within the workplace. On the other hand, IST therapists do not make many decisions in therapy based on the name of the problem or diagnosis. The diagnostic label certainly carries some information, and in some cases, it strongly suggests a course of action. For example, a client diagnosed with schizophrenia will need to be receiving psychiatric care. Or, when a client begins therapy with a pre-existing diagnosis of borderline personality disorder, the therapist may be on the lookout for problem sequences that may develop in the therapeutic relationship. All that said, IST bases the actual therapy on the specific problem sequences and constraints identified in the process of therapy. In the case of depression, the question isn't what is to be done for depression, but what is to be done for this client's specific patterns of action, meaning, and emotion (that have been classified as depression). Thus, a diagnosis does not modify the problem-solving steps of the essence.

Some agencies require extensive social histories and formal initial assessments. These requirements do not fit naturally with the IST guideline that defines assessment as an ongoing process that is inseparable from intervention. Although IST therapists may naturally be inclined to collect less information upfront, a requirement to collect more information can be easily accommodated. Useful information is collected in history taking and formal assessment, and the therapist can develop ways to be more systemic about what is collected and tailor some of the questions to IST. For example, in addressing the section of an assessment that describes the presenting problem, there is an opportunity to track a problem sequence(s). Then, when the assessment is done, the therapist can pick back up with the problem sequences that have been defined. The task for the IST therapist after the initial assessment period is to enter the IST essence diagram and, despite the wealth of information collected, simplify the therapy and work on a solution sequence. Information collected earlier in the formal assessment period can be reintroduced as needed over the course of therapy to identify constraints in what may become a more complex case formulation.

Case Management and Support Services

IST therapists also may work in community-based programs that provide case management and support services. These jobs may involve reaching out to economically disadvantaged or vulnerable populations who may or may not be immediately inclined to work on the relational or psychological concerns that therapists are most familiar with. Some of these clients may present with more basic and essential needs for food, shelter, income, physical safety, or the need to access appropriate health services. In IST, these needs can be the presenting problem. In other words, the caseworker focuses on what brings the client in and what they need. IST concepts and principles can be applied to these needs that are often associated with what therapists may think of as social service or social work. Further, applying IST to case management and support services reveals a less rigid boundary between case management and therapy. This is consistent with the traditional and enduring social work value of working with the person-in-the-situation (Richmond, 1922) and with the family therapy tradition of seeing people in context.

Drawing on the notion of a hierarchy of needs (Maslow, 1954) and the ideas of an IST theorist (Pinsof, 1995), Kilpatrick and Holland (2005) proposed approaching family assessment and intervention based on the level of need presented by the family. Their model posits that in some cases, basic human needs require intervention prior to clients identifying or focusing on the types of issues more typically identified as the province of therapy (e.g., family structure, interpersonal issues, or inner conflicts). This is not an all-or-none distinction, as people who are homeless or hungry may be quite aware of interpersonal struggles and their internal processes, but the model developed by Kilpatrick and Holland (2005) predicts that their immediate motivation with respect to services will tend to be the fulfillment of their basic needs. Working directly with clients on these needs can build the alliance and may open the path to work on issues more traditionally associated with individual, couple or family psychotherapy.

Case management has been described as "a collaborative process that assesses, plans, implements, coordinates, monitors, and evaluates the options and services required to meet the client's health and human service needs" (Commission for Case Manager Certification, n.d.). IST provides a systemic way of thinking about this process, conceptualizing basic needs as the presenting problem and the initial basis for the therapeutic alliance. The IST-trained caseworker or therapist assesses needs and determines what can be done to address them. Locating resources and accessing services are the equivalent of solution sequences on the essence diagram. The caseworker acknowledges client strengths and empowers clients to access resources that are identified, but as clients are constrained from navigating the systems and resources, the caseworker will facilitate access more directly and advocate on their clients' behalf.

These activities are established procedures of the case management process, but IST tools can enhance the process with the concepts of sequence and constraint and the use of the blueprint. The blueprint can be used to evolve collaborative conversations with clients that lead to accessing resources, building relationships, and better understanding the constraints. With respect to basic needs, the caseworker can identify sequences of interaction between the family and other systems in order to refine how resources are accessed and managed. The caseworker might say, "As you did not see Dr. Costanza for your appointment last week, I wonder if some things got in the way of that. Can we talk about it?" Specific constraints are identified within individuals ("I could not get out of bed"), within families ("my son was out late last night, we argued and I didn't sleep much"), in the community ("the nurse at that office disrespects me"), and at the level of society (under-funded public medical system). As constraints are identified and addressed, this work is not easily distinguished from therapy. The alliance that develops from meeting clients where they are and responding to their needs with respect and reliability may lead to a level of trust that allows the client to present other issues such as relational concerns, child-focused problems, depression, or substance abuse.

It is also essential within IST to recognize that there are more pervasive societal and community constraints that have to do with institutionalized racism, economic inequality, and lack of access to power and resources. The caseworker or therapist obviously cannot solve these issues, but they can acknowledge them and establish themselves as allies in the struggle for equality and inclusion. "I hear that it does not feel right to have to travel that far, taking two buses and a train to see Dr. Costanza, and then having to wait so long when you get there. I am with you on that. Your healthcare should be more accessible. Let's look at the options again."

Inpatient Psychiatric and Residential Programs

IST was developed in an outpatient psychotherapy context. It has been adapted to community-based settings and school-based programs. As a generalized, comprehensive, integrative approach, it can be adapted to any context. IST can also provide organizing principles for a practice or agency. One could suggest that inpatient psychiatric and residential settings could be organized around IST principles and methods, but this has not been done. The complexity of these systems, especially that of a hospital setting, could constitute constraints to this happening. That being said, therapists in these settings certainly can utilize IST, a case in point being the work of Whittaker (2018) who has described the utilization of IST in a psychiatric hospital in Norway. Interestingly, Whittaker found that inpatient work at the Family Unit at Modum Bad typically shifts more readily to drawing interventions from lower on the matrix since the outpatient work, a precondition of admission, has not successfully addressed the complex problem sequences and related constraints (K. J. Whittaker, personal communication, January 10, 2020).

Adaptation of IST to psychiatric hospitals and residential settings may face challenges. First, the length of stay in the program will have a profound influence on what can be done. In the case of shorter stays, IST work with problem and solutions sequences can be conceptualized as a short-term approach with the idea that the more continuous work on complex webs of constraint will be provided on an outpatient basis. Residential programs and hospitals permitting longer stays provide more opportunities for ongoing work, which may allow shifts down the matrix, as needed. Second, programs may not be structured to provide sufficient opportunities for family members to engage in family therapy. This would concern an IST therapist, who hopefully can find enough flexibility in the system to allow more family sessions to be conducted. If this proves difficult to do for scheduling or other reasons, the therapist can advocate to establsih family therapy as a priority of the program. Third, placement in these programs is sometimes mandated or all-but-mandated, so some of the principles discussed in the section of this chapter on mandated treatment may apply.

An inpatient or residential program provides a milieu for patients/clients that is a function of an overall philosophy and approach as well as the characteristics of staff and their working relationships. It is a system, a therapist system (as described in Chapter 2). An outpatient practice is also a system, of course, but often the therapists in the practice are relatively autonomous in their clinical work. To work in an inpatient or residential program is to work as part of a team of professionals that develops rules and boundaries for communication and coordination of their efforts within the program as a whole and with respect to their various contacts with individual patients. This means that there is significant communication among staff regarding each case. They may have different roles (e.g., psychiatrist, supervisor, therapist, group therapist, and mental health technician), but they have the opportunity to share views on treatment issues and discharge planning. This can be beneficial for patients and staff, of course, but it does mean that the therapist must coordinate their hypothesizing and planning closely with the other professionals.

Therapist Considerations

Each client system is unique, having its own set of evolving sequences, strengths, and constraints. Problem sequences in one family may be similar to those in others, but they are not actually the same, and the nature of the constraints that govern apparently similar sequences are highly variable from case to case. The IST therapist works within the concepts, principles and methods of IST, to collaborate in designing a pathway for therapy that fits the clients' goals and patterns. So, it can be said that each pathway for therapy, though governed by IST principles and procedures, is unique. The course and nuances of therapy also derive from the unique nature of the therapist. The therapy system (the combination of therapist and client systems) creates a once-in-a-lifetime experience.

Therapist Style and Preferences

In IST, there is no one correct way to approach a certain type of presenting problem and no one way to work with a particular client system. Guided by the IST perspective, informed by science, and practicing the art of therapy, the IST therapist tailors the therapy to the client system. Rather than asking clients to fit a model of therapy, the therapy is made to fit the clients. If the therapy can be tailored to a client system in multiple ways, then it follows that there is room for variability in how a therapist intervenes. Although each IST therapist is collaborative, mindful of the alliance, and faithful to IST's pillars, concepts and integrative procedures, they will also bring their unique style, specific training, and preferred ways of fulfilling IST strategies. As IST therapists develop, they will develop their own conversational style, which is an expression of who they are. Some may have more engaging and expressive styles. It is who they are. Others may be more reserved and methodical in their approach. It is who they are. They bring their evolving selves and preferred interventions to the work. They find their own fit within IST. This is expected and it is consistent with findings that therapists tend to find the approach to therapy that fits for them (Simon, 2003).

All IST therapists seek to be prepared to address a wide variety of constraints, though some will be drawn more to certain strategies and interventions within the IST planning metaframeworks based on the training they have received and preferences they develop. For example, all will need to help clients modify constraining meanings (strategy). Some therapists will tend to address this strategy with interventions learned from narrative therapy. Others may favor interventions drawn from cognitive-behavioral therapy or strategic therapy. Another example would be the strategy of conversing with clients about whether they are ready to make certain changes. Some therapists may prefer motivational interviewing for this purpose and others may tend to utilize circular questioning (Tomm, 1987). The idea that strategies can be addressed in a variety of ways is consistent with the systemic principle of equifinality (Von Bertalanffy, 1968), which states that the same end state can be reached in multiple ways.

Importantly, one cannot master all of the interventions that can be integrated into IST; therefore, some selection of interventive preferences is expected and necessary. It is part of the development of a therapist that takes place with continued clinical practice and continued training. As clinicians progress in their careers, their experience with clinical cases will call out for new learning. This will guide the training or supervision they seek. Additionally, and importantly, a continuous practice of reflecting on one's work is essential to support the professional development of a therapist throughout their professional lifecycle (Ronnestad & Skovholt, 2003, 2013). This reflection will support the development of expertise, personal style, interventive preferences, and the use of self. The use of self suggests something deeper than style or preferences; it refers to the development of what has been called the person-of-the-therapist.

Person of the Therapist

IST, resting on its philosophical pillars, provides a way to think about patterns in human systems including the constraints that exist at various levels of the system. Its integrative structures and diagrams demonstrate that IST is planful and logical. It is indeed an approach that invites therapists to think carefully about the therapy. However, there is a heart as well as head in it. Therapy is a person-to-person experience in which the person-of-the-therapist is as important as the methods employed. The therapist brings empathy and emotional intelligence to the process and seeks to establish a therapeutic relationship in which the clients feel understood, respected, and cared about. In addition to developing a personal style and a set of interventive preferences, therapists are presented with the opportunity to develop greater self-knowledge from the practice of examining their own reactions to the experiences reported by their clients. A therapist's own experiences, reactions, memories, relational patterns, and emotions impact the conduct of therapy and contribute to the one-of-a-kind relational pathway of therapy with a particular individual, couple, or family.

The terms *use of self* (Satir & Baldwin, 1983) and *person-of-the-therapist* (Aponte, 1982; Aponte & Winter, 2013) are roughly synonymous. Both acknowledge the importance of the personal and professional development of the therapist and the influence of the human qualities of the therapist on the conduct of therapy. Person-of-the-therapist is arguably a somewhat broader term that includes methods of self-development, including the Person-of-the-Therapist (POTT) Model and its supervision instrument (Aponte & Carlsen, 2009). In this approach, therapy is conceptualized as both technical (model, interventions) and personal (trust, empathy, relatedness). Students or supervisees are supported in identifying their signature relational/psychological issues (signature themes) and the cultural dimensions of their lives that are likely to affect their clinical work. The object is to begin to establish "a familiarity, comfort with, and command of these issues" (Aponte & Carlsen, 2009, p. 397) and take responsibility for managing them so that (in IST language) they do not *constrain* the conduct of therapy and can be harnessed as *strengths* in service of the personal human connection made with clients.

The essential context for POTT training is clinical practice. The therapist-in-training utilizes a questionnaire to consider and record their reflections on cases that they see. The questionnaire prompts focus on the clinical challenges of the case, the way the challenges impact the therapist, and how the therapist can bring this awareness to the therapy. The therapist reflects on this process and discusses it with their supervisor. As is the case in IST supervision (He et al., 2021), this component of the personal work targets the therapist's functioning as a clinician and is clearly distinguished as supervision and not psychotherapy for the therapist. Further fit with IST is the focus on getting "out of their own way in doing therapy" (identifying and removing therapist constraints) and on using "what they master about themselves in active constructive ways" (accessing strengths) (Aponte & Carlsen, 2009, p. 398).

IST's strength guideline (see Appendix B) and its clear preference for attempting to construct solution sequences can be applied to the development of the person-of-the-therapist as well. Given the discovery of a personal issue that may be impacting the therapy, the supervisor may ask the therapist to bypass the issue and perform an intervention (and acquire the skill) that their personal issue might otherwise prevent. In other words, can the therapist, upon reflection, recognize the constraining issue and operate as the case requires given its presence, and perhaps learn to use the internal reaction to better understand and perform their work? In this way, and in parallel to IST clinical work, a straightforward, action-oriented approach to supervision is preferred before suggesting a more intensive intervention, such as the therapist-in-training beginning their own psychotherapy. If the therapist-in-training is not already in their own personal psychotherapy, the failure of straightforward interventions to adequately address what constrains their work can provide the supervisor with justification for the recommendation that the therapist-in-training begin psychotherapy.

For example, Dee was working with a family consisting of a mother, a father, and a 10-year-old son. In the first session, the discussion of the presenting problem (son's underachievement) led to the father becoming angry and berating the child. At that moment, Dee felt overwhelmed and frozen. She did not know what to do, and she was emotionally flooded. The father finished his tirade and Dee gathered herself to summarize the session and scheduled the next session. Dee felt shaken by the experience. She discussed the session in supervision and for the sake of the therapy she and her supervisor, Ellen, agreed that it would be necessary to interrupt the berating and refocus the session (a solution sequence for the therapist's work). Next, given how overwhelmed Dee had been, Ellen asked her to discuss how she would feel about doing this and whether something might get in the way of doing it. Dee shared her experience in her family of origin which included a father who would berate the kids at times, especially her little brother. She felt terrible about this at the time but did not speak to it. Her older sister had the role of trying to get her father to stop. Given this insight, Ellen coached her to see the pain of the father and son, to commit to interrupt the berating, and to do so in a direct but non-judgmental way. Dee role-played this with Ellen and mentally rehearsed it several times. She began the second session ready to control the process of interaction, join the father in his concern about his son, and stop the berating that was occurring in the session. When the father became critical, she found her voice and interrupted him (solution sequence and competency) which proved easier than she anticipated. She led a discussion on the father's passion and discussed the effects of his passion on his son and on their relationship. There was a lot of work ahead for this family, but Dee was setting a tone for the sessions to follow. Dee felt empowered, though she realized that this person-of-the-therapist issue was one that would require continued work. IST strongly supports the general idea that therapists-in-training enter psychotherapy; however, given a constraint such as the one Dee struggled with, the first line intervention was not to recommend therapy but to work on empowering her to do what she needed to do in the session. If Dee continued to struggle with the issue of managing conflict in session or stopping a parent from berating a child, the supervisor could suggest that this issue be explored in the therapist's own therapy. In this way, the therapist's own development in IST follows the failure-driven guideline and, in doing so, works with the question of "what do we do when what we are doing is not working?"

Conclusion

IST is not a model of therapy. Rather, it is a systemic perspective for integrating therapy models, common factors, best practices, and research findings to develop a therapy that fits the unique needs and patterns of a client system. The actual course of therapy is a function of IST's tenets and methods, of course, but it is also a function of a once-in-a-lifetime collaboration of one therapist and one client system. For the therapist, every case is a new adventure with twists and turns on the road ahead that cannot be anticipated.

As discussed in this chapter, the course of therapy in IST is influenced by pathways created by variations in clients' presenting concerns and circumstances, the context of the therapy, and the characteristics of the therapist, including the style of relating, preferences for intervening, and deeper issues related to the person-of-the-therapist. Therapists, themselves, will have their own developmental pathways. They may seek mastery within IST, but IST itself is not designed to be mastered. Rather, it provides a vehicle for ongoing study and reflection—a framework for lifelong learning. As depicted in Figure 11.1, IST's *loaded blueprint* uses the blueprint components to organize and house the universe of possible concepts, strategies, interventions, and skills available in the field of therapy, but as a practical matter, therapists build their own personal blueprint by filling this figure with the concepts, strategies, interventions, and skills that they learn. This practical, personal blueprint is enriched by clinical practice, training, reading, and consultation or supervision. The knowledge and skill acquired by the therapist are not purely technical, however. They are expressed and delivered through the therapist's unique self in the context of an evolving therapeutic alliance. The ongoing

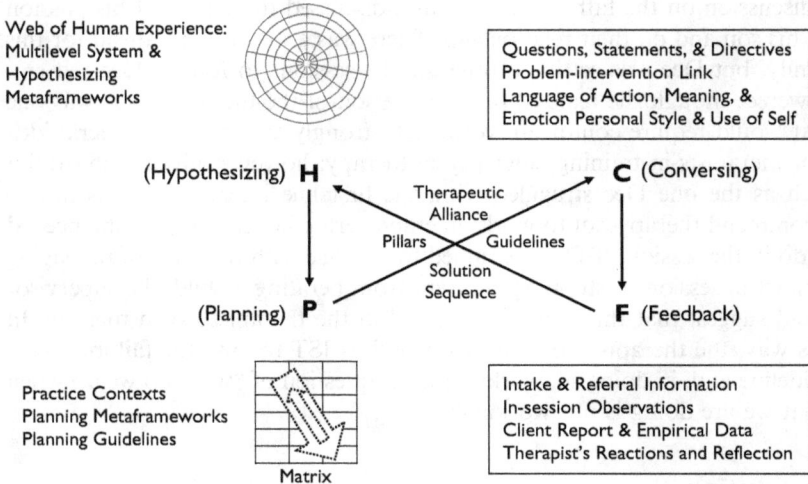

Web of Human Experience:
Multilevel System &
Hypothesizing
Metaframeworks

Questions, Statements, & Directives
Problem-intervention Link
Language of Action, Meaning, &
Emotion Personal Style & Use of Self

(Hypothesizing) **H**   **C** (Conversing)

Therapeutic
Alliance

Pillars   Guidelines

Solution
Sequence

(Planning) **P**   **F** (Feedback)

Practice Contexts
Planning Metaframeworks
Planning Guidelines

Intake & Referral Information
In-session Observations
Client Report & Empirical Data
Therapist's Reactions and Reflection

Matrix

Figure 11.1 The loaded blueprint. Adapted from "Integrative Problem-Centered Metaframeworks Therapy II: Planning, Conversing, and Reading Feedback," by D. C. Breunlin, W. Pinsof, W. P. Russell, and J. Lebow, 2011, Family Process, 50(3), p. 334. Copyright 2011 by John Wiley & Sons. Adapted with permission.

acquisition of knowledge and skill needs to be accompanied by continuous development of the person-of-the-therapist, as therapy is ultimately a relational practice.

Exercises

1   Think of a case you have seen (or a person you have known) that has very different political views than you do. Imagine the person strongly presenting a viewpoint in a therapy session. What feelings and thoughts do you have? Consider what you need to do internally in order to interact with them in therapy. What can you access within yourself to find a connection with this person?

2   Develop a conceptualization of a case from an IST perspective. Consider a problem sequence and at least two constraints. Imagine (or role-play) how you will discuss this case with a colleague who does not practice IST. For this imagery or role-play, pick a real or imaginary colleague who organizes their thinking about cases by identifying a problem by name (depression, anxiety, conflict) and seeking an intervention for that problem before considering the clients' actual sequences of action, meaning, and emotion. Describe

your IST formulation to that colleague using the specificity of a problem sequence as a starting point. Be mindful to respect the other clinician's view and maintain a good working alliance with them.

3   Think of a case you have seen that involved a relational or personal issue that paralleled what you have experienced while growing up. With respect to this parallel, what did you experience as you worked with the clients? Consider how that feeling or reaction may have impacted or limited your range of responses to the client(s). How did you deal with the situation? Looking back, would you have done something differently?

Alternate scenario for exercise 3 for those not currently seeing clients:

Consider a struggle or stressor you have experienced in family life. Are there strong feelings associated with remembering this hardship? Do you have beliefs or values that have come from it? Imagine that you are seeing a family with similar issues. How would you be affected as a family member begins to talk about the issue? How will your feeling or reaction limit your range of responsiveness to that family?

4   A father in a divorced family has been alienated from the children ages 9 and 11 for some years. The children refuse to see him. The mother maintains that the children are afraid to see their father, but he suspects their mother plays a role in their reluctance. There is no history of physical or sexual abuse. There had been a contentious divorce. The father asks the court to support him in having visitation with the children. The court orders that the father and children attend therapy together to deal with what keeps the children from wanting to see the father. The father calls to schedule an appointment. In discussion with a colleague or by means of making some notes, take a systemic perspective and consider who you will meet with in the initial weeks of the therapy and in what order. What will be the alliance challenges? How will you frame the therapy for mother, father and children? In particular, consider how you will want to discuss the therapy with the mother who is being required to bring the children to sessions.

References

Aponte, H. J. (1982). The person of the therapist: The cornerstone of therapy. *Family Therapy Networker, 46*, 19–21.

Aponte, H. J., & Winter, J. E. (2013). The person and practice of the therapist: Treatment and training. In M. Baldwin (Ed.), *The use of self in therapy* (3rd ed., pp. 141–165). Routledge.

Aponte, H. J., & Carlsen, C. J. (2009). An instrument for person-of-the-therapist supervision. *Journal of Marital and Family Therapy, 35*(4), 395–405. 10.1111/j.1752-0606.2009.00127.x

Baker, K. A. (1999). The importance of cultural sensitivity and therapist self-awareness when working with mandatory clients. *Family Process*, *38*(1), 55–67.

Barsky, A. E. (2010). Assumed privilege: A double-edged sword. In S. K. Anderson & V. A. Middleton (Eds.), *Explorations in diversity: Examining privilege and oppression in a multicultural society* (pp. 139–148). Cengage Learning.

Commission for Case Manager Certification. (n.d.) *Definition and Philosophy of Case Management.* https://ccmcertification.org/about-ccmc/about-case-management/def inition-and-philosophy-case-management

He, Y., Hardy, N. & Russell, W. P. (2021). Integrative systemic supervision: Promoting supervisees' theoretical integration in systemic therapy. *Family Process*, 61, 58–75.

Kilpatrick, A. C., & Holland, T. P. (2005). *Working with families: An integrative model by level of need* (4th ed.). Allyn.

Lebow, J., & Rekart, K. N. (2007). Integrative family therapy for high-conflict divorce with disputes over child custody and visitation. *Family Process*, *46*(1), 79–91.

Lincourt, P., Kuettel, T. J., & Bombardier, C. H. (2002). Motivational interviewing in a group setting with mandated clients: A pilot study. *Addictive Behaviors*, *27*(3), 381–391.

Maslow, A. H. (1954). The instinctoid nature of basic needs. *Journal of personality*, *22*, 326–347. 10.1111/j.1467-6494.1954.tb01136.x

Miller, W. R. & Rollnick, S. (2012). *Motivational interviewing: Helping people change*, (3rd ed.). Guilford.

Miller, W. R. & Rose, G. S. (2009). Toward a theory of motivational interviewing. *American Psychologist*, *64*(6), 527–537.

Pinsof, W. M. (1995). *Integrative problem centered therapy: A synthesis of biological, individual and family therapies.* Basic Books.

Pinsof, W., Breunlin, D. C., Russell, W. P., & Lebow, J. (2011). Integrative problem-centered metaframeworks therapy II: Planning, conversing, and reading feedback. *Family Process*, *50*, 314–336. 10.1111/j.1545-5300.2011.01361.x

Pinsof, W. M., Breunlin, D., Russell, W., Lebow, J., Rampage, C., & Chambers, A. (2018). *Integrative systemic therapy: metaframeworks for problem solving with individuals, couples, and families* (1st ed.). American Psychological Association. 10.1037/0000055-000

Richmond, M. (1922). *What is social case work?* Russell Sage Foundation.

Ronnestad, M. H. & Skovholt, T. M. (2003). The journey of the counselor and therapist: Research findings and perspective on professional development. *Journal of Career Development*, *30*, 5–44.

Ronnestad, M. H. & Skovholt, T. M. (2013). *The developing practitioner.* Routledge.

Rooney, R. H. (2009). Task-centered interventions with involuntary clients. In R. H. Rooney (Ed.), *Strategies for work with involuntary clients.* Columbia University Press.

Satir, V., & Baldwin, M. (1983). *Satir step by step: A guide to creating change in families.* Science and Behavior Books.

Simon, G. M. (2003). *Beyond technique in family therapy: Finding your therapeutic voice.* Allyn & Bacon.

Tomm, K. (1987). Interventive interviewing: Part II. Intending to ask lineal, circular, strategic, or reflexive questions? *Family Process, 27*, 1–15.

Von Bertalanffy, L. (1968). *General systems theory: Foundations, development, applications.* Braziller.

Whittaker, K. J. (2018). Flere perspektiver i ett: En introduksjon til integrativ systemisk terapi. *Fokus på familien, 46*(03), 180–187.

Appendix A

IST Tables of Strategies and Intervention Resources

Action Planning Metaframework

Strategy	Intervention Resources
Identifying and interrupting the problem sequence	• This book, Chapter 4 • Pinsof et al. (2018), Chapter 3 • Fishbane (2007, 2016) • Szapocznik and Hervis (2020) • Haley (1991)
Identifying a solution sequence and encouraging clients to implement it	• This book, Chapters 5 and 6 • Pinsof et al. (2018), Chapter 3 • Solution-focused questions (de Shazer et al., 2007) • Opposite action (Linehan, 2015)
Creating enactments	• This book, Chapter 5 • Nichols and Colapinto (2017) • Fishman (2013), Minuchin and Fishman (1981)
Modifying patterns of leadership and/or boundaries	• Boundary marking (Fishman, 2013; Minuchin & Fishman, 1981) • Unbalancing (Fishman, 2013; Minuchin & Fishman, 1981) • Clarifying and empowering leadership (Breunlin et al., 1997)
Developing between-session behavioral experiments ("homework")	• Homework (Kazantzis & L'Abate, 2007) • Directives (Russell, 2017) • Assigning homework (Dattilio, 2002) • Family dinners (Fishel, 2016) • Brief Strategic Therapy Szapocznik and Hervis (2020)

(Continued)

Strategy	Intervention Resources
Modifying communication patterns	• Time out for couples (Pinsof et al., 2018, pages 303-307; Markman et al., 2010) • Problem-solving and emotional expression for couples (Dadras, 2011) • Reflective listening (Markman et al., 2010) • Repair attempts (Gottman & Gottman, 2018) • Soften start-ups (Gottman & Gottman, 2018) • Repair and de-escalate (Gottman & Gottman, 2018)
Facilitating behavioral exposure	• In vivo exposure (Lang & Helbig-Lang, 2012) • Imaginal exposure (Koerner & Fracalanza, 2012) • Virtual reality exposure (Garcia-Palacios et al., 2001) • Exposure and response prevention (Rowa et al., 2007)
Facilitating behavioral activation	• Hopko et al. (2006) • Jacobson et al. (2001) • Kanter et al. (2010)
Reinforcing behavior	• Premack principle (Johanning, 2005) • Reinforcing desired interpersonal behavior in session (Kohlenberg & Tsai, 2007) • Behavior exchange (Jacobson & Christensen, 1996)
Developing adaptive routines	• Spagnola and Fiese (2007) • Fiese (2006)
Facilitating rituals	• Fiese (2006)
Evoking absent family members	• Empty chair technique (Kellogg, 2004; Elliot et al., 2004)
Spatializing the client system	• Family sculpting (Semmelhack, 2018; Papp et al., 2004)
Encouraging the practice of the problem to modify view or demonstrate control of the problem.	• Prescribing the symptom (Ruby, 2018; Haley, 1991) • Restraining change (Ruby, 2018) • Role-playing negative behavior (Jacobson & Christensen, 1996)

Meaning/Emotion Planning Metaframework

Strategy	Intervention Resources
Identifying thoughts, feelings, beliefs, and narratives that constrain implementation of a solution sequence	• This book, Chapter 7 • Pinsof et al. (2018), Chapters 4 and 5 • Circular questioning (Brown, 1997; Tomm, 1988) • Vulnerability cycle work (Fishbane, 2013) • Cognitive behavioral therapy-couples (Dadras, 2011; Epstein & Baucom, 2002; Baucom et al., in press) • Cognitive behavioral therapy (Beck, 2011) • Cognitive restructuring (Clark et al., 1999)
Identifying, accessing, and/or heightening contextually adaptive thoughts/meanings	• Reframing (Family Therapy survey texts; Watzlawick et al., 2011; Minuchin & Fishman, 1981) • Positive connotation (Bischof et al., 2017) • Externalizing the problem (White, 2000; White & Epston, 2004) • Circular questioning (Brown, 1997; Tomm, 1988) • Socratic questions (Overholser, 2018) • Unified detachment (Jacobson & Christensen, 1996) • Identifying exceptions (Trepper et al., 2007). • Solution-focused miracle & scaling questions (de Shazer et al., 2007) • Motivational interviewing (Miller & Rollnick, 2012) • Unified detachment (Cordova et al., 1998) • Cognitive behavioral therapy-couples (Dadras, 2011; Epstein & Baucom, 2002; Baucom et al., in press) • Cognitive behavioral therapy (Beck, 2011)
Addressing meaning with metaphors, analogies, or stories	• Metaphors (Martin et al., 1992) • Stories, metaphor (Freedman & Combs, in press; Combs & Freedman, 1990)
Facilitating the development and utilization of adaptive narratives	Narrative therapy references: • Freedman & Combs (in press) • White (2007) • Madigan (2011) • McAdams and Janis (2004)

(Continued)

Strategy	Intervention Resources
Accessing and/or heightening contextually adaptive emotions	• Accessing primary emotion (Pascual-Leone & Greenberg, 2009) • Johnson et al. (in press)
Emotion psychoeducation	• Pascual-Leone and Greenberg (2009) • Linehan (2015) • Linehan and Wilks (2015)
Regulating constraining emotions	• Emotion regulation (Gross & Thompson, 2007) • Distress tolerance (Linehan, 2015)
Facilitating healthy and direct emotional expression	• Pascual-Leone and Greenberg (2009)
Addressing readiness to change	• Motivational interviewing (Miller & Rollnick, 2012) • Restraining change (Ruby, 2018)

Complex Meaning/Emotion Planning Metaframework

Strategy	Intervention Resources
Facilitating grief and the adaptation to loss	• Walsh and McGoldrick (2004) • Neimeyer (2016) • Kosminsky (2016) • Worden (2009)
Identifying and transforming emotion recognition and management in addiction	• Emotion regulation for alcohol use disorders (Stasiewicz et al., 2018)
Identifying and transforming meaning in addiction	• Bacon (2019) • McCrady et al. (in press)
Facilitating forgiveness	• Christensen et al. (2014) • Greenberg and Iwakabe (2011) • Hargrave and Zasowski (2017)
Facilitating acceptance of challenging circumstance(s)	• Acceptance and commitment therapy (Hayes et al., 2012) • Radical acceptance (Linehan, 2015) • Emotional acceptance through greater self-care (Jacobson & Christensen, 1996)

(Continued)

Strategy	Intervention Resources
Exploring and integrating traumatic experiences	• Barrett and Fish (2014) • Herman (2015) • van der Kolk (2015) • Courtois and Ford (2016) • Eye Movement Desensitization and Reprocessing (Leeds & Shapiro, 2000; Shapiro, 2017) • Prolonged exposure (Peterson et al., 2019) • Addressing emotional upheaval following an affair (Baucom et al., 2009; Gordon et al., in press) • Trauma model of infidelity (Glass & Wright, 1997)

Biobehavioral Planning Metaframework

Strategy	Intervention Resources
Biobehavioral psychoeducation	• Psychoeducation (Lucksted et al., 2012) • Medical family therapy (McDaniel et al., 2014) • Family-focused treatment for bipolar disorder (Miklowitz et al., 2008) • Neuroeducation (Fishbane, 2007, 2013)
Exercise and fitness	• Exercise for mood and anxiety disorders (Otto & Smits, 2011)
Making a lifestyle change	• Smoking cessation (various methods) • Alcohol/drug use reduction (various approaches)
Relaxation and body awareness	• Mindfulness meditation practices (Tang, 2017) • Progressive muscle relaxation (McCallie et al., 2006) • Sensate focus IIII (Nelson & Hunt, 2016) • Yoga • Tai-chi
Biofeedback	• Biofeedback (Walsh, 2010; Schwartz & Andrasik, 2003)
Psychotropic medication	• Referral and coordination of care with a psychiatrist, APRN or a prescribing psychologist

(Continued)

Strategy	Intervention Resources
Physical Assessment	• Referral and coordination of care with a primary care physician, APRN or a PA
Sharing medical information with loved ones	• Facilitating direct discussion of a medical condition • Planning a conjoint medical visit • Shared reading
Neuropsychological evaluation/ counseling	• Referral and coordination of care with a clinical psychologist
Nutritional/allergy evaluation and intervention	• Referral and coordination of care with a dietician
Addiction evaluation detoxification and treatment	• Referral and coordination of care with a detox center or addiction treatment facility

Family of Origin Planning Metaframework

Strategy	Intervention Resources
Identify current problem sequences in an adult client's family of origin that constrain the implementation of a solution sequence	• Pinsof et al. (2018) • Bowen (2004) • Fishbane (2015, 2016, In press)
Identifying and working with the intergenerational transmission processes	• Detailed genogram analysis (McGoldrick et al., 2008) • Neurobiological-relational interventions (Fishbane, 2016, 2015) • Interpreting family-of-origin issues in relation to romantic attachment (Nichols, 2003) • Relational ethics (Boszormenyi-Nagy & Krasner, 1989)
Facilitating differentiation of self within the family of origin	• Schnarch (2009) • Bowen (2004) • Nichols (2003)
Changing a family of origin pattern with between-session experiments	• Coaching (Bowen, 2004) • Fishbane (2016, 2015)

(Continued)

Strategy	Intervention Resources
In session work with family-of-origin members	• Framo (1992) • Fishbane (2016, 2015)
Reconnecting distant or estranged family of origin member	• Assisting client with letter writing or emailing • Invitation to a session • Forgiveness work (see complex meaning/emotion strategies)

Internal Representation Planning Metaframework

Strategy	Intervention Resources
Helping clients identify internal representations of themselves and others	• Internal family systems (Schwartz 2013) • Object relations (Siegel, 2015; Siegel, In press)
Helping clients understand how internalized representations constrain implementation of the solution sequence within the current client system.	• Pinsof et al. (2018) • Internal family systems (Schwartz, 2013) • Object relations (Siegel, 2015; Siegel, In press)

Identifying and working with parts of self	• Internal family systems work (Anderson et al., 2017; Schwartz, 2013)
	  o Naming and accessing parts as managers, firefighters, exiles
	  o Identifying and accessing the self
	  o Diagraming the internal family system

Facilitating self-leadership	• Internal family systems work (Anderson et al., 2017; Schwartz, 2013)
	  o Evoking the self to nurture an exiled part
	  o Strengthening the leadership of the self
	  o Room technique with enactment of self and a part

Helping clients take responsibility for their internalized representations	• Interpreting projective identifications (Siegel, 2015)
Identifying key events associated with the development of the internalized representations	• Retrieving parts that are "frozen in time" (Schwartz & Sweezy, 2020) • Object relations (Siegel, 2015)

(Continued)

Strategy	Intervention Resources
Making the unconscious conscious	• Dream interpretation (Foulkes, 1994; Levy, 1996) • Interpretation of latent content (Levy, 1996) • Identifying slips of the tongue (Levy, 1996)
Transference interpretation	• Mentalizing the relationship (Bateman & Fonagy, 2010)
Helping clients understand and cope with the internal representations of other family members	• Vulnerability cycle (Scheinkman & Fishbane, 2004) • Object relations couple & family therapy (Siegel, 2015) • Internal family systems (Schwartz (2013)
Helping clients see how certain internal representations can be beneficial.	• Internal family systems (Schwartz (2013) • EMDR resource-building (Shapiro, 2017; Leeds & Shapiro, 2000). • Vulnerability cycle (Scheinkman & Fishbane, 2004)

Self Planning Metaframework

Strategy	Intervention Resources
Helping clients understand how the vulnerability of self-constrains implementation of the solution sequence	• Intersubjective self-psychology (Hagman et al., 2019) • Transference-focused psychotherapy (Stern et al., 2013) • Functional analytic psychotherapy (Kohlenberg & Tsai, 2007) (Note: Functional analytic therapy does not posit a self per se.)
Developing and tolerating dependency and emotional intensity with the client	• Intersubjective self-psychology (Hagman et al., 2019) • Self-psychology (Lessem, 2005)
Deepening the bond component of the alliance with the client through effective use of self	• Engaging in empathic attunement with clients (Hagman et al., 2019) • Monitoring transferences of twinning, mirroring, and idealizing (Hagman et al., 2019) • Functional analytic procedures (Kohlenberg & Tsai, 2007)

(Continued)

Strategy	Intervention Resources
Using the vicissitudes of the therapist-client relationship to strengthen the vulnerable clients' selves	• Self-psychology (Hagman et al., 2019; Lessem, 2005)) • Functional analytic psychotherapy (Kohlenberg & Tsai, 2007)
Transmuting internalizations	• Identifying minor, nontraumatic breaks in empathic bond and interpreting them (Hagman et al., 2019; Lessem, 2005)
Modeling rupture-repair skills within the therapeutic relationship	• Self-psychology (Hagman et al., 2019) • Safran et al. (2011)
Reinforcement of adaptive interpersonal behaviors as they occur in session	• Functional analytic procedures (Kohlenberg & Tsai, 2007)

Notes

1   The above lists of strategies and interventions are not meant to be exhaustive. IST is an open system of knowledge that accommodates new strategies as well as idiosyncratic strategies and interventions if they address a specific hypothesis, consider the impact on the alliance, are consistent with IST guidelines, and observe the principles of ethical practice.

2   The column, *intervention resources,* points the reader toward interventions they may want to learn. This column provides citations for relevant models, specific interventions, and IST procedures.

3   To use an intervention, a therapist must learn it well enough for its proper utilization. Many interventions can be learned and readily imported into an integrative therapy, but in the case of interventions embedded in complex models such as internal family systems, object relations and self-psychology, significant training will be required to use those interventions. Similarly, substantive training is required before borrowing a substantial module of work from any model of therapy.

References

Anderson, F. G., Sweezy, M., & Schwartz, R. C. (2017). *Internal family systems skill training manual: Trauma-informed treatment for anxiety, depression, PTSD & substance abuse.* PESI Publishing.

Andolfi, M. (2017). *Multi-generational family therapy: Tools and resources for the therapist.* Routledge.

Bacon, M. (2019). *Family therapy and the treatment of substance use disorders: The family matters model.* Routledge.

Barrett, M. J., & Fish, L. S. (2014). *Treating complex trauma: A relational blueprint for collaboration and change.* Routledge.

Bateman, A., & Fonagy, P. (2010). Mentalization based treatment for borderline personality disorder. *World Psychiatry, 9*(1), 11–15. 10.1002/j.2051-5545.2010. tb00255.x

Baucom, D. H., & Epstein, N. (1990). *Cognitive-behavioral marital therapy.* Brunner/Mazel.

Baucom, D. H., Snyder, D. K., & Gordon, K. C. (2009). *Helping couples get past the affair.* Guilford.

Baucom, D. H., Epstein, N. B., Fischer, M. S., Kirby, J. S., & LaTaillade, J. J. (In press). Cognitive-behavioral couple therapy. In J. Lebow & S. Snyder (Eds.), *Clinical handbook of couple therapy* (6th ed.). American Psychological Association

Beck, J. S. (2011). *Cognitive behavior therapy: Basics and beyond* (2nd ed.). Guilford Press.

Becvar, D. S., & Becvar, R. J. (1999). *Systems theory and family therapy* (2nd ed.). University Press of America

Bischof, G. H., Helmeke, K. B., & Lane, C. D. (2017). Positive connotation in couple and family therapy. In J. Lebow, A. Chambers, & D. C. Breunlin (Eds.), *Encyclopedia of couple and family therapy.* Springer.

Boscolo, L., Cecchin, G. F., Hoffmann, L., & Penn, P. (1987). *Milan systemic family therapy: Conversations in theory and practice.* Basic Books.

Boszormenyi-Nagy, I., & Krasner, B. (1989). *Between give and take: A clinical guide to contextual therapy.* New York: Brunner/Mazel.

Bowen, M. (2004). Family reaction to death. In F. Walsh, & M. McGoldrick (eds.), *Living beyond loss: Death in the family* (2nd ed.) (pp. 47–60). W. W. Norton.

Breunlin, D. C., Schwartz, R. C., & Kune-Karrer, B. M. (1992). *Metaframeworks: Transcending the models of family therapy.* Jossey-Bass.

Breunlin, D. C., Schwartz, R. C., & Mac Kune-Karrer, B. M. (1997). *Metaframeworks: Transcending the models of family therapy.* Revised and Updated. Jossey-Bass.

Brown, J. (1997). Circular questioning: An introductory guide. *Australian and New Zealand Journal of Family Therapy, 18*(2), 109–114.

Chon, T., & Lee, M. (2013). Acupuncture. *Mayo Clinic Proceedings, 88*(10), 1141–1146. 10.1016/j.mayocp.2013.06.009

Christensen, A., Doss, B. D., & Jacobson, N. S. (2014). *Reconcilable differences: Rebuild your relationship by rediscovering the partner you love—without losing yourself* (2nd ed.). Guilford Press.

Christensen, A., Jacobson, N. S., & Babcock, J. C. (1995). *Integrative behavioral couple therapy.* Guilford.

Clark, D. A. (2013). *Cognitive restructuring.* The Wiley Handbook of Cognitive Behavioral Therapy. 10.1002/9781118528563.wbcbt02

Clark, D. A., Beck, A. T., & Alford, B. A. (1999). *Scientific foundations of cognitive theory and therapy of depression.* Wiley.

Combs, G., & Freedman, J. (1990). *Symbol, story, and ceremony: Using metaphor in individual and family therapy.* W. W. Norton.

Cordova, J. V., Jacobson, N. S., & Christensen, A. (1998). Acceptance versus change interventions in behavioral couple therapy: Impact on couples' in-session communication. *Journal of Marital and Family Therapy*, *24*(4), 437–455. 10.1111/j. 1752-0606.1998.tb01099.x

Courtois, C. A., & Ford, J. D. (2016). *The treatment of complex trauma*. Guilford Press.

Dadras, I. (2011). Cognitive-behavioral therapy with couples and families: A comprehensive guide for clinicians. The Guilford Press.

Dattilio, F. M. (2002). Homework assignments in couple and family therapy. *Journal of Clinical Psychology*, *58*(5), 535–547. 10.1002/jclp.10031

de Shazer, S., Dolan, Y., Korman, H., McCollum, E., Trepper, T., & Berg, I. K. (2007). *More than miracles: The state of the art of solution-focused brief therapy*. Haworth Press.

Elliot, R., Watson, J. C., Goldman, R. N. & Greenberg, L. S. (2004). *Learning emotion-focused therapy: The process-experiential approach to change*. American Psychological Association.

Epstein, N. B., & Baucom, D. H. (2002). *Enhanced cognitive-behavioral therapy for couples: A contextual approach*. American Psychological Association.

Fiese, B. H. (2006). *Family routines and rituals*. Yale University Press.

Fishbane, M. D. (2007). Wired to connect: Neuroscience, relationships, and therapy. *Family Process*, *46*, 395–412.

Fishbane, M. D. (2011). Neurobiology and family processes. In F. Walsh (Ed.), *Normal family processes: Growing diversity & complexity* (4th ed.). Guilford.

Fishbane, M. D. (2013). *Loving with the brain in mind: Neurobiology of couple therapy*. W. W. Norton.

Fishbane, M. D. (2015). Couple therapy and interpersonal neurobiology. In A. S. Gurman, J. Lebow, & D. Snyder (Eds.), *Clinical handbook of couple therapy* (5th ed.). Guilford.

Fishbane, M. D. (2016). The neurobiology of relationships. In J. Lebow & T. Sexton (Eds.), *Handbook of family therapy* (4th ed.). Routledge.

Fishbane, M. (In press). Intergenerational factors in couple therapy. In J. Lebow & S. Snyder (Eds.), *Clinical handbook of couple therapy* (6th edition). American Psychological Association.

Fishel, A. K. (2016). Harnessing the power of family dinners to create change in family therapy. *Australian and New Zealand Journal of Family Therapy*, *37*, 514–527. 10.1002/anzf.1185

Fishman, H. C. (2013). *Intensive structural therapy: Treating families in their social context*. Basic Books. (Original work published 1993).

Foulkes, D. (1994). The interpretation of dreams and the scientific study of dreaming. *Dreaming*, *4*(1), 82–85. 10.1037/h0094402

Framo, J. L. (1992). *Family-of-origin therapy: An intergenerational approach*. Routledge.

Freedman, J., & Combs, G. (1996). *Narrative therapy: The social construction of preferred realities*. W. W. Norton.

Freedman, J., & Combs, G. (In press). Narrative couple therapy. In J. Lebow & S. Snyder (Eds.), *Clinical handbook of couple therapy* (6th ed.). American Psychological Association.

Garcia-Palacios, A., Hoffman, H. G., See, S. K., Tsai, A., & Botella, C. (2001). Redefining therapeutic success with virtual reality exposure therapy. *Cyberpsychology & behavior*, *4*(3), 341–347. 10.1089/109493101300210231

Glass, S. P., & Wright, T. L. (1997). Reconstructing marriages after the trauma of infidelity. In W. K. Halford & H. J. Markman (Eds.), *Clinical handbook of marriage and couples interventions* (pp. 471–507). John Wiley & Sons Inc.

Gordon, K. C., Mitchell, C. E., Baucom, D. H., & Snyder, D. K. (In press). Infidelity. In J. Lebow & S. Snyder (Eds.), *Clinical handbook of couple therapy* (6th edition). American Psychological Association.

Gottman, J., & Gottman, J. S. (2018). *The science of couples and family therapy: Behind the scenes of the love lab*. W. W. Norton.

Greenberg, L. S. (2010). *Emotion-focused therapy: Theory and practice*. American Psychological Association.

Greenberg, L. S., & Iwakabe, S. (2011). Emotion-focused therapy and shame. In R. L. Dearing & J. P. Tangney (Eds.), *Shame in the therapy hour* (pp. 69–90). American Psychological Association. 10.1037/12326-003

Gross, J. J., & Thompson, R. A. (2007). Emotion regulation: Conceptual foundations. In J. J. Gross (Ed.) *Handbook of Emotion Regulation* (pp. 3–24). Guilford Press.

Hagman, G., Paul, H., & Zimmermann, P. B. (2019). *Intersubjective self psychology: A primer*. Routledge.

Haley, J. (1991). *Problem-solving therapy* (2nd ed.). Jossey-Bass.

Hargrave, T. D., & Zasowski, N. E. (2017). *Families and forgiveness: Doing therapy in the four stations of forgiveness*. Routledge.

Hayes, S. C., Pistorello, J., & Levin, M. E. (2012). Acceptance and commitment therapy as a unified model of behavior change. *The Counseling Psychologist, 40*(7), 976–1002. 10.1177/0011000012460836

Herman, J. (2015). *Trauma and recovery: The aftermath of violence – from domestic abuse to political terror*. Basic Books.

Hopko, D. R., Robertson, S. M. C., & Lejuez, C. W. (2006). Behavioral activation for anxiety disorders. *The Behavior Analyst Today, 7*(2), 212- 232. 10.1037/h0100084

Jacobson, N. S., & Christensen, A. (1996). *Integrative couple therapy: Promoting acceptance and change*. W. W. Norton.

Jacobson, N. S., Martell, C. R., & Dimidjian, S. (2001). Behavioral activation treatment for depression: Returning to contextual roots. *Clinical Psychology: Science and Practice, 8*(3), 255–270. 10.1093/clipsy.8.3.255

Johanning, M. (2005). Premack principle. In S. W. Lee (Ed.), *Encyclopedia of school psychology* (pp. 395–396). SAGE Publications.

Johnson, S. M., Wiebe, S. A., & Allan, R. (In press). Emotionally focused couple therapy. In J. Lebow & S. Snyder (Eds.), *Clinical handbook of couple therapy* (6th ed.). American Psychological Association.

Kanter, J., Manos, R., Bowe, W., Baruch, D., Busch, A., & Rusch, L. (2010). What is behavioral activation? A review of the empirical literature. *Clinical Psychology Review, 30*(6), 608–620. 10.1016/j.cpr.2010.04.001

Kazantzis, N., & L'Abate, L. (Eds.) (2007). *Handbook of homework assignments in psychotherapy: Research, practice and prevention*. Springer.

Kellogg, S. H. (2004). Dialogical encounters: Contemporary perspectives on "chairwork" in psychotherapy. *Psychotherapy, 41*(3), 310–320. 10.1037/0033-3204.41.3.310

Koerner, N., & Fracalanza, K. (2012). The role of anxiety control strategies in imaginal exposure. In P. Neudeck, & H. U. Wittchen (Eds.), *Exposure therapy* (pp. 197–216). Springer. 10.1007/978-1-4614-3342-2_12

Kohlenberg, R. J., & Tsai, M. (2007). *Functional analytic psychotherapy: Creating intense and curative therapeutic relationships.* Springer.

Kosminsky, J. R. (2016). *Attachment-informed grief therapy: The clinician's guide to foundations and applications.* Routledge.

Lang, T., & Helbig-Lang, S. (2012). Exposure in vivo with and without presence of a therapist: Does it matter? In P. Neudeck, & H. U. Wittchen (Eds.), *Exposure therapy* (pp. 261–273). Springer. 10.1007/978-1-4614-3342-2_15

Leeds, A. M., & Shapiro, F. (2000). EMDR and resource installation: Principles and procedures for enhancing current functioning and resolving traumatic experiences. In J. Carlson & L. Sperry (Eds.), *Brief therapy with individuals & couples* (pp. 469–534). Zeig, Tucker & Theisen.

Lessem, P. A. (2005). *Self psychology: An introduction.* Rowman & Littlefield.

Levy, S. T. (1996). *Principles of interpretation: Mastering clear and concise interventions in psychotherapy.* Jason Aronson.

Linehan, M. (2015). *DBT skills training manual* (2nd ed.). The Guilford Press.

Linehan, M., & Wilks, C. R. (2015). The course and evolution of dialectical behavior therapy. *American Journal of Psychotherapy, 69*(2), 97–110. 10.1176/appi.psychotherapy.2015.69.2.97

Lucksted, A., McFarlane, W., Downing, D., & Dixon, L. (2012). Recent developments in family psychoeducation as an evidence-based practice. *Journal of Marital & Family Therapy, 38*(1), 101–121. 10.1111/j.1752-0606.2011.00256.x

Madigan, S. (2011). *Narrative therapy.* American Psychological Association.

Markman, H. J., Stanley, S. M., & Blumberg, S. L. (2010). *Fighting for your marriage* (3rd ed.). Jossey-Bass.

Martin, J., Cummings, A. L., & Hallberg, E. T. (1992). Therapists' intentional use of metaphor: Memorability, clinical impact, and possible epistemic/motivational functions. *Journal of Consulting and Clinical Psychology, 60*(1), 143–145. 10.1037/0022-006X.60.1.143

McAdams, D. P., & Janis, L. (2004). Narrative identity and narrative therapy. In L. E. Angus & J. McLeod (Eds.), *The handbook of narrative and psychotherapy: Practice, theory, and research* (pp. 331–349). Sage. 10.4135/9781412973496.d13

McCallie, M. S., Blum, C. M., & Hood, C. J. (2006). Progressive muscle relaxation. *Journal of Human Behavior in the Social Environment, 13*(3), 51–66. 10.1300/J137v13n03_04

McCrady, B. S., Epstein, E. E., & Holzhauer, C. G. (In press). Alcohol problems in couples. In J. Lebow & S. Snyder (Eds.), *Clinical handbook of couple therapy* (6th ed.). American Psychological Association.

McDaniel, S. H., Doherty, W. J., & Hepworth, J. (2014). *Medical family therapy and integrated care* (2nd ed.). American Psychological Association.

McGoldrick, M., Gerson, R., & Petry, S. S. (2008). *Genograms: Assessment and intervention.* W. W. Norton.

Miller, W. R., & Rollnick, S. M. (2012). *Motivational interviewing: Helping people change.* Guilford Press.

Miklowitz, D. J., Axelson, D. A., Birmaher, B, George, E. L., Taylor, D. O., Schneck, C. D., Beresford, C. A., Dickinson, M., Craighead, W. E., & Brent, D. A. (2008). Family-focused treatment for adolescents with bipolar disorder: Results from a 2-year randomized trial. *Archives of General Psychiatry, 65*(9), 1053–1061. 10.1001/archpsyc.65.9.1053

Minuchin, S. & Fishman, H. C. (1981). *Family therapy techniques*. Harvard University Press.

Neimeyer, R. A. (Ed.) (2016). *Techniques of grief therapy: Assessment and intervention*. Routledge.

Nelson, M., & Hunt, Q. (2016). Sensate focus. In J. Carlson & S. B. Dermer (Eds.), *The SAGE Encyclopedia of Marriage, Family, and Couples Counseling* (pp. 1494–1497). Sage.

Nichols, W. C. (2003). Family-of-origin treatment. In T. L. Sexton, G. R. Weeks, & M. S. Robbins (Eds.), *Handbook of family therapy* (pp. 93–114). Routledge.

Nichols, M., & Colapinto, J. (2017). Enactment in structural family therapy. In J. Lebow, A. Chambers, & D. C. Breunlin (Eds.), *Encyclopedia of Couple and Family Therapy*. Springer. 10.1007/978-3-319-15877-8_969-1

Otto, M. W., & Smits, J. A. J. (2011). *Exercise for mood and anxiety: Proven strategies for overcoming depression*. Oxford University Press.

Overholser, J. (2018). *The socratic method of psychotherapy*. Columbia University Press.

Papp, P., Silverstein, O., & Carter, E. (2004). Family sculpting in preventive work with "well families". *Family Process, 12*(2): 197–212. 10.1111/j.1545-5300.1973.00197.x

Parry, A., & Doan, R. E. (1994). *Story revisions: Narrative therapy in the postmodern world*. Guilford.

Pascual-Leone, A., & Greenberg, L. S. (2009). Dynamic emotional processing in experiential therapy: Two steps forward, one step back. *Journal of Consulting and Clinical Psychology, 77*, 113–126.

Peterson, A. L., Foa, E. B., & Riggs, D. S. (2019). Prolonged exposure therapy. In B. A. Moore & W. E. Penk (Eds.), *Treating PTSD in military personnel: A clinical handbook* (pp. 46–62). Guilford.

Pinsof, W., Breunlin, D., Russell, W., Lebow, J., Rampage, C., & Chambers, A. (2018). *Integrative systemic therapy: Metaframeworks for problem solving with individuals, couples, and families* (1st ed.). American Psychological Association. 10.1037/0000055-000

Rowa, K., Antony, M. M., & Swinson, R. P. (2007). Exposure and response prevention. In M. M. Antony, C. Purdon, & L. J. Summerfeldt (Eds.), *Psychological treatment of obsessive-compulsive disorder: Fundamentals and beyond* (pp. 79–109). American Psychological Association. 10.1037/11543-004

Ruby J. (2018). Paradox in strategic couple and family therapy. In J. Lebow, A. Chambers, & D. Breunlin (Eds.). *Encyclopedia of couple and family therapy*. Springer. 10.1007/978-3-319-15877-8_296-1

Russell, W. P. (2017). Directives in couple and family therapy. In J. Lebow, A. Chambers, & D. C. Breunlin (Eds.), *Encyclopedia of couple and family therapy*. Springer. 10.1007/978-3-319-15877-8_520-1

Safran, J. D., Muran, J. C., & Eubanks-Carter, C. (2011). Repairing alliance ruptures. *Psychotherapy, 48*(1), 80–87. 10.1037/a0022140

Scheinkman, M., & Fishbane, M. (2004). The vulnerability cycle: Working with impasses in couple therapy. *Family Process, 43*(3), 279–299. 10.1111/j.1545-5300. 2004.00023.x

Schnarch, D. (2009). *Intimacy & desire: Awaken the passion in your relationship*. Beaufort Books.

Schwartz, R. (2013). *Evolution of the internal family systems model*. Center for Self Leadership.

Schwartz, R., & Sweezy, M. (2020). *Internal family systems therapy* (2nd ed.). Guilford.

Schwartz, M., & Andrasik, F. (2003). *Biofeedback: A practitioner's guide* (3rd ed.). Guilford.

Semmelhack, D. (2018). Sculpting in family therapy. In J. Lebow, A. Chambers, & D. C. Breunlin (Eds.), *Encyclopedia of couple and family therapy*. Springer. 10.1007/978-3-319-15877-8_189-1

Shapiro, F. (2017). *Eye movement desensitization and reprocessing (EMDR) therapy: Basic principles, protocols, and procedures* (3rd ed.). Guilford Press.

Siegel, J. P. (2015). Object relations couple therapy. In A. S. Gurman, J. Lebow, & D. Snyder (Eds.), *Clinical handbook of couple therapy* (5th ed., pp. 224–245). Guilford.

Siegel, J. P. (In press). Object relations couple therapy. In J. Lebow & S. Snyder (Eds.), *Clinical handbook of couple therapy* (6th ed.). American Psychological Association.

Spagnola, M., & Fiese, B. H. (2007). Family routines and rituals: A context for development in the lives of young children. *Infants & Young Children, 20*(4), 284–299. 10.1097/01.IYC.0000290352.32170.5a

Stasiewicz, P. R., Bradizza, C. M., & Slosman, K. S. (2018). *Emotion regulation treatment of alcohol use disorders: Helping clients manage negative thoughts and feelings* (1st ed.). Routledge.

Stern, B. L., Yeomans, F., Diamond, D., & Kernberg, O. F. (2013). Transference-focused psychotherapy for narcissistic personality. In J. S. Ogrodniczuk (Ed.), *Understanding and treating pathological narcissism* (pp. 235–252). American Psychological Association.

Szapocznik, J., & Hervis, O. (2020). *Brief strategic family therapy*. American Psychological Association. 10.1037/0000169-000

Tang, Y. (2017). *The neuroscience of mindfulness meditation: How the body and mind work together to change our behaviour* (1st ed.). Springer International Publishing. 10.1007/978-3-319-46322-3

Tomm, K. (1988). Interventive interviewing: Part III: Intending to ask lineal, circular, strategic, or reflexive questions? *Family Process, 27*(1), 1–15. 10.1111/j.1545-5300.1988.00001.x

Trepper, T. S., Dolan, Y., McCollum, E. E., & Nelson, T. (2007). Steve De Shazer and the future of solution-focused therapy. *Journal of Marital and Family Therapy, 32*(2), 133–139. 10.1111/j.1752-0606.2006.tb01595.x

van der Kolk, B. (2015). *The body keeps the score: Brain, mind, and body in the healing of trauma*. Penguin Books.

Walsh, J. A. (2010). Biofeedback: A useful tool for professional counselors. Retrieved from http://counselingoutfitters.com/vistas/vistas10/Article_47.pdf

Walsh, F., & McGoldrick, M. (2004). *Living beyond loss: Death in the family* (2nd ed.). W. W. Norton.

Watzlawick, P., Weakland, J. H. & Fisch, R. (2011). *Change: Principles of problem formation and problem resolution*. W. W. Norton. (Original work published 1974).

White, M. J. (2000). *Reflections on narrative practice*. Dulwich Centre.

White, M. J. (2007). *Maps of narrative practice*. W. W. Norton.

White, M. J., & Epston, D. (2004). Externalizing the problem. *Relating Experience: Stories from Health and Social Care, 1*, 88.

Worden, J. L. (2009). *Grief counselling and grief therapy: A handbook for the mental health practitioner* (4th ed.). Routledge.

Integrative Systemic Therapy Guidelines for Practice

Integrative Systemic Therapy Guidelines

1.	The problem centered guideline	All interventions should be linked, in some way, to the client system's presenting problems or concerns.
2.	The strength guideline	Until proven otherwise, it is assumed that the client system can use its strengths and resources to lift constraints and implement adaptive solutions with minimal and direct input from the therapist.
3.	The social justice guideline	Posits that the therapist attends to cultural contexts of membership (intersectionality), inclusion, and social justice issues at each step of the problem-solving process.
4.	The assessment and intervention "inseparability" guideline	Assessment and intervention are two inseparable and co-occurring processes that span the course of therapy and lead to increasingly refined hypotheses and therapeutic plans that facilitate problem resolution.
5.	The sequence replacement guideline	The primary task of the therapist is facilitating the replacement of the key problem sequences with alternative, adaptive sequences that eliminate or reduce the problem.
6.	The empirically informed guideline	The practice of psychotherapy must be continually informed with empirical/scientific data in order to be maximally effective and efficient.
7.	The educational guideline	Therapy is an educational process in which therapists give away their skills, knowledge, and expertise as

(Continued)

Integrative Systemic Therapy Guidelines

	quickly as clients can integrate them.
8. The cost-effectiveness guideline	Therapy begins with less expensive, more direct, and less complex interventions and moves to more expensive, indirect, and complex interventions as needed.
9. The interpersonal guideline	When possible and appropriate, it is always better to do an intervention, regardless of its nature, within an interpersonal as opposed to an individual context.
10. The temporal guideline	Therapy generally begins with a focus on the here-and-now and progresses to a focus on the past as more complex and remote constraints emerge within the therapy.
11. The failure-driven guideline	Therapeutic shifts occur when the current interventions fail to modify the Web sufficiently to permit implementation of the adaptive solution to the presenting problem
12. The alliance-priority guideline	Growing, maintaining, and repairing the therapeutic alliance takes priority over the principle of application (planning matrix arrow) unless doing so fundamentally compromises the efficacy and/or integrity of the therapy.

Note: From "Integrative Problem-Centered Metaframeworks Therapy I. Core Concepts and Hypothesizing." by D.C. Breunlin, W. Pinsof, W.P. Russel, and J. Lebow, 2011. *Family Process, 50*, p. 301. Copyright 2011 by Wiley Reprinted with permission.

Index

For Product Safety Concerns and Information please contact our EU
representative GPSR@taylorandfrancis.com
Taylor & Francis Verlag GmbH, Kaufingerstraße 24, 80331 München, Germany